FROM THE CONSCIOUS INTERIOR TO AN EXTERIOR UNCONSCIOUS

LINES OF THE SYMBOLIC SERIES

Edited by Danielle Carlo and Ian Parker

FROM THE CONSCIOUS INTERIOR TO AN EXTERIOR UNCONSCIOUS

Lacan, Discourse Analysis and Social Psychology

David Pavón Cuéllar

Edited by Danielle Carlo and Ian Parker

Routledge
Taylor & Francis Group
LONDON AND NEW YORK

First published 2010 by Karnac Books Ltd.

2 Park Square, Milton Park, Abingdon, Oxfordshire OX14 4RN
52 Vanderbilt Avenue, New York, NY 10017

Routledge is an imprint of the Taylor & Francis Group, an informa business

First issued in hardback 2019

British Library Cataloguing in Publication Data

A C.I.P. for this book is available from the British Library

ISBN-13: 978-1-85575-794-3 (pbk)
ISBN-13: 978-0-367-32463-6 (hbk)

Typeset by Vikatan Publishing Solutions (P) Ltd., Chennai, India

CONTENTS

ACKNOWLEDGMENTS

I especially thank Ian Parker for his initiative and support. I would also like to express my gratitude to Ksiezniczka Bieszczad, Rukmini Bose, Danielle Carlo, Jean-Pierre Cléro, Mario Alberto Cortez Rodríguez, José Luis García Castellano, Franz Gleiger, Eduardo González Di Pierro, Francisco Javier and the other members of the Popular Revolutionary Army (EPR) of Mexico, Elisabeth Lage, Pia Leighton, Mariola López Albertos, Adelio Melo, Viviana Pilar Melo Saint-Cyr, the Psychophores of Paris, François Regnault, José Manuel Sabucedo Cameselle, Wiola Slaska and María Luisa Vega.

PREFACE

This book weaves together into a multi-layered text three strands of work; Lacan's contribution to a theory of language, political engagement with those who aim to go beyond interpretation of the world to changing it, and insightful review of contradictions and gaps in studies of discourse in social psychology. It is tempting to treat these three strands as if they were the three rings of a Borromean knot, as if a failure to respect the linkage between them would lead to disaster. In truth, sad to say, research in each of those three strands of work in the English-speaking world has often been undertaken in such a way as to hermetically seal off each strand, to treat it as if it were independent of the other two. Attempts to connect them so far have been faltering and uncertain, and we have had to wait for David Pavón Cuéllar to show us how this work could be done.

Here we have a detailed review and synthesis of Lacanian concepts which lead us through the development of a distinctive approach to language and clarification of confluence and divergence with other theoretical traditions. The illustrative example text which at first glance seems to be little more than a fragment of speech becomes, as the line of the book unfolds, a window onto the world of political action, a world in which an ostensibly academic theory of language is brought to life. If that were not enough, there is in the text and in the densely referenced footnotes an articulation of the arguments in relation to the field of 'discourse analysis' in social psychology. Those interventions in that field of research will energise and at last make relevant 'social psychology' to those concerned with social-political phenomena as such and those working in the individual-clinical domain. In sum, what Pavón Cuéllar has given us here is a work of scholarship and commitment, one that can be read from at least three vantage points, one that will enrich at least three areas of debate. But this is not a definitive text. It is even better than that, for it now opens the way for further exploration of Lacanian theory, politics and discourse, and will serve as an indispensable point of reference for a new generation of researchers.

Psychoanalytic clinical and theoretical work circulates through multiple intersecting antagonistic symbolic universes. This series opens connections between different cultural sites in which Lacanian work has developed in distinctive ways, in forms of work that question the idea that there could be single correct reading and application. The Lines of the Symbolic series provides a reflexive reworking of psychoanalysis that translates Lacanian writing from around the world, steering a course between the temptations of a metalanguage and imaginary reduction, between the claim to provide a god's eye view of psychoanalysis and the idea that psychoanalysis must everywhere be the same. And the elaboration of psychoanalysis in the symbolic here grounds its theory and practice in the history and politics of the work in a variety of interventions that touch the real.

Ian Parker

ABOUT THE AUTHOR

David Pavón Cuéllar is professor of psychology and philosophy at the Universidad Michoacana de San Nicolás de Hidalgo (Morelia, Michoacán, Mexico). He also taught in the Department of Psychoanalysis at the University of Paris VIII (Saint-Denis, France). Besides books and papers on guerrilla warfare, he has recently published a number of articles on discourse analysis (*Revista Latinoamericana de Psicología*, 2009), political theory (*Araucaria, Revista Iberoamericana de Filosofía*, 2009), and Lacanian psychoanalysis (*Lettre Mensuelle de l'École de la Cause Freudienne*, 2005; *Letterina, Bulletin de l'Association du Champ Freudien*, 2006; *Dilema, Revista de Filosofía de la Universidad de Valencia*, 2007; *Filosofia, Revista da Faculdade de Letras da Universidade do Porto*, 2008; *Annual Review of Critical Psychology*, 2009).

INTRODUCTION

An application of Lacanian concepts to discourse analysis in social psychology

After the Revolution, which lasted from 1910–1921, the Institutional Revolutionary Party (PRI) came to power in Mexico. It established a corrupt and repressive regime that ran the country, without a break, until the year 2000, when the rightist National Action Party (PAN) won the elections. Before this long-awaited victory of the Opposition, there were 50 years of protest demonstrations against the PRI government. Some were peaceful, others were violent. Many guerrilla leaders became legendary figures. This is the case for Rubén Jaramillo, Arturo Gámiz, Genaro Vásquez, Lucio Cabañas, and recently Subcomandante Marcos, of the Zapatista Army of National Liberation (EZLN).

In June 1995, 17 peasants were killed by the police somewhere near Acapulco. A year later, in the same place, the members of the Popular Revolutionary Army (EPR) made their first appearance. They were hooded and armed with AK-47 guns. They declared that they came to avenge the victims of the government and bring about a second revolution, the definitive proletarian one. During the next three years, the members of the EPR, the *Eperrists*, braved the Mexican Army several times. A large number of fighters were killed.

In 1997, I met with an Eperrist to ask his opinion of the EZLN (Pavón Cuéllar & López Albertos, 1998). After this encounter, in collaboration with María Luisa Vega, I began a long electronic interview with the EPR (Pavón Cuéllar & Vega, 1998, 1999a, 1999b, 2003). The interview started in Spain, continued in Portugal, and in 1999, inside an underground shelter in the suburbs of Mexico City, led to a face-to-face encounter with five hooded Eperrists.

In this book, I will use a fragment from the electronic interview with the EPR. I will systematically use it as an example to illustrate my application of Lacan in the field of discourse analysis in social psychology. The fragment is an answer from an Eperrist named Francisco Javier to a question posed by María Luisa Vega about "the possibility of harmonization, in the life of an Eperrist, between familiar obligations and revolutionary activities". Here is the answer:

> "Family is one of the fundamental pillars for the construction of the new society and the new man. This is so, as it represents the germ of the future education, which has to be based on instruction and communication of proletarian ideology, culture and values that will contribute to man's development and total fulfilment. Hence the importance and significance of marriage for the revolutionaries, as a starting point for the establishment of family and thereby for the constitution of society. From our revolutionary point of view, couple relations have to be based on love. For us, love is not only an identification in the perception of the world, in the way of life and in the social objectives, but it is also the most important moral conquest of our time, that is, individual sexual love as the foundation of monogamous family. This love leads to mutual respect and to faithfulness from conviction, or to a dissolution of the couple when the feeling disappears. We would not be consistent revolutionaries if our conceptions of marriage and the couple were not based on love, respect and faithfulness."

We will continually come back to this fragment. It will be a sort of experimental field where I will put my reflections to the test. It will be also the one concrete case to exemplify the proposal of the book.

***

What I am proposing here is *an application of Lacanian concepts to discourse analysis in social psychology*. We can grasp the significance of this proposal by getting a general view of its parts and their combination:

- *Application.* It is an application in the sense of its functional usage that allows us to act on something, just as we *apply* tools to solve a problem, a certain strategy to clear up an issue, a treatment to cure an illness.
- *Application of concepts.* The application is strictly conceptual, but each concept will logically involve its epistemological conception, its theoretical conceptualization, its methodological function and its practical functioning.
- *Application of Lacanian concepts.* In order to apply the Lacanian concepts, it will be necessary to make way for them between other concepts that fight, or could fight, for the ground of the application. Those other concepts will come mainly from phenomenology, semiology, psychoanalysis, Marxism, cognitivism, constructionism and deconstruction.
- *Application of Lacanian concepts to discourse analysis in social psychology.* Discourse analysis will not be regarded only as a theoretical and methodological perspective, but also as a spontaneous activity that is knowingly or unknowingly executed by those who study attitudes, categories, representations or constructions. As social psychologists move towards their objects through discourse, they are directly concerned with discourse analysis.

My proposal is not without precedent. It is actually preceded by two generations of intense work. The first one was French and clearly Marxist and Althusserian (Pêcheux, 1969, 1975a, 1975b; Pêcheux & Fuchs, 1975). The second one is mainly British and rather multifaceted (Parker, 1997b, 2000, 2001, 2003, 2005a; Frosh, 2002; Frosh et al., 2003; Georgaca, 2005; Hook, 2003, 2008; Branney, 2008). Just like those who precede me, I think that discourse analysts should take Lacan seriously. They should recognize the intrinsic value of his approach to discourse (e.g., Pêcheux, 1975b; Parker, 2005a), or at least the cultural and psychological importance of what is disclosed by his approach (e.g., Parker, 1997b, 2000; Dunker & Parker, 2009). Despite such importance, several psychologists do not want to hear a word about Lacan. They refuse to *see* Lacan. This refusal cannot always be rationally explained by the 'fundamental incompatibility' between psychology and Lacan, the inflexible psychoanalyst, 'who operates as the antithesis of psychology' (Parker, 2003, pp. 95, 110). The refusal is often irrational. It is often motivated by phobic reactions to the real that shows through the old worn mirror reflecting the 'distorted representations of psychoanalysis in psychology textbooks' (Parker, 2000, p. 335). At least for health reasons, it would be advisable to cure such a phobia. That does not entail either closing our eyes to the incompatibility between psychology and psychoanalysis, or abjuring social psychology to join those psychoanalysts who were characterized by Moscovici (1985), rightly or wrongly, as 'priests prostrated before the image of the creator of their doctrine' (p. 291).

Even if my purpose here is not to abjure any discipline, I assume the need to change social psychology so as to open it to Lacanian psychoanalysis. Thus, I regard as an actual need what Hook (2008) considers a virtual necessity, namely, that 'it is the conceptual domain of the social psychological itself that needs to be broadened, revised, even radically so, if that is what is required for it to productively engage with advances in Lacanian thought' (p. 69). Before that revision, it is extremely difficult for a social psychologist to think with concepts, such as Lacanian ones, that result from a 'work entirely conceptually independent of the assumptions that psychologists make about the human subject' (Parker, 2003, p. 111).

In order to avoid fruitless difficulties, this book is positioned out of the conceptual domain of the social psychological. What is proposed here comes from the outside of this *conscious interior*, that can only be broadened and revised from the outside, from the exteriority which is denoted by the *exterior unconscious* of Lacan.

On the *exterior* of the *conscious interior*, this book has not only the position of discourse analysis 'as an alternative' to 'cognitive social psychology' (Potter & Wetherell, 1987, p. 157), but it also takes up the position of Lacanian psychoanalysis 'as an alternative to psychology' (Parker, 2003, p. 96). In this position, the body of the text is reserved for Lacanian psychoanalysis and for the diverse means of applying it to contemporary social psychology. As for this psychology, even turned against itself and even impregnated by Lacan, it is relegated to the footnotes, together with digressions and excursions into all sorts of questions related to the proposed concepts.

The book's twofold organization is intended to keep a vital separation and a beneficial tension between the fields of psychology and psychoanalysis. As a matter of fact, both fields present already essential 'differences over conceptual focus and methodological grounding, over ontological and epistemological claims' (Parker, 2008, p. 148). Furthermore, psychoanalysis and psychology are already separated enough in the reality of their social practices and institutional locations, associations and scientific meetings, academic journals and other forms of the exercise of power and the transmission-accumulation of knowledge. This physical gap is emphasized, inside the book, in the form of the separation between the footnotes and the body of the text. Nevertheless, despite this separation, there will be a permanent interaction between psychoanalysis and psychology. The two fields will be defined by this interaction, which embraces the application of Lacanian concepts to social psychology.

It is an unquestionable fact that Lacanian psychoanalysis offers concepts that can be applied to discourse analysis in social psychology. However, as Branney (2008) has noticed, 'Lacanian psychoanalysis does not offer a comprehensive theory, and it would be difficult to select any concepts that could either introduce Lacanian psychoanalysis or provide the foundation of data analysis' (p. 584). Faced with such a difficulty, here I select only those concepts that have been permanently prioritized by Lacan himself in his different approaches to discourse: the real, the imaginary and the symbolic; the signifier, the signified and the signification; the full word and the empty word; the enunciation and the statement; the subject as a signifier; the unconscious as discourse; the representative of the subject; the discourse of the master; the symbolic being of word and the real lack of being in word; the interpretation and the understanding.

Since this book is situated in the perspective of Lacanian psychoanalysis, the proposed concepts shall not be treated as psychological notions. Following the line indicated by the most important work preceding my proposal (Parker, 2005a), the concepts shall not be treated as 'empirical definable substances' that would constitute 'a fully formed theory of discourse', a 'sure-fire way of analyzing discourse', or a 'fixed method for reading text'—which would indeed be 'anathema to Lacanian psychoanalysis' (pp. 166–167). If, in this book, Lacanian concepts are applied to methods of discourse analysis, this does not mean they can form 'a *method* that might be applied' to analyze any kind of discourse (p. 167). By their own nature, they cannot be coordinated in a simple general method. Even so, they can be used as conceptual coordinates to orient particular methods adapted to fit different discourses. As such, they are designed 'to be suggestive rather than prescriptive' and 'to be explicated and warranted each time for each piece of analysis' (p. 178). Only under these conditions can the proposed Lacanian concepts bring into being alternative, innovative, and subversive methodological tools. Integrated into what Parker terms 'Lacanian Discourse Analysis' (pp. 165–166), these tools can be useful to radically reform discourse analysis in social psychology. They can also be helpful to deepen and sharpen it, but only by setting boundaries to it. Involving necessarily these boundaries, the conceptual application of Lacan will inevitably restrict discourse analysis. This restriction will be intrinsic to each concept. So it will automatically be identified when specifying the concepts in the chapters of the book.

CHAPTER ONE

The symbolic and the imaginary

The book starts, in this chapter, with a differential definition of three psychic dimensions, the *real*, the *imaginary*, and the *symbolic*. Concentrating on the distinction between the symbolic and the imaginary, I use it to distinguish between what must be analyzed and what should rather be avoided by a Lacanian Discourse Analysis. In this analysis, the avoidable imaginary side of discourse will offer us nothing more than vague similarities between analogous mental entities. As for the unavoidable symbolic order, it will appear to us as composed of rigorously analyzable identities and differences between discrete literal elements.

Imaginary representations in the mirror of discourse

To 'understand anything' about Lacanian theory, we should first learn to differentiate between its 'three systems to guide ourselves by' (Lacan, 1953–1954, 24.02.54, p. 119). These systems are the *symbolic*, the *imaginary* and the *real*. They represent for Lacan (1953c) the 'essential registers of human reality' (p. 13). In order to distinguish these 'three quite distinct registers' (ibid.), we will first begin with the 'methodological distinction' between 'the symbolic and the imaginary in their relationship to the real' (Lacan, 1966a, p. 198).

Let us read our fragment of discourse: "Family is one of the fundamental pillars for the construction of the new society and the new man".[1] An image of the pillar comes to our mind. It is a vertical support that is used for a construction. We can imagine all of this. We can also imagine that Francisco Javier has in his mind an image that is similar to ours. However, the fact remains that his image is not our image. There is not a shared social imaginary representation, but two individual representations. Unlike the external words, which may be identical (word "pillar" = word "pillar"), those internal images can be merely similar (one image of a pillar ≅ another image of a pillar), but they are essentially distinct, because similarity is never enough to erase a distinction and make an identity.[2]

When analyzing the imaginary in our fragment of discourse, an ordinary empiricist psychologist will not be consistent with his empiricism if he does not recognize the existence of at least two distinct images: the one in his mind, and the one of Francisco Javier, 'understanding man' of my 'country', in his 'mind' (Locke, 1690, III, II, §4, p. 282).[3] There are these two images because the Eperrist cannot impose his image as the only one. He cannot even share it. He cannot *communicate* it, because every 'image' is a 'single experience' that 'lodges in an individual consciousness and is, strictly speaking, incommunicable' (Sapir, 1921, p. 12).

Francisco Javier cannot give us access to his mind. He cannot communicate his image. So we cannot know his image, but only ours. We certainly are right in supposing that there is a similarity between his image and ours, in the sense that the 'imaginary' is precisely 'the supposition that there is a similarity' (Milner, 1983, p. 7). Anyhow, our image is not his, but ours. It is our image reflected in the mirror of discourse.[4]

When discourse is analyzed through the imaginary, it becomes a mirror that reflects the imaginary representations of the one who analyzes it. These representations do not reside in discourse, but in the analyst. They belong to his imaginary kit. They have nothing to do with a so-called *mental representation* of the one who enunciates discourse. Until there is proof of the contrary, we must accept that this representation is not objectively analyzable. To compensate, the analyst can always analyze his own representations. These are certainly analyzable. In fact, they are systematically analyzed by a number of cognitive psychologists.

Contrary to those cognitive psychologists who stand in front of their mirrors for life, Lacanian discourse analysts prefer to break these mirrors of cognition.[5] Fortunately, there is not only the mirror. The imaginary is not the only thing that I can analyze in discourse. The fact that 'the analyzable meets the imaginary' does not mean that 'the imaginary is the analyzable' (Lacan, 1953c, p. 23).

The symbolic value and the imaginary equivalence

We admitted that there is a similarity between my image of the pillar and the one of Francisco Javier. This similarity lies in the fact that both of us imagine the same thing. Just as I imagine the pillar, so does Francisco Javier. This is easily explainable. We both imagine the same pillar because we are both under the influence of the same word "pillar".

The similarity between the two images of a pillar depends on the identity of the same word, "pillar", which is identical for me and for Francisco Javier. As Wittgenstein (1969) noticed, 'it is not a similarity' which turns the images into *images of a pillar* (V, §62, p. 139). If they are both images of a pillar, it is because 'I say it' (ibid.). It is because I ascribe the same word "pillar" to both images.

Between my image and the image belonging to Francisco Javier, the only necessary similarity rests on the word "pillar", which is identical for both of us. What is *equivalent* between the two images belonging to the two individuals is this *social identity* of the same symbolic *value*. Now this value, unlike the image, is discrete and not analogical. This means that the word, contrary to the image, cannot be *similar* or *analogous* to other words, but only *identical* to itself and *different* from other words.

Imaginary equivalence	*Symbolic value*
Similarity (based on identity)	Identity (base of similarity)
Analogical entities	Discrete entities
$(a+b_1) \cong (a+b_2)$	$a = a \neq b$
Image (b_1) of the pillar (a) ≅ image (b_2) of the pillar (a)	"pillar" (a) = "pillar" (a) ≠ "family" (b)

The 'symbolic value' of the word "pillar" determines an 'imaginary equivalence' between two images of the pillar (Lacan, 1953c, pp. 19, 24). *Between the image of the one who expresses a discourse and the correlative image of the one who analyzes the same discourse, the hypothetical similarity involves an imaginary equivalence founded on the real identity of the same symbolic value.* In our fragment of discourse, this value is the word "pillar" [a], which remains always identical to itself [a = a] and different from any other word [a≠b], for instance the word "family" [b]. This working of discrete identities and differences between symbolic values [a = a≠b] is easily distinguishable from the imaginary functioning of analogical resemblances or similarities between images [$(a+b_1) \cong (a+b_2)$]. In this imaginary functioning, my image of a pillar ($a+b_1$) is just *like* another image of a pillar ($a+b_2$). But such a likeness is not an identity. This 'kind of accuracy of images' is not valid for 'words' (Plato, *Cratylus*, 432c-d). Cognitive psychological exactness is not acceptable to Lacanian Discourse Analysis.

The real structure of the symbolic

When we distinguish the image of a pillar, we know that it is an image of a pillar, and not an image of a family, because the image *tells us that*. But it does not tell us with words, of course. As Wittgenstein (1969) argued, for the image 'to explain itself through a language would represent a detour' (IX, p. 114). When we perceive a pillar, we do not see the word "pillar". We recognize the contour of the image and not the six letters of the word. Nevertheless, the contour of the image has the symbolic value of the word. When we see something indistinguishable in the distance or through a haze, we can only imagine a pillar when we *read*, on the deep and hazy sheet of reality, the contour of that which has the symbolic value of the word "pillar". This is particularly true when we read the word "pillar" on a sheet of paper. In this case, we imagine a pillar because we interpret the six letters of the word "pillar".

When we listen to or read a discourse on any shallow or deep page of our world, the symbolic precedes and determines the imaginary. This does not suppose, however, that in writing or talking the imaginary precedes and determines the symbolic. Even if someone, such as Francisco Javier, seems to be talking with the aim of outlining the imaginary shape of a "construction of the new society", it must be granted that this "construction" is not imaginary in itself. The "new society" is built of words and relations between words. Its architecture is essentially symbolic. It results from a material and structural symbolization. It is a sort of architectural writing carried out by a symbolic archi-worker (*arkhi-tektôn*).

Here it is hard to avoid Derrida's 'mythical archi-writing (*archi-écriture*)', as the 'blind spot of all cogitations about writing' (Lacan, 1970–1971, 10.03.71, p. 78). Since the symbolic is intrinsically conditioned by symbolization, one can certainly agree with Derrida (1967) when he regards the archi-writing as the 'condition of the linguistic system' (p. 88) and the 'base' of 'language' (p. 75) and 'speech' (p. 82). This is true, but only provided that the archi-writing, as the 'condition for all other differences' (p. 95), is a mere symbolic differentiation from the real. Take for example the symbolic differentiation of the "consistent revolutionary" from Francisco Javier, as a condition for symbolic differences between a "man" and the "new man", a "family" and the "monogamous family", etc. All these differences between symbolic entities require an opening to symbolization of the real. They necessitate an initial symbolic differentiation from the real. Assimilated to this differentiation, the archi-writing can be also assimilated to the '*différance*' of Derrida, that is to say, the 'pure movement which produces differences' (p. 92), including the difference between differences and identities, identities which produce similarities by 'reducing differences' (p. 83).

Real	*Imaginary*	*Symbolic*
Beyond description	Within description	Discourse, description
Thing to be described	Thing which is described	Words that describe

Even supposing that a discourse exists for the purpose of describing a thing, it must be admitted that the discursive existence of the thing (the symbolic existence of the word "family") begins where the description differentiates itself from the thing to be described (the real family). After this symbolic differentiation, the thing is lost forever in discourse. It is impossible to recover it by an accurate description of something identical to it. The identity of the real thing becomes indescribable. Discourse can describe merely something similar to it (an imaginary family). That is easily understandable. Description can only make use of words. Yet these words cannot describe without determining that which is described. This is why the determined image described by a discourse could never correspond to the undetermined thing being described.

The thing within description is not the real thing. So there is no realistic descriptive discourse. The impression of 'realism' is 'a mere effect of discourse' (Lacan, 1966c, p. 225). In a sense, symbolism is the single universal style of discourse. Because of this symbolism, a Lacanian does not claim to be able to attain, through discourse, something real behind and before discourse. Such a real 'escapes us' and remains 'beyond reach' (Lacan, 1953c, 53, p. 13). It is, for example, the family that Francisco Javier would try in vain to describe for us. That real family could never completely fit its description. It is beyond description. It remains far away behind the words that we analyze. These words talk to us about another family, an imaginary one, which concerns only ourselves. In point of fact, the only family that concerns both Francisco Javier and us is the symbolic "family" of discourse. But this shared *word* is not the *thing*. It is not the thing that Francisco Javier would probably try to share with us. That is more than a word. Unfortunately, that is none of our business.

If Lacanian Discourse Analysis leaves aside the indescribable extra-discursive real thing, it is not with the intention of concentrating on a described imaginary thing within discourse. When this intra-discursive thing can be analyzed, it is irrelevant, because it concerns merely those who analyze discourse. Otherwise, when the imaginary thing concerns the producer of discourse, it is not more accessible than the real thing, since it is concealed by discourse, which is *always* a 'cosmetic writing' of words that 'have nothing to do with their content' (cf. Barthes, 1957, p. 137). That explains also the unanalyzable character of the real thing behind discourse. In both cases, communication is obstructed by the cosmetic and symbolic character of discourse.

Cosmetic writing breaks off any kind of non-symbolic identity between the two sides of discourse, the one of the speaker and the one of the analyst. These two sides are thus differentiated. They are differentiated by the same movement that differentiates the symbolic from the real. So the archi-writing manifests itself in cosmetic writing. The symbolic differentiation from the real entails a separation between the writer and the reader. This separation reveals the 'spacing' of Derrida (1967, pp. 99–101).

Viewed from a Lacanian standpoint, the spacing is a rupture in the real identity. It is a symbolization that hollows out the real and opens what we usually call 'real space' (Lacan, 1975–1976, 10.02.76, p. 86). Between the writer and the reader, this space is the symbolic place of discourse. It comprises the space of pages and paragraphs, the sold advertising space in a newspaper, as well as the web space, but also corridors and rooms of a building, streets and neighbourhoods in a city or in a dreamland, and even open spaces and geographical environments. In any case, the real space is a discursive context where the analyst can meet the enunciator of a discursive text. Therefore, it is a matter for discourse analysis, whose 'findings' may then be of a 'psychogeographical' nature (Debord, 1955).

Lacanian Discourse Analysis takes all the real space, and everything in it, as an analyzable discursive context. Here the so-called *real space* is nothing more than a *symbolic place* that we fill with an *imaginary reality*. Thus space 'straddles imaginary and symbolic' (Miller, 2006–2007, 17.01.07, p. 6). It constitutes the essence of 'reality' as the 'junction of symbolic and imaginary' (06.12.06, p. 11). As for the real, it is just the spacing by symbolization. It is the 'opening to being' where space spreads as a 'construction' (29.11.06, p. 6). In this opening 'by the symbol' (ibid.), the real turns into *the real of the symbolic*. Everything develops into discourse. The discursive construction of space includes all other constructions, for example "the construction of the new society" by Francisco Javier and his friends. Just as any other construction, this one takes place in the analyzable space of discourse, in this 'purely verbal construction' which has been 'spelled in three dimensions' (Lacan, 1975–1976, 10.02.76, p. 86).

Before the discursive construction of the three-dimensional space, there is only the void of the real that has been emptied by the symbol. From a Lacanian point of view, such a void constitutes the indeterminate real background of imaginary reality. Against this background, reality is constructed by discourse. Its construction arises from its floating determination by its symbolic architecture. Now, since the real is empty, this architecture also represents the only foundation of reality. It is the real structure that holds up reality by organizing the real emptiness that is filled by reality.

The archi-writing carves a structure in the real. Then this written structure organizes the real emptiness. Finally, this emptiness takes the symbolic form of the structure. In this way, the real emptiness becomes the structured real of the symbolic. We shall see later how this real plays a part in the enunciation and the literal articulation of discourse. We will not examine what takes place in this real of the symbolic, namely the release of enjoyment, the movement of drives, the excitement of desire, the cause of anguish, and the incitement to irrational or unfounded violence. However, one must be aware that all of this *occurs* in the interstices of discourse. All of this happens in the same empty real structure of the symbolic. The experience of all of this gives us an idea about the only real identity that we ever know in discourse, that is, the real emptiness of the symbolic.

In discourse, the empty structure of the symbolic is the only real stuff. It is the foundation of everything. It is the insubstantial substance of both symbolic values and imaginary mirror equivalences. While the symbolic determines the imaginary, the real of the symbolic supports the symbolic and the imaginary. This is why Lacanian Discourse Analysis cannot disregard, in discursive material, either the symbolic differences or the real or literal identity of the symbolic differences. Both are crucial in discourse. If the symbolic is decisive, its real structure is fundamental.[6]

The fundamental real and the determining symbolic

The symbolic is not only decisive for the imaginary, but it also has a real structure that is fundamental for everything. Besides this, the symbolic is made up of discrete relations which can be directly scrutinized. This being so, Lacanian Discourse Analysis must concentrate on the symbolic and its real structure in order to:

- Work with the accuracy and distinctness of discrete relations (symbolic differences and identities) and avoid the imprecision and vagueness of analogical associations (imaginary likenesses and similarities).
- Describe what is determining (the symbolic) and so explain what is determined (the imaginary).

- Consider what is founding (the real of the symbolic) and not only what is founded (the symbolic and the imaginary).
- Stay close to that which is directly accessible and analyzable (that which relates to the symbolic) and stay away from that which always escapes us (the real in itself).

In Lacanian Discourse Analysis, one can usually overlook both the inaccessible real of the real and the derived and mirrored imaginary. However, one cannot miss either the determining symbolic or the fundamental real of the symbolic. Thus, discourse must be approached from the angle of the real spacing and the resultant symbolic space. All this is what we usually call *the structure*, which is composed of its real emptiness and of symbolic relations, discrete differences and identities, or rather differences between identities, since identities are just simple entities whose only symbolic value is to be different from other entities.

Instead of wasting time looking for imaginary similarities beyond discourse, Lacanian analysts may confine themselves to examining evident real gaps and symbolic differences in discourse.[7] So they may restrict analysis to the situation and variation of discrete values. Unlike traditional and cognitive psychologists, Lacanian analysts are not obliged to imagine a unifying mental content that fills the emptiness of discourse and brings together its diverse elements. The aim of Lacanian Discourse Analysis is not to fill the real 'void' of 'the symbolic' with a 'consistency affected with the imaginary' (Lacan, 1975–1976, 09.12.75, p. 36), for example the *pillared consistency*, firmness or cohesion of the "monogamous family" of Francisco Javier. Instead of this conjectural and even fictional consistency, what should count here is the literal and factual inconsistency of expressions such as the "monogamous family".

What really matters to Lacanians is the literal foundation and factual distinction of each symbolic value. Their central subject is the structure of values and not the conjecture of equivalences between these values. After all, these imaginary equivalences are always based on the real structure of symbolic values. By knowing the values, we know what determines the equivalences. By looking at their structure, we look at their real foundation.

Although Lacanian Discourse Analysis can include incidental explorations of the imaginary, these must always take the real and the symbolic into consideration. If I am interested in the image of the family that Francisco Javier conjures up for me, I can only understand it by analyzing real gaps and symbolic differences between "family" and "individual sexual love", "marriage" and "monogamous family", "familiar obligations" and "faithfulness from conviction", etc. In this case, my image is also explained by my particular position in relation to "family" and "love", "marriage" and "monogamy", "obligation" or "conviction". All this is important so far as discourse analysis can be seriously affected and obstructed by the imaginary of the analyst and by everything that determines it outside the analyzed discourse. In fact, the imaginary must primarily be approached to be avoided. Its exploration must be subordinated to the analysis of the symbolic and the real of the symbolic. In any case, Lacanian analysts should never devote themselves to the imaginary to such a point that literal discourse is forgotten.

The unimaginable real and the imaginary reality

If usually we speak only about our 'own imaginations' (Locke, 1690, III, II, §5, p. 282), a Lacanian perspective gives priority to what we speak over what we imagine. However, what we imagine, in this perspective, is nothing less than the entire reality. *We imagine reality*. Lacan (1953c) also says that we 'hallucinate' our 'world' (p. 18). Therefore, the reality of this world is not 'real', but 'illusory' (ibid.). Although it seems to be 'really given' (1958b, p. 169), reality must be clearly distinguished from the 'pure and simple real' (1953c, p. 18). Reality has nothing to do with this real. *The real* of Lacan begins only beyond reality and behind the mirror in which reality appears. Between this reality and the real, the only quality in common is the 'solidity' and the 'impassable' character (1967a, p. 354).

Unlike the real, reality is not real, pure or simple. It is not exterior, but interior. From the Lacanian point of view, reality is always an inner reality. It consists of the contents of the mind, the content of discourse, the meaning of the word, the stuffing of psychology handbooks. It is composed of cognitions, representations, categorizations, etc. It is what we imagine, that which is decided by discourse, that whose foundation is precisely the real. So it is not the real.[8] *Unlike the unimaginable, unfounded and indeterminate real, reality is imaginary, determined by the symbolic and founded on the real of the symbolic.*

On the foundation of the real structure, the symbolic determines the entire reality. Discourse generates the things around us. As Humboldt (1821) noted a long time ago, 'objects' are 'created by words' (pp. 121–122). It is 'within language' where the entire reality arises as the 'total image of objects' and 'invisible affinities' and 'connections' between 'objects' (p. 159). Lacan (1967b) would remark that 'language puts objects in reality' (p. 250). Following a 'transcendental principle of sign constitution of objects', we may say here that 'signs' constitute 'objects' of reality (Melo, 2000, p. 158). In Lacan's terminology, the 'symbol constitutes human reality' (1953c, p. 55). 'It is the world of words that creates the world of things' (1953a, p. 274). In Francisco Javier's "perception of the world", for instance, the real world is created by being perceived as a real world through the *symbolic grid* of "proletarian ideology, culture and values", which determines "the perception of the world, the way of life and the social objectives". Here, 'perception takes on its characteristic of reality only through symbolic articulations that interweave it with a whole world' (Lacan, 1956b, p. 390). If perception creates its own reality, it is because of the symbolic that acts through perception.[9] In this way, the imaginary reality is created by the symbolic. The word creates the world's image.

Concerning the idea that the word creates the world's image, Schaff (1964) notes that 'the creator of the world's image is a world's creation' (p. 203). So he assumes that words would be created by a world, a sort of real world, a 'social and historical' world (ibid.). Here it can be objected that such a world consists of nothing more than 'words' (Lacan, 1953a, p. 259). Besides these words of language, the reality of the world is nothing but our image of the world in 'the mirror' of 'language' (cf. Schaff, 1964, pp. 205–218). Therefore, despite Schaff, this language does not 'reflect reality', but it 'creates reality' (ibid.). The imaginary reality of the world is created by language. It is created *ex nihilo* by the symbolic.

Let us take the case of Francisco Javier. His words form part of the symbolic that executes the creation of the imaginary reality, for example through "the construction of the new society". If Lacanian Discourse Analysis leads to this revolutionary discursive "construction", it cannot give access to the imaginary outcome for

Francisco Javier. Actually, this access is strictly forbidden to us. We could never know the reality that is imagined by our fellow human beings. This mental reality stays in the depths of 'individual consciousness' (Sapir, 1921, p. 12). It cannot be reached from here. So it does not exist for us. It has not been created for us, even though we have access to the symbolic creation of it.

The relative autonomy of the imaginary

To 'understand how man agreed about the sense of the first words', it is not enough to 'observe that people pronounced words in circumstances in which each one must relate the same words to the same perceptions' (Condillac, 1746, IX, §80, p. 269). First of all, perceptions are never the same for me and for my neighbour. As long as his neighbouring position is not exactly my position, his perceptions are not exactly my perceptions. But even if we admitted that we could share the same perceptions, it would be difficult to conceive of those circumstances in which the same word would be related to the same perception. Aside from the act of thinking, writing or pronouncing the same word "pillar" ten times, I cannot conceive of any other circumstance in which ten identical occurrences of the same word "pillar" would be related to ten similar perceptions of an image of a pillar. Even from the perspective of Condillac, there is only the word that can establish its connection with the perception. When the perception is missing or lacking, the word can always produce it in order to establish or re-establish its connection with it. In this way, I now perceive an image of a pillar that is determined, through my perception, by the word "pillar" and the symbolic environment in which I am thinking about it.

Imaginary reality is constantly determined, through perception, by the word and its symbolic environment. The consequence, as we shall see later, is the transformation of imaginary reality into a 'constituted element of the symbolic code' (Lacan, 1958b, p. 168). Thus, the permanent determination of the imaginary by the symbolic is also a general symbolization of the imaginary. The human 'imaginary' is always and everywhere 'symbolized' (1953c, p. 47).

Once symbolized, the image of a pillar is no less symbolic than the word "pillar". Nevertheless, the imaginary can be relatively autonomous, independent from the symbolic. It can even prevail over the symbolic. The fact remains that this quantitative prevalence does not suppose a qualitative inversion of the logical relation between the symbolic and the imaginary. The symbolic will always determine the imaginary. As the value of an imaginary reality is always a symbolic value, a strengthening of this reality is just a reinforcement of its symbolic value. So the prevalence of the imaginary is a symbolic prevalence. Likewise, its independence is also symbolic.

In the Lacanian perspective, everything human is both determined by the symbolic and situated in a symbolic environment. Lacan's 'human order' is a 'symbolic order' (Althusser, 1964, p. 38). This being so, we cannot conceive of a non-symbolic human imaginary. Such an imaginary would be intrinsically contradictory.

To conceive of an imaginary that is totally freed from the symbolic, we should think about a non-human imaginary, for instance the one that is at work in the analogical communication of bees, which functions by a 'signalling of the location of objects' (Lacan, 1956a, p. 19). As 'first tentative of symbolic behaviour', the signalling imparts a proto-symbolic, 'socialized value' to a 'displaced segment', which 'is used by the animal group as a reference mark for a collective behaviour' (1953c, p. 22). Lacan (1956a) finds a human equivalent of this imaginary 'communication' in the 'communion established between two people in their hatred directed at a common object' (p. 19). This hatred would be an elementary human aversion that signals, by a displacement, the hated position of the object.[10] Yet, in human hatred, the symbolic regains control of the imaginary and 'introduces a new reality into the animal reality' (Lacan, 1953c, p. 56). Once we are in this new reality, the hated position in a *natural space* becomes a symbolic position in a *cultural environment*. This can be seen in the hated position of the Institutional Revolutionary Party (PRI) in relation to the Popular Revolutionary Army (EPR) of Francisco Javier. If the "institutional revolutionary" is hated by the "popular" one, it is because of the opposition between the structural positions of both revolutionaries. The "institutional revolutionary" is thus hated because of his position in the cultural environment of the structure. This is the position which is signalized by the hatred of the guerrilla. As a symbolic position, it can be everywhere in the natural space. Therefore, it cannot really be *signalized*, such as bees signalize the spatial position of a field of flowers. Instead, the human hated position must be *signifierized* through discourse, as we will see later. For the time being, we need only to know that *signifierization* locates the hated position in the real structure of the symbolic, which reorganizes everything in space and opens up the only universe where a human being can survive.

In human language, there is not only the 'artificial reproduction' that is characteristic of animal communicative displacement of a natural space (Lacan, 1953c, p. 63). Nor is there only the 'voice used to indicate where pleasure and displeasure are' (Aristotle, *Politics*, I, 2, 1253a). The voice of Francisco Javier, for example, does not work just to signalize a pleasing left position and a displeasing right position, but it also incorporates a third symbolic dimension in which the left and the right are not just physical sides in the natural space, but rather structural points in a cultural environment where we find the "consistency", the "conviction" and many other landmarks. In this environment where we live, the "pleasing" and "displeasing", as well as the "right" and "left", become words of 'a discourse which is used' to locate the structural positions of what is convincing and unconvincing, consistent and inconsistent, 'fair' and 'unfair' (Aristotle, *Politics*, I, 2, 1253a).

Despite the submission to the symbolic, sometimes the human imaginary attains an almost animal stage of autonomy. This may occur even in discourse. It was perhaps the case of the 'first human words', in which 'the hatred' for the same 'aggressor' might be independent of his 'unfair' character (cf. Rousseau, 1781, p. 43). In this instance, hatred would have been a simple feeling of 'repulsion' for an aggressor whose 'fairness' or 'unfairness' was not yet decided (ibid.). This situation might still exist when discourse is deficient in the symbolic mediation that decides the difference between fairness and unfairness. Without this mediation, there is just a binary logic of attraction and repulsion, excommunication of the aggressor and communion-communication of his victims, dissimilarity of the former and similarity of the latter. When coming across this kind of logic, our discourse analysis may exceptionally stop neglecting the imaginary.[11]

Independently of its usual practice, Lacanian Discourse Analysis must be prepared to deal with an imaginary discursive reality that occasionally attains a relative autonomy within the bounds of its symbolic determination.

In that eventuality, we must drastically change our approach to discourse. Instead of overlooking or avoiding the imaginary, we must systematically look for discursive traces of its binary logic. We must search for those twofold alignments of words that merely signalize a single line of vision (the flower) in relation to the own line (the bee). Here is a typical analyzable expression of the relatively independent imaginary, which is still never analyzable in itself, but only through the symbolic material of discourse. Actually, we often encounter such an expression within simplistic and dogmatic discourses that reduce every three-dimensional structural difference to the same two-dimensional mirror polarization of similarity-dissimilarity, identity-disparity, integration-disintegration, confusion-distinction, we-others, friends-enemies, agreement-disagreement, right-wrong, right-left, good-evil, etc. Here, in this binary logic, something unfair or inconsistent would automatically be reduced to the pole of wrongness and otherness. In a revolutionary discourse, the idea of a "consistent revolutionary" would be a tautology, since a true "revolutionary" would be always "consistent". An inconsistent revolutionary would be a false revolutionary. He would be wrong and unfair. He would also be other than us, an enemy, with whom we disagree. Obviously, this imaginary functioning always plays an important part in all moral and political discourses, and specially in situations of relative imaginary independence, for example in the mirror polarization of integration-disintegration inherent in nationalist discourses that realize 'archaic fantasies of dismemberment' related to the 'first perception of corporal identity in Lacan's mirror stage' (Lakhdari, 2003).

By achieving the imaginary integration of *what we are,* the mirror surface of discourse may cover up the real separation between individual subjects, between the writer of a discourse and *people like him,* but also between the writer and his readers. The result is an imaginary collective identity, for instance the ideal identity of the "consistent revolutionaries" such as Francisco Javier. In this way, the imaginary makes it possible to 'bring together an indefinite number of subjects in a common ideal' (Lacan, 1956a, p. 19). This is how individuals congregate simultaneously *around* an 'ideal-ego', such as the "consistent revolutionary" of the EPR, and *against* an 'alter ego', such as the "inconsistent revolutionary" of the PRI, which suffers from the 'aggressiveness' of the 'ideal-ego' (1953c, pp. 34–35).

Notes

1. I will employ double inverted commas to quote Francisco Javier's discourse, as well as any other literal word used to exemplify the application of Lacan to discourse analysis. As for Lacan and other authors, their words will always be in single inverted commas.
2. The social character of representations is based merely on that 'similarity' (Harré, 1985, p. 149). For lack of a real *identity* that gives substance to society, the psychology of social representations reduces the social field to an 'aggregate of people' who are only 'united' by that 'similarity' (ibid.).
3. 'The references to the subject in this book as 'he' (rather than 'he or she', or some other similar formulation) are designed to reveal rather than conceal assumptions about gender in the language we use to describe ourselves. There is a good deal of conceptual work to be done regarding this, and such work would question and take forward Lacanian analysis (work that was, unfortunately, beyond the scope of this book). To cover over this question in the main text would jar with quotations from Lacan (in which dominant ideological conceptions of gender are alive and well). It is work that cannot be solved by merely replacing masculine gendered nominations for the subject with those that pretend to be 'gender neutral'.
4. This reflected image proves the 'reflective properties' of a discourse where psychologists find an imaginary depth to be filled with psychic contents (Bromberg & Trognon, 2000, p. 295). This is how discourse becomes a sort of mirror. When psychologists are perspicacious enough to break the mirror, they immediately try 'to reorganize the pieces of the broken mirror' (Ghiglione, Matalon & Bacri, 1985, pp. 16–17).
5. In this way, they take a firm stand on the side of certain 'anti-cognitivist' discourse analysts (Hepburn & Potter, 2003, pp. 192–193).
6. Studied by cognitive psychology, the correlative imaginary is simply determined by the symbolic and supported by the real of the symbolic. It neither supports nor determines anything. Yet it facilitates both the symbolic determination and its real foundation. It facilitates them by causing a 'misrecognition' of them. The imaginary involves by definition this 'misrecognition of the symbolic network which determines us' (Žižek, 1999a).
7. With Ian Parker (2005a), we can compare this 'focus on differences' to 'one of the founding principles of discourse analysis in psychology, in which the analyst looks to the variability in accounts rather than divining a deeper unitary principle that would bring diverse statements together' (p. 168).

8. Pêcheux and Fuchs (1975) describe this 'reality', very accurately, as opposed to 'the real', as 'imaginary' and 'determined', as a 'mirror play' and a 'subjective variable' made up of 'attitudes, representations' (p. 15).
9. From a 'semiotic perspective', Camus (1999) would observe that 'perception is an activity because it is attribution/construction of signification' (p. 277). From a Lacanian perspective, we would qualify this by saying that perception is an activity *of the symbolic signifier* that may involve an attribution/construction of *an imaginary signification*.
10. This signalization corresponds approximately to the communication of a cognitive attitude of aversion. The attitude *marks* discourse. Here is a particular imaginary situation that would confirm the social psychological representation of 'a linguistic behaviour which is marked by the cognitive activity of a social subject that marks his attitudes on his statements' (Bromberg & Trognon, 2000, pp. 294–295).
11. On the subject of this 'mode of interaction in which relations of similarity and opposition are constituted and reproduced', Parker (2005a) already emphasizes the necessity for a 'discourse analysis of *imaginary* aspects of interaction' that 'would pick up those specific kinds of textual operations that hold antagonistic positions in relation to each other' (p. 171).

CHAPTER TWO

The signifier and the signified

This chapter focuses on the active and determining power of the symbolic order within discourse, in the form of a real *signifying structure* that is ordered by the *signifier* and opposed to a *signified* that is not exactly real, but rather imaginary, as well as passive and determined. Assuming this Lacanian reversal of the traditional signifier and signified positions, I argue that the imaginary cannot be avoided in discourse analysis if we accept even the merest idea of signification. Instead, I offer the Lacanian concept of *signifierization.* In the light of this concept, we will see how the imaginary signification of a social reality covers up the fact of its symbolic signifierization. When being *signifierized,* the so-called signified reality is absorbed into discourse and becomes a new signifier of the signifying social structure. This way of looking at discourse and society will lead us to a critique of Barthes and semiology. In this critique, the logical working of the symbolic signifiers will be opposed to the semiological, mythological functioning of imaginary signs, significations and signified realities.

Necessary determination and impossible signification

The imaginary is determin*ed*, while the symbolic is determin*ing*. In Lacan's terminology, we can also state that the imaginary is signi*fied*, while the symbolic is signify*ing*. However, the two statements are not interchangeable. The *determination* does not correspond exactly to the *signification*. Determination is real, effective and necessary. Conversely, signification is imaginary, ineffectual and simply impossible. In fact, signification is impossible precisely because determination is necessary.

The symbolic hypothetically determines the same thing that it signifies. However, if this is so, the thing cannot be signified, since it is not the thing to be signified anymore, but rather it becomes a thing that has been determined and then changed into another thing. Once the first thing is transformed by the symbolic, it is changed into a determined thing that has nothing to do with the thing to be signified. This undetermined thing disappears without being signified. It has no time to be signified. Before being signified, it becomes another thing. Accordingly, there is an *impossibility of signification* that results precisely from a *necessity of determination*.[1] Signification is impossible because it cannot exclude a determination of the signifiable thing by the signifying symbolic. Such a determination neutralizes the thing to be signified. Consequently, it also impedes signification or meaning, which becomes unreal, illusory, and purely imaginary.

Even if the symbol cannot signify the thing that it must determine, the symbolic is nevertheless signifying and not only determining. In this sense, each symbol is a signifier or a set of signifiers. The fact remains that these signifiers do not signify anything. As Lacan explains, 'every true signifier is, as such, a signifier that signifies nothing' (1955–1956, 11.04.56, p. 210).

As a true signifier, a symbol does not signify anything, but it simply signifies. The verb *signify* is here an intransitive verb. As we already know, the thing to be signified (the direct object of the verb) cannot be signified, but only determined. Being determined by the symbol, the thing is only 'symbolized' (Lacan, 1953c, p. 47). It becomes a new symbol among all the other symbols of the outside world. Each one of these symbols is a signifying symbol. Each one is a signifier. It always signifies, but it always fails to signify something. Therefore, as will be seen, the signifier is unconscious.

Its conscious signification is just imaginary. Contrary to the signifier, which is a material thing, the signified is just an ideal thing.

Since everything signifies around us, the signifier is around us everywhere. It corresponds to each one of the material things we perceive in our outside world. It is everything in Francisco Javier's "perception of the world". It is the symbolized object of every perception, sensation or impression, vision or sound. It is not only the word "family", but also the symbolized image of a family, whether in person or in a picture. Similarly, the signifier is not only the sound of the word "birdsong", but also the symbolized sound of a real or imaginary birdsong. Both are symbolic signifiers that go into one's ears. In this way, they differ from 'the imaginary, as signified', which has 'nothing to do with one's ears, but only with the reading of that which we hear of the signifier' (Lacan, 1972–1973, 09.01.73, p. 45). This reading interprets the signifier. It understands it. It assigns an imaginary mental signification to the sound of the material signifier.

Imaginary signified	*Symbolic signifier*
Ideal	Material
What would be communicated and understood	What is heard and spoken
Passively determin*ed* (past participle)	Actively determin*ing* (present participle)

In speech, the material signifier is articulated and heard, while the ideal signified would be communicated and understood. Apparently, the central aim of speech is this understanding of the signified, which also seems to entail an understanding between persons. From this point of view, speech may even be defined as an 'understanding-oriented activity' (Habermas, 1988, pp. 67–68). Far from this definition, a Lacanian separates imaginary understanding and 'speech, that is, the symbol' (Lacan, 1953c, p. 16). As noted above, the symbol signifies, but it does not signify anything, so there is nothing here that can be understood. There is no authentic understanding that proceeds from the spoken symbol. Instead of an authentic understanding, there is a misunderstanding. There is a fictitious understanding of an imaginary signifi*ed*, which is passively determin*ed*, distort*ed*, chang*ed*, replac*ed*, reconstitut*ed*, re-creat*ed*, symboliz*ed* (the passivity being indicated by the past participle). And all this is accomplished by the signify*ing* symbolic, which is actively determin*ing*, distort*ing*, etc. (the activity being designated by the present participle).

Even if the symbolic is continuously signifying, the concept of *signifier* is not contained in the one of *symbolic*. When we state that *a symbol is a signifier*, we are specifying the concept of *symbol*. In Lacan's work, this specification arises from a 'logical chain' that begins with 'discrete elements', then regards them as 'linguistic elements', and finally separates 'sense' from them (Juignet, 2003). All this follows the early theoretical evolution of Lacan, who has 'increasingly promoted the notion of the signifier in the symbol' (1956a, p. 61). This promotion stresses the active determining and signifying aspect of the symbolic. It can be considered a 'structuralist' promotion of the 'dynamic ensemble' of signifiers (Mukarovsky, 1929, p. 54). In this ensemble, signifiers are distinguished from symbols by their activity, relativity, multiplicity, and overdetermining capacity. This capacity resumes all the specificity of signifiers, as it designates the concurrent, synchronized and coordinated determination by multiple, relative, and active signifiers. In Lacanian Discourse Analysis, this overdetermining capacity of signifiers justifies a choice of complexity, flexibility, probability, uncertainty, and undecidability.[2] Naturally this choice could never be justified by the simple determining capacity of a symbol that may be alone, static, and absolute. Instead, this symbol could ultimately justify an analytical choice of rigidity and irrevocability.

In the linguistic theory of Sapir (1921, 1931a, 1931b, 1933), which is strikingly consonant with our Lacanian perspective, the signifier would not be a 'symbol attached' to a 'single image', to a 'single perception', or to a 'single experience', but a 'simplification of experience' into 'delimited classes of experience' (1921, pp. 12–13). This simplification takes place in language. A signifier is not only a symbol, but a symbol that belongs to the symbolic system of language. As a 'linguistic symbol' (p. 17), the signifier is a 'symbol' among other 'symbols' and within a 'flow of speech' that involves 'mutual relations' between its elements (p. 13). All this can be regarded, of course, as an 'actualization' of the 'tendency of looking to reality in a symbolic way' (1931a, p. 40). The fact remains that such an actualization must be organized by a 'language' (ibid.). As constituent elements of this organizing language, the signifiers are 'organized symbols' (Lacan, 1953c, p. 26). They are organized 'in a language' (ibid.). Therefore, they obey 'the structure of language' (ibid.). In this structure, the "pillar" of Francisco Javier is not merely the absolute symbol of the family, but it is also a signifier in relation to "faithfulness", "monogamy" and the other signifiers of the structure. The multiplicity of these signifiers overdetermines the family in different ways and not only in a single symbolic way.

Like symbolic determination, structural overdetermination impedes a real signification. Instead of achieving this signification, the signifying structure overdetermines that which should be signified. Therefore, the signification fails, since the overdetermined thing is no longer the thing to be signified. The signifying structure is thus unconscious, in the sense that it lacks a real conscious signification. This signification is just imaginary. In truth, it is composed of unconscious signifiers. As we shall see later, these *words without meaning* are *the truth* of the cognitive, mental meaning, which forms part of the unconscious structure of language.

While cognitive psychology explains language by cognition, Lacanian psychoanalysis puts language forward to explain cognition as well as cognitive psychology. This applies to psychology in general. As Lacan (1950) remarks, 'language determines psychology more than psychology explains language' (p. 128). Put differently, 'language does not come within the framework of the subject, but the subject is determined by the acts of language, that are deeper than the subject' (Cléro, 2008, p. 171). Determined by language, the subject *has* the psychology *of* language. The psyche lies in the signifiers. Individual psychic consciousness belongs to the trans-individual unconscious structure of language. It is this exteriority of language that externally shapes and arranges the internal cognitions of cognitive psychology.[3] It is this same exteriority that deeply moves and orchestrates the superficial behaviours of behavioural psychology. Now, as this determining exteriority comprises all crossable or inhabitable places around us (e.g., underground shelters, houses, streets, cities, countries, dreamlands), its psychoanalytical study is not unrelated to a 'psychogeography' defined as 'the study of the precise laws and specific effects of the geographical environment, consciously organized or not, on the emotions and behaviours of the individuals' (Debord, 1955). Actually, psychogeographers and psychoanalysts intend to explain the exterior causes (the laws of the environment) and their primary effects (the enforcements of the laws), while behavioural and cognitive psychologists confine themselves to explaining the secondary effects (the effects of the enforcement) as conditioned behaviours or signified cognitions.

While behavioural psychology focuses on conditioned behaviours, cognitive psychology prefers to study signified cognitions. Until quite recently, this study was remarkably predominant in psychology. The signified was the main topic of psychology. It was *the thing* of psychology. This was only natural, since *naturally*, 'when one talks about the signified, one thinks of the thing' (Lacan, 1953–1954, 23.06.54, p. 376). Nevertheless, in the eyes of Lacan, this first impression is erroneous. Even before defining 'the Thing' as 'the beyond-of-the-signified' (1959–1960, 09.12.59, p. 67), Lacan states that 'the signified is not the thing' (1953b, pp. 149–150), that is, it does not correspond to 'the thing in its raw state, already there, given in an order open to meaning' (1955–1956, 01.02.56, p. 135).

Let us take the case of Francisco Javier's "pillar". The signified pillar is not a real thing out there. It is not a building block outside discourse. Nor is it the real family of the Eperrist. The so-called signified pillar is, rather, another signifier. It can also *be* a concept, an idea, or an image, of course, but only for the one who wants to regard the signifier as a concept, an idea, or an image. Actually, the signified pillar can be everything one wants. It can be everything one imagines. However, all of this is just imaginary. Furthermore, these images are only for somebody specific. They are not the same for anybody else. Nor are they the signified pillar in itself. In itself, this pillar *is not*; it is not a signified pillar, but a signifying pillar, that is, a new signifier that relates to the signifier "pillar". Just like the first signifier, the second refers to a third that refers to a fourth and so on. This is why a dictionary cannot give a definite conscious signified, but only new signifiers that refer to other signifiers ("pillar", which refers to "support", which refers to "sustain", and so on). Moreover, in real language, this reference entails an overdetermination that continuously changes the value of the signifiers (the value of "sustain" is thus altered by its relation to the "pillar" as a "family" for the "construction of the new society" by a "revolutionary"). Here is the unstable and inexhaustible unconscious structure of language, which could never be definitely and entirely explored by a Lacanian Discourse Analysis.

Each signifier can be fixed in a conscious definite and definitive signified. The fact remains that such a signified is just imaginary. In truth, it is a symbolic signifier. Even when it is *imaginarized*, it still has the symbolic value of a signifier in the signifying structure. It is always a signifier that refers to another signifier. Now, to *make sense*, the signifier pretends to refer to a signified. This 'imaginary' signified is precisely that which 'makes sense' (Lacan, 1975–1976, 13.04.76, p. 131). However, in order to make sense, the signified should 'be of value' (Barthes, 1957, p. 196). Its imaginary reality should have a symbolic value, or a position in the signifying structure.

The symbolic value of an imaginary reality can be described as *the signifying truth of a signified illusion*. It is the genuine reference of the signifier that we find in a discourse. It is what we usually call *the sense of the word*. As a symbolic value of an imaginary reality, this sense is situated 'between imaginary and symbolic' (Lacan, 1975–1976, 17.02.76, p. 92). It is the 'copulation' of 'symbolic and imaginary' (16.03.76, p. 121).

Meaning	*Sense*
Imaginary reality with a symbolic value	Symbolic value of an imaginary reality
It can be represented, but it cannot be transmitted	It can be transmitted, but it cannot be represented

As a symbolic value of an imaginary reality, the sense is the 'attribute' of the signified (Deleuze, 1969, p. 99). Simultaneously, as the symbolic value of the real word in its literality, the sense is the 'expressible' aspect of the signifier (ibid.). In short, the sense expressed by the signifier is the symbolic value that is attributed to the imaginary reality of the signified. Contrary to this inexpressible reality of meaning and signification, its symbolic value can be expressed. It can be transmitted or communicated. As *exchange value*, it can even be exchanged and put into circulation. It is the transmissible symbolic representative of the untransmittable imaginary reality. So it can represent this reality. Yet it cannot be represented. Just as is the case for the 'logic form' of Wittgenstein (1921), the Lacanian symbolic value 'cannot be represented' by 'discourse', but it can 'represent reality', because it is 'what a discourse has in common with reality' (4.12, p. 83).

The symbolic value joins the real signifier of discourse and the imaginary reality of the signified. This junction is the 'sense' (Wittgenstein, 1921, 4.022, p. 75). It is the sense 'expressed' by discourse (4.121, p. 84). It is, for instance, the figurative sense of a "pillar" as a family. This sense is expressed by Francisco Javier's discourse. It can also be detected by Lacanian Discourse Analysis. It is the *familiar* symbolic value of both the word "pillar" and its imaginary meaning. This value is the only thing we can discern in the reality described by Francisco Javier. Here is our only positive knowledge about the cognition that would be operating behind discourse. Unfortunately, our knowledge refers merely to the trans-individual exchange value of a precise element in this individual cognition. We can just get to an unconscious symbolic value of the conscious imaginary reality, but we cannot approach *the reality of this mental reality*. Put differently, we can reach the sense of the word, but we cannot recognize its meaning. We can estimate the symbolic value of this meaning, but not the meaning itself. Although we distinguish the *familiar* figurative sense of the word "pillar", we will never know exactly what it means for Francisco Javier. We will never attain the imaginary signified of the symbolic signifier that we analyze.

The inaccessibility of the signified should not suggest to us that it corresponds to the real inaccessible thing. In itself and for the one who enunciates discourse, the signified is not the thing that would be designated by discourse. The signified does not belong to the real order of 'designation' (Lacan, 1953c, p. 27). Nor is it an element of the symbolic order created by a real symbolization or 'signifierization' (1962–1963, 13.03.63, p. 204). Instead, its right place is in the imaginary order of meaning or 'signification' (1953–1954, 23.06.54, p. 376). Now, as Wittgenstein (1949) notices, this 'signification hides the functioning of language with a haze that makes impossible the clear view of it' (§5, p. 29). To clear this imaginary haze of meaning, we must bring it back to the symbolic value of sense.[4]

As a matter of principle, Lacanian Discourse Analysis must reduce the unanalyzable imaginary to the analyzable symbolic. The 'signified' of the signifier must be reduced to the 'sense' of the word (Lacan, 1953b, p. 149). Here the sense indicates something that is shared between the signifier and the signified. It is a point where their respective functions intersect. It is a junction between the symbolic and the imaginary. As we know, this junction is nothing more than the signifying symbolic value of the imaginary reality of the signified. In this imaginary reality, the symbolic value is the only thing we can analyze. Yet this thing is not the signified of the interpreted signifier, but it is rather another signifier. It is the signifying aspect of the signified. It is the truth of the signified. This truth does not lie, for instance, in the image of the family evoked by Francisco Javier through the word "pillar", but in the "family" of this image. In other words, the truth does not lie in the imaginary signified that is called to mind by the interpreted signifier, but in an interpretative signifier that is positively related to the interpreted signifier. This interpretative signifier underlies the signified that is imagined by both Francisco Javier and the one who analyzes his discourse. Between their respective minds, the only possible connection is the signifier of the signified (the symbol "family") and not the signified of the signifier (the image of the family). This mental signified cannot be communicated.

When the one who analyzes discourse runs across a mental signified, he must be aware that it is not something that has been communicated by the analyzed discourse. Accordingly, it must not be analyzed as a meaning of discourse, as it does not come from discourse, but from the analyst of discourse. It is his imaginary representation of the meaning of discourse. We can accept this representation as the meaning of discourse, of course, but only so long as we specify that it is its meaning for the analyst of discourse. This imaginary meaning is the only mental information that can be reached by the one who analyzes discourse. Unfortunately, my own mind is the only accessible mind, and it is not exactly my own, as will be seen later.

The mental meaning imagined by the analyst of discourse is always *his* meaning, which is reflected in the analyzed discursive word. Even if this meaning may be similar to the one imagined by the enunciator of discourse, it is not identical to it. Nor is it identical to the real unimaginable thing objectively denoted by discourse. This is the thing to be signified, but it is not signified. As discussed above, this thing cannot be signified. The only signifiable thing is an imaginary representation of the real thing. Yet the presence of this undetermined thing stays always behind the mental mirror of its determined representations. It stays always beyond the signified imagined by both the analyst and the enunciator of discourse.

The 'Thing' is by definition 'the beyond-of-the-signified' (Lacan, 1959–1960, 09.12.59, p. 67). Nevertheless, 'in its original sense it concerns' also 'the notion of a proceeding, deliberation, or legal debate' (p. 43). Etymologically, the *Thing* is the case (*causa*) before the court (in Latin), or the *Thing* of a meeting or assembly (in Saxon), that is, the focus of discussion, the subject of every predicate, the core issue or centre of gravity of all signifiers. *The Thing is this*. If such 'a Thing could be signified, then it would be that which every signifier signifies' (Pavón Cuéllar, 2005, p. 13). Now, since *the Thing* is the real thing, its signification implies a designation. So we can say that all signifiers try to designate *the Thing*. In a sense, language is an attempt to designate it. Yet this attempt is in vain. Lacan (1953–1954) describes the attempt as 'a lure, because it is quite clear that language is not made to designate things' (23.06.54, p. 376).

In the focal point of the lure of language, *the Thing* is a void that consumes all attempts to designate it. These attempts are in vain, but they persist. Paradoxically, they still persist precisely because they are always in vain. The determining signifiers proliferate since the void of the undetermined signified is unfathomable. As long as the real thing cannot be signified, there cannot be a successful real signification that brings to an end the multiplication of the signifiers.[5]

Signification is not successful since the real thing to be signified is rather overdetermined and changed into another thing before being signified. This is why the so-called signified is just imaginary: an imaginary representation of the real thing that is no more. Instead of this undetermined thing, there is now the overdetermined thing, which constitutes the truth of the representation, that is, the signifying symbolic value of its signified imaginary reality. Here, as always, the symbolic governs the imaginary. Overdetermined by the structure, each signifier, in turn, determines its representation as a signified. In fact, this symbolic determination of the imaginary is just a ramification of the structural overdetermination of each signifier. The imaginary form of the signified is basically overdetermined by the real structure of the symbolic signifier. When I read Francisco Javier, for instance, I imagine a family which is formed and informed by the matrix of related signifiers in both the text I read ("monogamous" or "proletarian") and the context through which I read it ("father" or "poor" in the structure of my symbolized psychoanalytic knowledge, childhood memories, and class prejudices).

Even when I perceive a *real family* out there, my perception is overdetermined by the real structure of the signifier, which functions as an *a priori* condition of the experience of reality. In order to study such a transcendental relation of the signifier to the signified, we would need a semiotic reinterpretation of Kantian philosophy (Melo, 2000). This would lead us to a kind of 'transcendental semiotics' (pp. 378–379) about 'transcendental modes' treated as 'pure signifiers' (pp. 443–478) that would precede and govern the signified by 'signi-fying objects' (p. 430) and 'pro-positioning things' (p. 478).

Overdetermination, symbolization, signifierization

Unlike the real eliminated by the symbolic, the imaginary reality of the signified would be transcendentally preceded and governed by its signifying symbolic value. By virtue of this value, there would be an instant reality for an individual subject, as well as the similarity or equivalence between different realities for diverse individual subjects, which would be based on the social identity of the same symbolic values. From the optimistic viewpoint of Searle (1995), the symbolic value would thus correspond to the 'function' by which there is a 'reality', a 'reality relating to the observer', a 'social reality' based on the 'collective intentional attribution' of a 'function' to entities without an intrinsic function (p. 29). Likewise, Barthes (1957) would regard the symbolic value, in a functional way, as a 'social use' that changes the 'closed' real of 'pure matter' into a reality 'open to social appropriation' (p. 194). By the same token, the Lacanian symbolic value transforms the closed real into an open reality. This transformation can be performed in a collective way too, but also in an individual way, and not necessarily in an intentional way, as Searle believes. Lacan, in opposition to both Searle and Barthes, does not postulate an essentially useful or functional character of the symbolic value. The only function of the Lacanian symbolic value is the *signifying function*. It is a *purely symbolic function*. It is 'a function in the mathematical sense of the word', as in the expression 'x = function of y', in which something is 'replaced' by something else (Lacan, 1968–1969, 23.04.69, p. 270). Rather than a *use value*, this *replacement function*, as symbolic value, constitutes the 'exchange value' of the signifier as a constituent element of language (1958–1959, 17.12.58). As for the supposed use value of this language, it designates the imaginary reality of the signified.[6]

Following the 'structuralism of Marx' (Lacan, 1968–1969, 04.12.68, pp. 64–65), a Lacanian Discourse Analysis must give priority to the symbolic 'exchange value' of the signifier over the imaginary 'use value' of the signified (1973e, pp. 68–69). In this way, 'the primacy the real has over thought is reversed in the relation of the signifier to the signified' (1959, p. 183). Contrary to the real structure of the symbolic, which has precedence over the symbolic value of my thoughts, the imaginary reality of the signified is subordinated to the symbolic value of the signifier. In order of precedence, there is first the real signifying structure of the symbolic, then the symbolic value of each signifier, and finally the imaginary reality of the signified. Put differently, there is first the fundamental arrangement of literal words, then their determining sense, and finally their determined meaning. But we must remember that this imaginary meaning has nothing to do with a real thing denoted by the word. The latter is undetermined and unattainable, while the truth of the former is a symbolic value overdetermined by a language and accessible through a discourse analysis.[7]

In truth, as a symbolic value, the imaginary reality of the signified is overdetermined by the signifying structure of a language. Thus, in a sense, the signifier is the *cause* of the signified. In spite of Barthes (1957), there is actually a 'causal process' between the two elements (p. 217). In this process, the signified is the effect of the overdetermination by the signifying structure. Cognitive meaning results from an existing configuration of words.[8] The signifier is prior to the signified.

Assuming the causal 'priority' of the 'signifier' over the 'effect of signifying' (Lacan, 1961, p. 181), Lacanian Discourse Analysis treats the signified as an 'effect of the signifier' (Lacan, 1972–1973, 09.01.73, p. 45). The effect is overdetermined by its cause. As we know, this overdetermination excludes all possibility of signification. Signification must preserve the thing to be signified, while overdetermination transmutes this undetermined thing into another determined thing. So overdetermination supposes a determining thing (a symbolic "family") that precedes the thing that is determined (the symbolic "pillar"). Signification, on the contrary, supposes a signifying thing (a realist "family") that follows the thing to be signified (the so-called *real family*, that is, the imaginary reality of the family). In Lacan's work, this signification, still surviving until 1958, must never be confused with overdetermination, which prevails from 1958 onward. Overdetermination is not a signification, but rather something that Lacan (1962–1963) names 'signifierization' (13.03.63, p. 204).

Signifierization is the point of arrival of a Lacanian theoretical route whose 'departing point' is the decision of 'going towards a signified which is determined by the signifier' (Miller, 2007–2008, 13.02.08, p. 10). Essentially, signifierization synthesizes determination and signification. Unlike signification, which simply refers to that which is preserved as a signified, signifierization determines that which is transformed into a signifier. Contrary to signification, which makes an imaginary signified of a symbolic signifier that is detached from the signifying structure, signifierization makes a symbolic signifier of an imaginary signified that is attached to the same structure.[9]

As discussed before, the verb 'signify' is 'intransitive' (Lacan, 1970a, p. 417). The signifier signifies, but it cannot signify anything. It can only *signifierize* something, that is, communicate its signifying function to that which is *signifierized*. According to Lacan (1962–1963), 'signifierization' is precisely the 'assimilation to the function of the signifier' (13.03.63, p. 204). Through this assimilation, 'language' does not 'superimpose' only '*a* logic' on *the* human world, but it imposes *the only* signifying and overdetermining logic of *a* human world (cf. Berger & Luckmann, 1966, p. 64).

Real	*Imaginary*	*Symbolic*
Realization	Imaginarization	Symbolization
Designation	Signification	Signifierization

Lacanian signifierization is at the same time a transmutation into a signifier, a fixation to the real structure of a symbolic system, and an imposition of the signifying and overdetermining logic of this structure. Before 1958, the theoretical precedent for this signifierization does not lie in an *imagination* or *imaginarization* indistinguishable from signification. Nor does it lie in a designation treated as *realization*. It rather lies in the *symbolization* or 'symbolizing' action of a symbol that 'symbolizes the image' (Lacan, 1953c, p. 47). Due to this action, the image acquires a symbolic value in language. In this way, it becomes 'something whose sense varies according to the place it occupies in the dialogue' (p. 25). Likewise, signifierization assimilates an image to discourse. It incorporates the imaginary form of the signified (an image of a pillar or a family) to the structure of the signifier (to the symbolic functioning of the "pillar" as a "family"). Signifierization is thus a kind of symbolization. It is a symbolization that communicates a signifying symbolic value to the imaginary reality of the signified.

In signifierization, the so-called *signified* (a pillar or a family) becomes a signifying thing (a "pillar" as a function of a "family"). Signifierization is precisely an action of a signifying cause ("family"), which generates a signifying effect ("pillar"). Like the God of Spinoza (1674), the cause is 'immanent but not transitive' (I, XVIII, p. 43). The signifier ("family") is present in its effect ("pillar" as a "family") just as the creator is present in his creature. Instead of a transcendent transition from the signifying cause ("family") to the signified effect (a real family), there is an immanent transmission of the signifying function ("…") from the signifying cause ("family") to the signifying effect ("pillar" as a "family"). This is why Lacan uses the verb *to signify* as an intransitive verb. It is intransitive because there is no transition of signification. This transition is just an ideal. In fact, there is only an 'intransitive materialization from the signifier to the signified' (Lacan, 1970a, p. 417). There is only the real transmission of a symbolic material being from the creator to its creatures, from the signifierizer to the signifierized, from the materializer to the materialized. Signifierization is therefore a kind of creation and materialization. It is the divine creation of matter, corresponding to the Freudian *Bejahung*: the affirmation that ensures the materialization of that which is affirmed. This can be illustrated by considering the affirmation of our "consistent revolutionary". Francisco Javier "would not be a consistent revolutionary" if his "conceptions" were not the affirmation of a "consistent revolutionary". This affirmation is already a materialization of the "consistent revolutionary".

More than materialization, signifierization may appear to be a process of formalization whereby 'matter takes the form of language' (Marx, 1846, p. 1061), or 'matter transcends itself in language' (Lacan, 1966b, p. 209), as soon as the material 'image' of 'meaning' acquires a linguistic or symbolic form (Barthes, 1957, pp. 195, 203). The fact remains that this symbolic form is the universal form of all human materiality. In our symbolic universe, all material forms are symbolic forms. The symbolic formalization is therefore a materialization. That being the case, if Barthesian meanings take a material form as images, they do so only insofar as they acquire a formal symbolic value. This value ("...") is the only matter of which they are made (the only matter in an image of a "pillar" as a "family"). The imaginary materialization is nothing but an effect of a symbolic formalization.

On the subject of signifierization, it would be possible to *lacanise* Barthes, but the conflict between him and Lacan would still persist. In the semiologist's 'signification' or 'semantizing', what is signified or *semantized* acquires an intelligible ideal 'form' which already implies a 'state of consciousness' (Barthes, 1964, pp. 41–43). In Lacanian signifierization, on the other hand, what is signifierized acquires the unintelligible material form of an unconscious signifier without conscious signification. Thus, when materialized in language, that which is signifierized 'becomes writing' at the very instant it becomes, not an intelligible 'significant thing', but rather a perceptible signifying thing (cf. Barthes, 1957, p. 195). This process of 'precipitation of the signifier' (Lacan, 1975–1976, 11.05.76, p. 144) constitutes the positive aspect of Derrida's (1967) 'archi-writing', as 'movement of the sign-function linking content to expression' (p. 88). In this process, signifiers intervene in the immaterial content and cause the signifying effect of its written material expression. Yet this effect can no longer be termed *signified*, as it is not what would have been expressed if the transition necessary for signification to occur had succeeded. The effect should rather be called *signifierized*, since it becomes a new signifier when an intransitive overdetermination fixes it to a signifying structure.

In the surrounding structure, everything has been signifierized. All things are signifying effects of signifying causes. It is always the instance of the signifier that drives real things to exist and 'come to signify' (Lacan, 1957–1958, 11.06.58, p. 449). Paradoxically, the only real things we know arise only from contact with 'discourse' (1953b, pp. 148–150). They are no more than literal 'words' or 'material elements' linked together by the structure (ibid.). They are things insofar as they are signifierized things. They become things as they are incorporated into a language. This is why language appears from the start as 'inherent in the nature of things' (Berger & Luckmann, 1966, p. 59).

In a Lacanian perspective, things *are* signifiers of a language. As for the signified imaginary reality of things, it depends on their signifying symbolic value. Signifierization necessarily underlies signification. There is the imaginary reality of the signified from the moment it is signifierized, that is, from the instant it has a signifying symbolic value. This value is the truth of reality. The signifier is the truth of the signified. It indicates its overdetermination by the signifying structure.

The so-called signified *is overdetermined by the concerted action of multiple signifiers. This overdetermination is also a symbolization and signifierization. The overdetermined thing is transmuted into a signifier and is thus assimilated into the real structure of the signifying symbolic values. Hence, it becomes the truth of the imaginary reality of the signified, that is, a derived signifying symbolic value which is imagined as the original signifiable real thing*. It is quite obvious that such a real thing is not so real. Its reality is just imaginary. It exists merely by a retrospective illusion in which the signifierization is taken as a signification and the discursive signifier is treated as a cognitive signified.[10]

The family Francisco Javier is talking about, for example, strikes us as being prior to its discursive existence as a symbolic "family". At first sight, it is as if the meaning were there, in the past, earlier than the word. On second thought, we realize that the meaning is effectively there, in the past, because it is put there by the word. What a discourse retrospectively means is thus retroactively determined by discourse.[11]

The symbolic system of discourse achieves a retroactive transformation of the real thing into a retrospective imaginary meaning. In other words, the signifier plays an 'active role in determining the effects by which the signifiable appears to succumb to its mark, becoming, through that passion, the signified' (Lacan, 1958a, p. 166). But in truth, as we know, this signified turns out to be signifierized by the signifier. This is only natural. Being a 'mark' of the signifier and not the signifiable itself, the signified has to be 'here in the position of the signifier' (Derrida, 1967, p. 108).

Lacanian discourse analysis and Barthesian semiological analysis

From 1958 to 1964, the signifier prevails more than ever in Lacan's work. Overdetermination and signifierization eat into meaning and signification. In the end, the corroded signified is no longer. It is absent. It is nothing but the reality of its representation. Accordingly, this reality is just imaginary. Although it seems to be the only real external reality, it is merely an imaginary internal reality. If this mental reality stands out as a physical reality, it is through the use of persuasion. After determining a meaning retroactively, discourse persuades us to believe that this meaning is a reality that was already out there before being determined by discourse. This is how the meaning becomes an imaginary reality. For this imaginary reality to be retrospectively perceived as a reality, discourse has to construct it retroactively *in the past*, but it also has to persuade us *at present* that its meaning is reality and that it had already existed before discourse. Thus the work of discourse is not only constructive, but also persuasive.[12]

Cognitive constructionist psychologists are able to recognize the persuasive character of discourse. But they cannot always resist persuasion. They often let themselves be persuaded by the same persuasion they recognize. They are thus misleadingly convinced that the constructed imaginary meaning is something absolutely real. More than 50 years ago, Politzer (1947) had already criticized such 'idealist psychology' as a 'realism' in which 'meanings explain realities' (II, VI, p. 137). Instead of going upstream to discover signifierization, this psychology keeps to a 'signification' that 'becomes a thing' (I, VIII, p. 50). This thing is still *the thing* of current cognitive constructionist psychologies. It is their imaginary reality. It is the 'spiritual reality' inherent in a reified 'meaning' composed of 'representations' and 'images' (I, VII, p. 42). As the '*sui generis* reality of inner life' (1928, II, I, p. 83), this mental reality is also the ideal content that cognitive psychologies find within discourse. It goes without saying that those idealist psychologies are incompatible with a Lacanian Discourse Analysis that focuses on the signifying materiality of discourse. To use this method, our psychology does not have to be 'idealist', but 'materialist', just as the 'concrete psychology' formerly proposed by Politzer (1928, 1947).

When we advance towards concrete psychology and Lacanian psychoanalysis, we also move from the imaginings about signification to the analysis of signifierization. As a result, we leave the psychological meaning effect to first approach its discursive causation and then its structural foundation.[13] In the end, we must examine the combination of discursive causation and structural foundation. This combination is precisely signifierization. It is the *structural real movement* that imposes a *discursive symbolic value* on that which can then become a *psychological imaginary meaning*.

If we treat the signifying symbolic value as a positioning function in the structure of language, we can describe the *signifierization* as 'the movement that imposes' this 'function *y* on the object *x*' (Searle, 1995, p. 98). This structural movement 'presupposes' evidently a 'linguistic system' (Chomsky, 1975, p. 54). It presupposes a symbolic system, as well as its real structure, the structure of language. In fact, at stake here is a movement characteristic of language and inherent in every discourse, for example that of Francisco Javier, which imposes the function "family" on the object "pillar", which thus becomes "a fundamental pillar for the construction of the new society". In this 'movement' that Searle (1995) regards precisely as the gesture that constructs society, '*x* is counted as *y*' (p. 107). The "pillar" is counted as a "family". The "pillar" is signifierized by the "family". Put differently, "pillar" = function of "family".

In Lacan (1968–1969), the 'mathematical' equation '*x* = function of *y*' expresses 'the concatenation between two signifying chains' (23.04.69, p. 270). The signifierizing chain *y* (family-society) is tied to the signifierized chain *x* (pillar-construction). To compose a signifying social structure, this concatenation has to be repeated countless times. Different signifying chains have to be tied and tied again in the fabric of society. It is a sort of sewing. As we shall see later, this needlework is the work of the unconscious, the same work that was made in the textile industry passionately studied by Marx (1867), as if by chance.

By using the *needleworkforce* of the proletarianized real subjects of society, the signifiers must be signifierized and re-signifierized again and again. According to Searle (1995), this 'iteration' would constitute 'the foundation of the logic structure of complex societies', in which the 'term *x*, situated on a high level, can be a term *y* of the low level' (p. 107). This is how a *signifierized* "pillar" can *be* a *signifierizing* "family", in the same way that this "family" can *be* a family in the flesh. This is also how the signifiers "conviction" and "obligation" on a high level can *be* the signifiers "revolutionary" and "interviewer" of the low level, just as these signifiers can *be* respectively two subjects of a lower level, namely Francisco Javier and María Luisa Vega, who meet one another in discourse. Here is the superimposition of levels that forms the history of a language that 'embodies society' (Humboldt, 1820, §19, p. 87). In this history, society 'is being reanimated or creatively reaffirmed from day to day by particular acts of a communicative nature' (Sapir, 1931b, p. 104). Through these acts, 'language', as a practice of signifierization, constitutes a 'force of socialization' (1933, p. 15).

We can base the above idea of historical socialization on a Lacanian alternative version of the well-known Barthesian diagrams regarding 'myth' as a 'semiological system' (Barthes, 1957, p. 200) and 'connotation' as a 'system of signification' (1964, p. 77). In our version of these diagrams, connotation will not be a *system of signification* anymore, but rather a *system of signifierization*. Instead of the 'semiological chain' which is 'built' from previous chains (ibid.), we will see a signifying chain built on successive levels by adding a new signifier (S2) to an old one (S1) every time. This signifierization, like the signification described by Barthes, functions as the opposite to metalanguage, which transforms the signifier into a signified. In the Lacanian system, as in the Barthesian one, something 'becomes a signifier' (Barthes, 1964, pp. 77–78). However, what becomes a signifier is not the same thing in the two systems. In the Barthesian system (Barthes, 1957, 1964), it is whether the 'sign', as the 'totality joining a concept and an image' (1957, pp. 199–202), or 'the signification', as a 'relation' between 'content' and 'expression' (1964, pp. 76–77). Instead, in the Lacanian system, what becomes a signifier is the signifiable *concept* or *content*, that is transformed into a signifying *image* or *expression*. Actually, the sudden signifierization, or appearance of a new signifier, precedes and impedes the accomplishment of a *signification* and the consequential existence of a *sign*. Instead of the mythological semantic relation between a signifier and a signified, there is here a logical syntactic relation between a signifierizer and a signifierized. Between these two signifiers, there is a real signifierization as an alternative to the imaginary signification of Barthes.

Signifier	Signified?	
Signifierizer Signifier (S1)	Signifierized Signifier (S2)	Signified?
Signifier Signifier (S1)	Signifierizer Signifier (S2)	Signifierized Signifier (S2′)
Signifying chain (signifierization)		

1. Signifier	2. Signified	
3. Sign? I. SIGNIFIER		II. SIGNIFIED
III. SIGN? Semiological chain (signification)		

Unlike the Barthesian Semiological Analysis, the Lacanian Discourse Analysis is not specially devoted to conjectural entities such as the sign, the signified, and the signification. Our analysis is, rather, dedicated to literal features directly analyzable in discourse, in particular the material occurrence of the symbolic signifier and the factual incidence of signifierization. When we analyze discourse, these features must be analyzed simply because they are indistinguishable from discourse itself. As an authentic discourse analysis, our analysis thus prioritizes discourse itself, that is, the signifying *container* or *form* of discourse as opposed to any kind of signified *content*.[14]

By focusing on the discursive form, Lacanian Discourse Analysis specializes in the only true 'content' of discourse (Lacan, 1968–1969,

11.12.68, p. 89). This content is not signified, but signifierized. It is contained in the sense that it is incorporated into the signifying structure. It is content as it fills and takes the form of its discursive matrix. But by taking this form, it automatically becomes discourse. And then, it is not only contained, but also containing. *It contains itself.*

Paradoxically, the true content of discourse is not inside discourse, but it is discourse itself. It is its inner surface and internal organization. It is this transparent or unconscious symbolic form of the container. So it is not the coloured or conscious imaginary content, which is determined, or shaped by its unconscious container, and which includes all the signified stuff of cognitive social psychology, namely social representations, attitudes, stereotypes, etc. In a Lacanian Discourse Analysis, all this can be disregarded. What must not be disregarded, however, are the signify*ing*, determin*ing* and contain*ing* form of discourse. This must be analyzed. In the words of Francisco Javier, for example, we must analyze:

- Not a supposed *representation* of the family as a single-parent family, but the evident symbolic value of this imaginary representation, that is, the signifying exchange value of the "monogamous family" in relation to "marriage".
- Not a positive *attitude* to monogamy, but the determining structural necessity of "monogamy" when "family is one of the fundamental pillars for the construction of society".
- Not the *stereotype* of revolutionaries as modernizers and innovators, but the triangular containing connection between the "consistent revolutionaries", the "new man", and the "family" as the "germ of future education".

Lacanian Discourse Analysis obliges us to analyze the signifying form of discourse. This obligation does not prohibit, however, an analysis of the signified content. We are allowed to analyze this content, of course, but on three conditions. Firstly, the signified content must be regarded as that which is determined rather than expressed by the signifying form.[15] Secondly, the signified content must be treated as a problem that should be analyzed to be eventually solved and, meanwhile, controlled and put into perspective. Thirdly, the content in question must not be considered absolutely and independently of the signifying form. For instance, we may imagine the paradoxical situation in which three somewhat abstract things, love, respect, and faithfulness, support the heavy concretion of the monogamous familiar pillar that in turn supports a new society. We may imagine all this, but we must not come to the conclusion that what is at stake here is a social representation of the family which would involve a positive attitude towards marriage and monogamy. In other words, we are not ethically allowed to raise what we imagine, through a scientific sublimation, to the unmerited dignity of the *general, objective, and predictable Thing* inherent in cognitive attitudes and representations (Pavón Cuéllar, 2007b, pp. 41–44).[16]

The pre-discursive real and the discursive construction of reality

There is often a real Thing prior to discourse. However, in discourse, that Thing is absent. It is *deleted* by discourse. After this deletion, all that remains of the real Thing, in discourse, is the real emptiness of a symbolic form that was supposed to contain and express the Thing. This emptiness of the signifying structure is the last remaining trace of the Thing to be signified. Unfortunately, this trace disappears behind the 'image' that seems to 'fill the emptiness' (Derrida, 1967, p. 208). We can then forget the absence of the Thing.

It is true that 'we can never infer', in the imaginary reality, the 'absence' of the 'signified thing' from the 'presence of the sign' (Arnauld & Nicole, 1683, p. 81). Nevertheless, in the symbolic universe, we can always infer the absence of the undetermined real Thing from the presence of the determining symbolic signifier. Unlike a sign of a thing that might be present somewhere, the signifier is present in the place of the Thing. The symbolic "pillar" as a "family" is present instead of a real pillar. The symbolic determination by the signifier replaces the real indetermination of the Thing. As a replacement for the Thing, the signifier excludes the presence of a Thing that should be absent to make way for it.

Being 'erased' by the signifier (Lacan, 1961–1962, 14.03.62), 'the Thing is that which in the real suffers from the signifier' (1959–1960, 27.01.60, p. 150). The 'killing of the thing' is necessary for the existence of the signifier (1953a, p. 317). The appearance of the signifier entails the disappearance of the Thing. According to Lacan

(1956a), the signifier would even be 'destined by nature to signify the cancelling out of what it signifies' (p. 33). This is quite true, as long as we remember that the undetermined Thing to be signified is cancelled because it cannot really be signified without being determined, eliminated and transformed into another thing.

Even from a Lacanian point of view, we may have the retrospective feeling that 'the signifier takes its material from somewhere in the signified, in living relationships which have been exercised or lived through' (Lacan, 1956–1957, 05.12.56, p. 53). For instance, we may feel that Francisco Javier produces his discourse from bits and pieces coming from past experiences within a real family. This feeling could be confirmed sooner or later. Now, as we shall see later, the retrospective feeling can only be confirmed retroactively. The confirmation *will have created*, in the past, the signified experiences which will confirm our feeling. To exist, those experiences must first be incorporated into the signifying structure. They must be signifierized in order to be signified and thus confirm our feeling.

Feeling: signified	*Confirmation: signifier*
Retrospective imaginary signification *vs.* unimaginable real thing	Retroactive symbolic signifierization *vs.* unsymbolizable real object

The signifier begins by signifierizing that which will be apparently signified. The signifying structure will have put in the past that which will be taken from the past. Retroactive symbolic signifierization precedes and determines any kind of retrospective imaginary signification. By way of example, we can imagine a childhood memory of Francisco Javier that would confirm that the "monogamous family" retrospectively signifies a single-parent family. Before this signification, the single-parent family of the childhood memory will have been incorporated retroactively into the signifying structure. Without this incorporation that we call *signifierization*, there cannot be any kind of signification. Actually, there cannot be anything. For the childhood memory to be something, it must first be in contact with signifierization. Once in contact, there are two possibilities. On the one hand, the real can be signifierized as a "single-parent" or "monogamous family" based on "individual sexual love". On the other hand, the real can 'resist signifierization' and become 'scraps' of the signifying symbolic fabric (Lacan, 1962–1963, 13.03.63, p. 204). At stake here would probably be something related to a polygamous family, or a confusion between marriage and family, or a certain individual sexual hatred. All this would involve, with regard to signifierization, a real unsymbolizable object which could not be retroactively signifierized. At the same time, with regard to signification, this object would correspond to the real unimaginable Thing that could not be retrospectively signified.[17]

Before being taken by the structure of the signifier, the Thing is practically nothing for the subject. It is not a conscious, internal, intelligible signified thing. Nor is it an unconscious, external, perceptible signifying thing. To become *a* thing, *the* Thing has to be annihilated. Its real nothingness must be neutralized to obtain something unreal, whether symbolic or imaginary. To open thus the civilized human world of things, the Thing has to be emptied. Once emptied, its emptiness can be structured. Then and there the literal signifiers 'appear' as 'pebbles' to 'fill this hole, this emptiness' (Lacan, 1956–1957, 15.05.57, p. 330). Here is the origin of the true discursive content that must be analyzed by Lacanian Discourse Analysis. This material content obviously has nothing to do with the ideal content of the mirror that is analyzed by traditional content analysis. First of all, this ideal content is not the real content of discourse. It is not in discourse, but in the mirror. In this mirror, the ideal content is a mental image that covers the real emptiness behind the mirror. On the contrary, the material content is the literal structure that organizes the same emptiness of discourse. But the organized emptiness is indistinguishable from its organizing structural content. It is actually this content that empties the insignifiable Thing. It is the same signifying material content of discourse, as discourse, that creates the signified ideal content in the mirror. The latter content is an effect of the former. The signified is 'the effect of discourse' (Lacan, 1972–1973, 09.01.73, p. 45).

The imaginary reality of the signified is overdetermined, as an effect of discourse, by the concerted symbolic action of the signifiers. From the nothingness of a pre-discursive real Thing, this overdetermination entails a discursive causation and construction of a supposed mental reality, which is habitually taken as the entire reality. Yet this mental reality is just our imaginary internal reality. As for the external reality, everyone must agree that it is not *mental*, but rather *physical*. In a sense, it is also *literal*. It is not the figurative, imaginary reality of the supposed signified inside us, but the literal, material, real structure of the symbolic signifiers around us. At least for each one of us, the external reality is nothing but *discourse*, in the most general sense of the word. In this sense, the external reality constitutes a meaningless discourse whose only meaning, an imaginary meaning, is supposed to lie in our minds. In itself, this perceptible discourse is meaningless, unintelligible, and unconscious. Yet it determines its imaginary meaning, its intelligibility, and its conscious representation. Like an empiricist, a Lacanian recognizes the precedence of a manifest physical experience that causes hypothetical mental entities. From our point of view, the ideal concept of a pillar is preceded by the empirical incident of stumbling upon a material "pillar", an inky or marbled "pillar", when exploring a Mexican revolutionary discourse, or a Greek antique ruin. In both cases, the signified concept is preceded by the signifying incident. The internal reality of the signified is actually constructed by the external reality of the signifiers. Now, *a* discourse, in the strict sense of the word, is nothing but a portion of this external *real reality*. As is, it has the power to construct the internal *imaginary reality*.[18]

The external discursive configuration functions as a matrix that gives a shape to the internal cognitive reality. This imaginary reality of 'thought' is cast in a 'mould' of 'language' (Sapir, 1921, p. 22). To be more specific, the symbolic unconscious container moulds the raw material of the real Thing into the imaginary reality of a conscious content. It is true that this cognitive content is not objectively contained, but only subjectively reflected in discourse by the one who imagines it. In truth, behind the mirror, the cognitive content is nothing but a discursive content. As a cognitive content, it is just imaginary. However, in any event, it is shaped by discourse. Its imaginary reality is a signification by signifierization, that is, a cognitive construction that is constructed by discourse. In this sense, the discursive construction of reality could be defined as *a discursive construction of a cognitive construction*. Lacanian discursive constructionism would thus explain and embrace a cognitive constructionism relegated to the sphere of the imaginary.[19]

Retroactively signifying social structure and retrospectively signified social reality

The symbolic hollows out the unbreathable compactness of the real. It opens, clears and ventilates the place where we live. This place becomes liveable. Its real emptiness is ordered following the structure of language. The interior spaces are furnished and decorated with an imaginary reality. Thanks to the enunciating workforce of the real subjects, a language may *pay*, with its symbolic values, for those furnishings and decorations. By using the same workforce, the language urbanizes and organizes the exterior social spaces. Thus, social reality is discursively constructed by the architecture of language.[20] Actually, behind the mirror, social reality is nothing but a symbolic system. The only real 'intersubjective relation' is the symbolic 'intersignifying relation' (Lacan, 1970–1971, 13.01.71, p. 10). The emptiness of the signifying social structure is the only real place where we can meet one another as signifiers relating to one another.

To become signifiers relating to one another, we should presumably enter into a *symbolic pact* that would institute and regulate our intersignifying relation. Our *society inside language* would be inaugurated by this pact, agreement, or convention. This idea may justifiably remind us of the theories about the contractual or conventional origin of human language and civil society. Following these theories, we may think of a sort of symbolic pact that would function as a prerequisite for the constitution of civil society inside human language. There is much evidence of this pact, namely in myths of origin, legends of the chosen people, gang commitments, customer loyalties, familiar obligations, complicity of couples, or engagement rings. In Francisco Javier's discourse, for example, the symbolic pact may be evidenced by the "significance of marriage" as "a starting point for the establishment of the family and thereby for the constitution of society". The same pact may be at stake in the "faithfulness from conviction" as an alternative to the "dissolution of the couple".

The term *symbol* originates in the Greek word *sumbolon*, which refers to a 'broken piece' of a real thing, a *Thing* whose pieces are shared between individuals and function as signs of recognition between them (Lacan, 1975–1976, 18.11.75, p. 19). In all probability, the complementary pieces of the Thing would correspond to the constituent elements of the real structure of the symbolic, that breaks the Thing into complementary pieces, words, *subjects*, or structural signifying positions. In human language and civil society, the complementary pieces would be incarnate literal symbols that remind us of the pact that makes possible the *sharing of the Thing*.

From the very beginning, 'symbol means pact' (Lacan, 1953a, p. 270). As symbols, the constituent elements of the structure are 'signifiers of the pact they constitute as the signified' (ibid.). Although the signifiers cannot signify the Thing, they can be signifiers of the pact. They can signify the broken Thing. Actually, this Thing is the only Thing that can be signified. In this sense, the signifying structure is the only signified Thing. The signifiers signify nothing but their structure.

By signifying the structure, each signifier ratifies and fulfils the symbolic pact. Furthermore, as a perceptible execution of the pact, each signifier can be considered a sign of recognition between the *subjects of the pact*. For instance, "love, respect and faithfulness" would allow the recognition between the "consistent revolutionaries" that are subjected to a particular pact. Now, before being recognized as subjects of this pact, the revolutionaries are already subjects of the pact, since they are already *subjected* to the real structure of their cultural environment. Only after this subjection to the broken Thing, can they attain *recognition* by us, or between them. At that moment, they can also establish *communication* of the pact. Francisco Javier communicates a clause of the pact, for example, when he explains to us that they "would not be consistent revolutionaries" if their "conceptions of marriage and the couple were not based on love, respect and faithfulness". In this sense, we can say that signifiers realize retrospectively *communication* of the structure and not only *recognition* of the structural positions. But before that, they must have realized a retroactive *subjection* of the subjects who are thus constituted by the structure by being positioned in it.[21]

Signified social reality	*Signifying social structure*
Retrospective objectivation	Retroactive subjection
Event of imaginary recognition and communication	Symbolic pact of recognition and communication

The signifying social structure can be defined, from a Lacanian point of view, as a symbolic pact of recognition and communication between those who are retroactively subjected, constituted and positioned by it. This pact precedes and determines the signified social reality, which can be in turn defined as a retrospectively objectified event of imaginary recognition and communication. Even when this event seems to be comparatively independent from the symbolic, as in the shared hatred of the same object, its way always has to be paved, in the human world, by at least one signifier that implies the symbolic pact. Without this signifier, there would be nothing social.

From the time when the signifier 'was born between those ferocious animals that were primitive humans', it has been a 'password' indispensable to reproduce the social structure, or the symbolic pact of recognition and communication, between the members of the same couple, family, cave, clan, class, tribe, nation, party, revolutionary group, etc. (Lacan, 1953c, p. 28). As a symbol, the signifier embodies this pact in the form of a signifying social structure. In this real structure, each piece of the broken Thing is a piece of society shared by its members. But the members of society are also pieces of society. The signatories to the social contract are already signifiers of the social structure. They are subjected to this structure. They are subjects of the symbolic pact.

Besides being subjects of the symbolic pact, the subjects communicate this pact. They communicate the structure. In fact, as the subjects are signifiers in the structure, their communication *of the structure* is nothing but a signifying relation *in the structure*. It is the structure that communicates through its subjects. The communication of the structure between subjects illustrates the necessary flow of information between the positions of the signifying structure of society. In this communication *of* the structure *by* the structure, the communicated information exclusively concerns the communication of information. It is not metalanguage, but language circling around itself. It is information on information. As Lacan (1953b) notes, 'inter-human communication' is 'information about information, a test of the language community' (p. 150). What is thus put to the test is not unrelated to Francisco Javier's "love". It amounts precisely to that which is 'expressed', a word, but also a 'feeling' whose 'sharing generates the family and the society' (Aristotle, *Politics*, 1253a).

Intransitive signifying action and imaginary signified object

In a Lacanian perspective, we communicate structural determinations and not mental significations. Put differently, communication is not an exchange of cognitive information between persons, but a transmission of discursive information between positions in the signifying social structure.[22] This discursive information is not composed of meanings, thoughts, ideas, or opinions, but of structural flexions, tensions and actions, functions and directions, distinctions and oppositions. All of this has nothing to do with cognition. It is not mental data, but an actual fact. It is not a signification that moves from one mind to another, but a signifierization of one signifier by another. What must be communicated here is not information in the psychological sense of the word.[23] It is, rather, the means of communication. Language must only communicate language. If so, from a psychological point of view, language must not communicate anything. We 'can be using language in the strictest sense with no intention of communicating' (Chomsky, 1975, p. 61).

A signifier communicates only itself *or* the signifying structure. It signifies only its symbolic value *or* the symbolic pact of recognition and communication. As in the case of the engagement ring, the signifier implies a convention about the relation between the signifier and the signified, the position and the structure, the ring and the engagement. This relation would ideally be the same for the two subjects. However, that is not the case, because the two subjects are themselves signifiers that have different positions in the *signified signifying structure*. Correlatively, this structure *is different for* the positions of each of them. So the two subjects must perceive a difference in the shared signified of all signifiers (i.e. the broken Thing, the symbolic pact, the signifying structure). This general difference entails specific differences in the relations between all the signifiers of the structure, including each signifierizer (e.g., a "pillar" or an "engagement ring"), and each signifierized, or alleged signified (e.g., "family" or "marriage"). These relations cannot be the same for two subjects. Furthermore, the relations change incessantly for each subject, as his structural position is not stable, or definitive. All this creates a situation in which:

- For the same subject, the same signifier cannot signify the same thing in two different moments. The same engagement ring engages to a different "faithfulness" during holidays and returning home. It does not entail the same "respect" night and day. It indicates a different "love" now and 50 years later. Besides that, the ring can also indicate hatred, unfaithfulness, or disrespect, as well as wealth or faith, hope or disappointment, life or death.
- At the same moment, the same signifier cannot signify the same thing for two different subjects. The same engagement ring can represent love for Francisco Javier and hatred for his wife, faithfulness for him and unfaithfulness for her, a revolutionary dowry for him and the reactionary "starting point for the establishment of a family" for her.

From the angle of a Lacanian Discourse Analysis, the relation between the analyzed signifier and the signified changes from one language to another, from one subject to another, from one moment to the next. There is here a variable multivocal relation that depends on the structural context, or, to be more specific, on the signifying positions of the subject who analyzes and the analyzed signifier in relation to one another, and to the other signifiers in the signified structure. Thus, there is no fixed univocal signifying relation. But the so-called *sign* precisely means this relation. Consequently, the sign does not mean anything. In a sense, there is no such thing as a *sign*. This sign is just as imaginary as the signification.

Real	*Imaginary*	*Symbolic*
Signifierization	Signification	
	Sign	
	Signified	Signifier

The sign and the signification are imaginary representations of the non-existent transition between the intransitive signifying action and the object of this action. Now, since this real signifying action is intransitive, its signified object is as imaginary as the sign and the signification. In other words, the signified is imaginary because it cannot *really* be signified by an intransitive signifying action. If the Lacanian verb *to signify* functions as a verb without a direct object, then the direct object of this intransitive verb can only be imaginary. The signified must be treated as an imaginary object of the signifying action. Besides this real action of the symbolic signifier, there is only the signifier of a 'language' which is 'devoid of signification' (Lacan, 1953c, p. 29). And without this signification, there is no such thing as a sign. Instead of a sign that represents a transitive signifying action between the signifier and the signified, there is a breakdown of the transition, an interruption of the signifying action, a 'cut' of the sign (Lacan, 1970a, p. 403), a 'real border' (p. 416), or a 'bar placed' by 'linguistics' between 'the signifier and the signified' (p. 403).

The Lacanian conception of the signifier is based on linguistic theories that place a bar between the signifier and the signified. Among those theories, there are the ones of Saussure and the Prague Circle, but also the ones of Locke, the Stoics and the Hermogene of Plato. Initially, thanks to that which was expressed by Hermogene and the 'Stoic wisdom', we 'distinguished between the signifier and the signified' (Lacan, 1973a, p. 515). In other words, we made a distinction between the 'signifying thing', or 'sound', and the 'signified thing' of our 'intellect' (Sextus Empiricus, *Against the Logicians*, 250, II, §11). Once distinguished, the signifier and the signified can no longer be confused in an imaginary analogical similarity. The liberated signifier must not imitate the signified anymore. The relation between the signifier and the signified is no longer an obligatory imitation, but a capricious convention. This progress from the 'mimologism' to the 'conventionalism' (Genette, 1976, pp. 59–60) is also the advancement from the confusion to the distinction between the imaginary and the symbolic. After this advance, the symbolic functioning of the signifier cannot be confused with the imaginary functioning of the signified to any further extent. So, moving with the times, Lacanian Discourse Analysis must analyze discursive conventional identities and oppositions which cannot be reduced to the old mirror of cognitive mimological similarities and dissimilarities. Likewise, in Platonic terms, our analysis of the signifierization as literal *methexis* (by which Francisco Javier partakes of the signifying structure of his discourse) cannot be confused with the psychological analysis of the signification as mental *mimesis* (by which the analyst's model would try to mimic the cognitive form of Francisco Javier's signified).

In the mimological view, every language is a sign language. The sign is explicit. It explicitly reproduces the signified. To be understood, this imaginary reproduction does not require either a convention or a symbolic pact of recognition and communication. Thus, in cognitive psychology, the obvious data-processing model of *cognition* does not need any pact of *recognition* (as if recognized cognitivists were not necessary to believe in their cognitive model). Moreover, this archaic mimological model, in contrast to the 'communicational model' of Habermas (1981), assumes an immediate communication, which already *is* comprehension, that dispenses with any kind of mediation, pact of communication, intercommunication, 'negotiation', or 'intercomprehension' (p. 111).

When we reduce every language to the imaginary mental transparency of a sign communication, we do not need to analyze the real structural transparency of an unconscious container hidden by the symbolic opacity of language.[24] With the clear exposure of a made-up cognitive content, there is no need for us to analyze discourse. It is not even necessary to read it, or interpret it. All we have to do is perceive the signs and understand them. All we need is 'someone to whom the sign makes a sign of something' (Lacan, 1953c, p. 28).

For the sign to be immediately understood, we only need someone overly clever who blocks the 'Stoic access' to linguistics (Lacan, 1972a, p. 489). Now, to undertake a Lacanian Discourse Analysis, we must go into and through linguistics. Therefore, we must begin by opening its entrance. We must clear this entrance of the desperately perspicacious semiologist or psychologist who is still blocking it. From our Lacanian point of view, the extreme perspicacity of this personage is nothing but 'foolishness' (1970a, p. 404). We must relieve ourselves of this foolishness, which is 'productive of myths' rather than 'mythological' (cf. Barthes, 1957, p. 214). We must stop mythically comprehending the incomprehensible, or imagining the symbolic, by persisting in discovering in every discourse the 'analogical' or 'mythical signification' (p. 212).

Before leaving linguistics, we must enter linguistics by differentiating the signifier from the sign. So, before undertaking a

Lacanian Discourse Analysis, we must provisionally recognize that the symbolic signifier, unlike the imaginary sign, is not natural but conventional, artificial, unjustified, non-analogical, arbitrary. This means that:

- The 'accuracy of the word' is 'a convention' (Plato, *Cratylus*, 384d).
- Some 'articulate sounds' correspond to some 'ideas' by a 'voluntary imposition' and not by a 'natural connection' (Locke, 1690, III, II, §1, p. 281).
- The signifying 'acoustic image' and the signified 'concept' are not linked by an 'internal relation' (Saussure, 1916, §136, p. 100).

Without an internal relation between the signifier and the signified, a linguist may study the signifier independently of the signified. In fact, he *must* concentrate on the *signifying word*. He must not keep any *signified world* in mind. This supposes that linguistics 'is not a conception of the world' (Milner, 1978, p. 59). Put differently, the linguistic theory about the word is not a philosophical theory about the supposed content of the word. Accordingly, discourse analysis, as a linguistic practice, cannot be merged into content analysis. Likewise, we cannot get confused between pre-linguistic cognitive psychology and linguistic discursive psychology. For instance, the former excludes Lacan, while the latter may lead us to Lacan. Nevertheless, in a Lacanian perspective, we cannot be completely satisfied with any of them. Of course, we may use Lacanian Discourse Analysis as part of a discursive psychology. Now, in so doing, we would only concentrate on the symbolic and disregard the real and the imaginary. This is quite legitimate, but our concrete psychology would thus be reduced to an abstract discursive psychology. Our post-linguistic method would also regress to the linguistic practice of traditional discourse analysis. Its Lacanian distinguishing feature would be forgotten.

To reach Lacanian Discourse Analysis, we must enter into linguistics, but we must also go through and out. We must go beyond the conventional and arbitrary sign. We cannot resign ourselves to a conventional and arbitrary connection instead of the 'real natural connection' between the signifier and the signified (Saussure, 1916, §140, p. 101). Neither can we be satisfied with an 'interdependence' in 'autonomy' instead of the 'absence of autonomy' between the 'two faces' of the sign (Jakobson, 1949, pp. 163–171). These linguistic ideas cannot be 'appropriate' for us (Lacan, 1972–1973, 09.01.73, p. 41). To be more specific, what cannot be appropriate for us is the mere existence of an interdependence or connection between the signifier and the signified. It is not enough to acknowledge the autonomy and arbitrariness of this relationship between the 'two faces' of the 'semiotic unit' (Jakobson, 1949, p. 163). In our perspective, there cannot simply be this relationship inherent in a 'sign' as a 'semiotic unit' that 'keeps us from grasping the signifier' (Lacan, 1970a p. 404).

In Lacan, the signifier has nothing to do with the sign as a semiotic unit.[25] Lacanian psychoanalysis rejects the idea of a *semiotic unit* that *unites* the signifier with the signified. Our perspective cannot be consonant with a 'semiology' that 'postulates' this 'relation between the signifier and the signified' (Barthes, 1957, p. 197). In our perspective, 'it is not only the arbitrariness of the sign, as Saussure said, but it is really a kind of independence' (Miller, 1996a, p. 17). It is impossible not to contrast this Lacanian one-sided independence of the signifier from the signified (and not vice versa) with the Jakobsonian *reciprocal interdependence between the two faces of the sign*. In fact, Lacan would not even regard the signifier and the signified as *the two faces of the sign*. Furthermore, we already know that the Lacanian relationship between the two elements is not a *semiotic signification*, but a syntactic signifierization by a signifier that incorporates the signified into the signifying structure. In this structure, as discussed before, the incorporated signified becomes a new signifier (a *signifierized*) structurally related to the incorporating signifier (the *signifierizer*). Now, unlike the imaginary signification, this real structural relationship cannot be arbitrary. It cannot be arbitrary precisely because of its structural necessity. In the structure, there is no room for arbitrariness.

Before	*Linguistics*	*Lacan*
Natural sign	Arbitrary sign	Arbitrating sign
Signified thing	Signified concept	Signified structure

Lacan ascribes the arbitrariness of the sign to the tyrannical power of a legislator, a founding master, in the *master discourse* denounced by the Saussurean *university discourse* (two discursive forms to which we shall later return). Instead of this linguistic arbitrary sign and the pre-linguistic natural sign, Lacan (1975–1976) offers a post-linguistic 'arbitrating sign' between 'two signifiers' (18.11.75, p. 19). The 'signified' is here the principle of 'arbitration' (ibid.). It is thus the symbolic pact of communication and recognition. It is not the concept or thing (a family) related to the signifier ("pillar" or "family"), but the *signified signifying structure* that arbitrates between the signifier ("pillar") and another signifier ("family") that we wrongly take for its signified.

Contrary to the irrational and even immoral arbitrariness denounced by Saussure, the arbitration involves a 'moral reason' of 'signification' that should satisfy the Cratyle of Plato as well as the Theophile of Leibniz (1704, III, II, I, p. 216). This *moral reason* also represents a *scientific reason*. The arbitrating sign might thus become a scientific rational replacement for a 'fantastic' and 'unscientific' arbitrary sign (Schaff, 1964, p. 201). With the hypothesis of the arbitration, Lacan (1972–1973) actually claims to put forward a 'scientific discourse' as an alternative to the 'master discourse' denounced by Saussure (09.01.73, p. 41). This Lacanian 'scientific discourse' assumes 'a signifier' that is 'not related to the signified', but only to the other signifiers of the structure (ibid.). Now, as those signifiers belong to a structure, their relations are arbitrated by the structure. Take for example the relation between the "family" and the "pillar", which is patently not arbitrary, but systematically arbitrated by the structure in which the family is "monogamous", has a "foundation", and is used for a "construction".

Assuming a signifier that is not dependent on the signified, the Lacanian scientific discourse may at first seem to be an 'insulating method' that 'treats the perceptible and the intelligible as closed and independent spheres' (Jakobson, 1949, p. 162). However, we see that, in Lacan, the intelligible signified sphere is not only dependent on the perceptible signifying sphere, but even reduced to it. After this reduction, there is no longer a perceptible sphere formed by signs that signify a closed and independent intelligible sphere. This intelligible imaginary sphere is opened, overdetermined, and signifierized by the signifiers. It becomes thus dependent on the perceptible symbolic sphere. The fact remains that this perceptible sphere is not symmetrically dependent on the intelligible sphere. Nor is it reduced to it. Just like the God of Pseudo-Dionysius in his asymmetrical relation to the created things, the perceptible signifying Thing of Lacan does not partake of the intelligible signified things that partake of it.

The Lacanian perceptible signifier does not communicate an intelligible signified to an intelligent analyst, but it simply refers to another perceptible signifier in order to communicate just itself *or* its symbolic value, that is to say, the signifying structure *or* the symbolic pact of communication. This pact makes possible an intelligible interpretation, but it is not intelligible in itself.[26] Likewise, the structure is not conscious. The communicating perceptible signifiers are unconscious or unintelligible. They are closed to the faculties of consciousness or intelligence. But at the same time they are completely open to the real signifying structure of those faculties. They are actually indistinguishable from this structure. And this structure, after all, is the only *truth* of consciousness or intelligence.

The sign as a perceptible signifier with an imaginary intelligible signification

During the 1950s and 1960s, Lacan stresses that 'a signifier is not the sign' (1961–1962, 06.12.61). Simultaneously, he gives 'the supremacy' to 'the signifier' (1956a, p. 20). Later, at the end of the 1960s, he puts forward a 'signifier logic' against the 'sign lure' (1970a, p. 413). In this lure, my intelligence is lured into the trap of the mirror. I take the perceptible signifier ("family") for a sign that *makes a sign* precisely out of the intelligible signified that I have in my mind (*my* family). By a strange coincidence, the signifier means exactly what I think. All this is obviously an illusion. I cannot even perceive either the subjective signified in my mind, or the objective signified of the signifier. Until there is proof to the contrary, those two imperceptible entities must be considered imaginary things. The only real things evident here are the perceptible elements of the signifier logic.

The perceptible elements of the signifier logic are the only real substratum of the sign lure. They are the real means that make it possible to create the illusion of signification. They are thus 'articulate distinct sounds used by man to signify his thoughts' (Arnauld & Lancelot, 1676, p. 24). By means of those sounds, Francisco Javier and his interviewer, María Luisa Vega, will think they are able to generate identical social 'significations' that they can 'share' (Habermas, 1984, p. 72). This *shared social identity* is unfortunately a mirror illusion 'formed through the reciprocal reflection of their expectations' (ibid.). However, contrary to all expectations, there is always a misunderstanding. The mirror of discourse cannot reflect the same image to different people. To be sure, different people have different expectations that generate different understandings. Take for example Francisco Javier, who is talking about "faithfulness by conviction", while María Luisa Vega is asking a question about "familiar obligations". Behind these symbolic differences, there is probably an imaginary similarity, but there is evidently not a real shared identity of signification. The only real shared identity here lies in the signifiers, such as "family" and "revolutionary", which remain the same, identical to themselves, even when they are shared, expressed or perceived, by different people. As discussed above, this real identity is the only foundation for the imaginary similarity. Besides this identity, if there is an understanding between the interviewer and the interviewee, it is clearly a misunderstanding. Actually, understanding is always a misunderstanding. This is why Lacanian Discourse Analysis, as will be seen in the last chapter of this book, excludes formally understanding from its modus operandi.

When a psychologist understands a word, he takes the signifier for a sign and he grasps the 'signification' that he imagines is 'contained in the word' (Arnauld & Lancelot, 1676, p. 24). However, this signification poses a problem, because it was not contained in the word before being put there by the imaginative psychologist. Therefore, as a posterior addition, the understood signification is not inherent in the analyzed word. It does not come from the mind of the person who pronounced or wrote the word. If we do not believe in telepathy, we must acknowledge that the mental signification cannot move from one mind to another. One of the analytical disadvantages of the sign is this *individual rooting* of its fixed signification.

Unlike the perceptible external signifier, the sign involves an intelligible internal signification which cannot be shared or socialized. Yet this signification is just imaginary. Therefore, in truth, the sign is nothing more than a signifier that can be shared or socialized. This signifier thus constitutes the real social structure of a signified social reality that is just imaginary. As a constituent element of this structure, the signifier can be analyzed as a social thing. In actual fact, it is the only social thing that we can analyze, and it does not contain anything for us, because we are nothing but another signifier in relation to it. We are, for example, a "familiar obligation" facing "faithfulness from conviction". We are probably also "bourgeois ideology" against "proletarian ideology". Those *class struggles* are logical relations between opposing signifiers that compose the real signifying social structure. Actually, as language, this structure consists of nothing more than signifiers and logical oppositions between signifiers. In this battlefield of class struggle, there is no place for understanding between classes. There is no place for communication. There is no place for the sign lure.

In the sign lure, the logical opposition between signifiers becomes a mythological amalgamation that unites a communicating signifier with a communicated signified. The ensuing 'semiotic unit' would thus 'attach language to the function of communication' (Lacan, 1970a, p. 404). This is deplored by Lacan. For him, language 'is not functional' (1956a, p. 26). It is not the 'functional system' of the Prague Circle (cf. Mathesius et al., 1929, p. 23). It is not composed of 'expressive means appropriate to their purpose' (ibid.). In the Lacanian structuralist perspective, the only purpose of language is language itself, or the enjoyment of language, as we shall see later. Besides this 'enjoyment value', the only value of language is the 'exchange value' of its signifiers (Lacan, 1966–1967, 12.04.67, 19.04.67). Its only real function is the signifying symbolic function, or *replacement function* (x = function of y, or "pillar" = function of "family"). Language does not fulfil another real function. It certainly does not fulfil a 'function of communication' (cf. Mathesius et al., 1929, p. 31).

At the time of the Prague Circle, Sapir (1931a) was already against the reduction of language to the 'function of pure communication' (pp. 40–42). He also showed how 'language plays an important role in situations that have nothing to do with communication' (ibid.). He mentioned, for instance, the 'autistic use of language by children', as well as a 'dinner' in which 'what really counts is not what we say, but the fact of saying something' (ibid.). Such situations demonstrate, according to Sapir, that 'language is much more than a simple technique of communication' (ibid.).

Like Sapir's language, Lacan's language is not a technique of communication. Nor is it a technique of something else. It is neither a strategic resource, nor a transmission channel, nor a form of expression, nor even a work instrument, such as a construction tool.[27] In short, language is not *a way of doing something to achieve something else*.[28]

In the Lacanian perspective, language is not functional. Nevertheless it functions. It signifies. We can even acknowledge that it communicates, provided that we know that it does not communicate a signified to a person, but a signifier to another signifier. Language communicates itself to itself. It functions as a 'monologue' (Miller, 1996b, pp. 13, 16). In the terms of the Prague Circle, we could say that language does not perform essentially a 'communicative function', but rather a 'poetical function', since it is 'always directed to itself' (Mathesius et al., 1929, p. 31). The words of Francisco Javier, for example, are not exactly directed to the interviewer, but to other words. Among those words, there is admittedly the interviewer, but this subject *is* a word, a signifier, a symbolic position in the real signifying structure of society. María Luisa Vega is precisely the position of "the interviewer", but also the position of "familiar obligations", and perhaps "bourgeois ideology", or even "society". Directed to these positions, Francisco Javier's signifiers are directed to language. In this way, they must ironically perform a 'poetical function' (Jakobson, 1936, p. 96). As for the 'communicative function' and the 'representative function', they are subordinated to this 'poetical function' (ibid.). Even if the signifier communicates itself and represents a subject for another signifier, what is essential here is the poetical relation between the two signifiers. Communication and representation are subordinated to this relation. They depend on it. They are determined by it.

The signifier communicates only to another signifier. Besides that, as discussed above, the signifier just communicates itself, or its symbolic value, or its communication to the other signifier, which amounts here to the same thing. Thus, regarding 'what it communicates', the signifier of 'language is not a signal, nor a sign, nor even a sign of a thing as exterior reality' (Lacan, 1953b, p. 148). It is rather a signifier that signifies to another signifier precisely its immanent relation to it. As a signifier, for instance, Francisco Javier may be considered a "conviction" that signifies to an "obligation" nothing but the signifying relation between "conviction" and "obligation". Put differently, the "consistent revolutionary" functions as a *revolutionary* "conviction" that refers to its *consistent* opposition to "obligation". In any case, this reference is not outside discourse. It is not a *reference* according to the strictest definition of the term. It does not denote either a pre-discursive real or an imaginary extra-discursive reality.[29] It is rather a '*connotation*' of other intra-discursive signifiers or symbolic values, as well as a '*denotation*' of the real structure of the symbolic, or the literal context of the discursive text, which includes the making of the pact that arbitrates between signifiers (cf. Mill, 1843, I, II, §5, pp. 20–26). As we shall see in chapter four, this real of the symbolic is an actuality inseparable from discourse. It is enunciation, overdetermination, and signifierization. It is also the passion of a signifier, but not the passion of a person. This is the only real that may be analyzed by Lacanian Discourse Analysis.

In the signifier logic, signifierization is a real process that underlies the symbolic fact of a signifying discourse. Contrary to the imaginary signification of the sign lure, this real process is not communicated as that about which we are speaking. Signifierization 'is not an effect of communication of speech, but of displacement of discourse' (Lacan, 1970a, p. 407). It is a discursive displacement that absorbs *something*. What is absorbed into discourse is always out there, but its position becomes a position in the signifying structure. The thing becomes a signifier of discourse. This is how a signifier signifierizes the thing to which it refers. By transforming this thing into a signifier, the reference to the thing represents a signifierization of that which becomes a new link of the signifying chain of discourse. Here the 'word *reference*' indicates 'what discourse constitutes as a link' (Lacan, 1972–1973, 09.01.73, p. 41). The family to which Francisco Javier refers is thus constituted as a "family" that discursively links the signifiers "obligation" and "conviction", that is, the respective links of the interviewer and the interviewee. Between these links, the link of "the family" functions as a *social link*. This kind of link is the only true social link that we can analyze in discourse. In general, it represents the symbolic pact of communication, or the signifying structure of society. In particular, it is a discursive link between two positions of this structure. In any case, this social link forms part of discourse, which is the only reference of the signifier. As Lacan (1972–1973) explains, the signifier 'refers only to a discourse' defined as 'the utilization of language as a link between those who speak' (09.01.73, pp. 41–42).

Parallelism between signifying elements and signified entities

Viewed from a Lacanian standpoint, 'the relation between the signifier and the signified is entirely included in the order of language' (Lacan, 1953b, p. 148). This being so, the relation cannot be interpreted according to the psychological parallelism between discursive and cognitive processes. In this 'parallelism of language and thought', we 'transform significations into processes', or 'the grammar into psychology', by using the grammatical form of discourse to infer a parallel psychological content (Politzer, 1947, I, VIII, p. 50). By contrast, in Lacanian Discourse Analysis we analyze the 'form' as 'content' (Lacan, 1968–1969, 11.12.68, p. 89), as the only content which is not imaginary.[30] In this content, which is still form and content in parallel, we again come across the parallelism between 'our mental discourse' and 'our verbal discourse' (Hobbes, 1651, I, IV, p. 28). But this parallelism is now established within discourse. It is not a parallelism between a grammatical discursive form and a psychological extra-discursive content, but instead a parallelism between a signifying discursive form and a signified intra-discursive content. To illustrate such a parallelism, Lacan (1956–1957) proposes the first *scheme of the parallels*, with the 'parallel superposition of the course of the signifier, or concrete discourse, and the course of the signified, as continuity of life experience or flow of tendencies in a subject or between subjects' (05.12.56, p. 47).

Parallels (1956–1958)

----------------------------------	Signifier (S-S)
----------------------------------	*signified* (s-s)

The parallelism does not imply a regular, invariable, and predictable correspondence between the signifier and the signified. Even if the signifier always refers to the structure in general, this reference crosses different structural positions and relations each time. The univocal reference to the structure involves a plurivocal structural mediation. The same signifier does not always refer to the same mediating signified. This can be seen in Francisco Javier's discourse, in which the same "family" can signify a "pillar" as well as a "germ". Similarly, "love" first signifies "an identification in the perception of the world", then a "moral conquest of our time" and the "foundation of monogamous family", and finally that which "leads to mutual respect", but also "to a dissolution of the couple". The same signifier thus signifies various and heterogeneous things.

The Lacanian signifying structure can be regarded as *the* symbolic pact of communication between the structural positions, but this pact is not 'a contract of contracts' that would ensure 'the unity of the signifier and the signified' (cf. Derrida, 1975, p. 493). According to Lacan, the 'scheme of the parallels supposes that a signifier of a thing can always become a signifier of another thing' (1956–1957, 05.12.56, p. 47). The scheme also implies the 'perpetual sliding of the signified under the signifier' (ibid.). Besides that, every signified is a signifier and each signifier can be signified. Each word can become a meaning that is always a word. The word "family" can become the figurative meaning of the word "pillar" whose literal meaning is the word "support". There is a permanent exchange here between the signifying and signified elements of the two parallels. The result is a mutual pollution and corruption of the syntactical and semantic levels.[31]

Despite the interference between the parallels, there is not an intersection, but a parallelism of 'two chains' at two different 'levels', namely, the 'superior level' of the 'signifier', and the 'inferior level' of the 'signified' (Lacan, 1957–1958, 22.01.58, p. 196). At this inferior level, we see the 'circulation of itinerant signified entities' (ibid.). These entities 'are always sliding' (ibid.). They are always sliding simply because there is a succession of signifying elements. This can be illustrated by considering how the breaking succession of photograms in a projector explains the changing continuity of the film on the screen. Likewise, when we are reading a novel *or* living a life, the imagined reality is constantly changing because words *or* moments come one after another. *As time passes, the imaginary signified entities are analogically and continuously moving in a function of the succession of moments in time or words in discourse. In parallel, at each word or moment, all the symbolic signifying elements are discretely and recurrently reorganized. While this reorganization requires an application of the structure of language, the resulting discursive chain makes possible the parallel experience of reality*. Assuming this to be true, Lacanian Discourse Analysis must distinguish systematically:

- *The structure of language*. It constitutes 'the synchronic structure of the material of language in so far as each element takes on its precise usage therein by being different from the others' (Lacan, 1956c, p. 411). This structure is organized and reorganized, at each moment, as a symbolic static or timeless order. Its principle is the *metaphor*, which functions with discrete differences. The 'metaphor' is thus 'not the same thing' as the 'analogy', which functions with analogical similarities (Lacan, 1953a, p. 261). This analogy slides through similar imaginary entities (e.g., the images of a *family* and a *fraternal society*), while the metaphor substitutes a symbolic element ("pillar") for a different symbolic element ("family"). In this way, the metaphor functions by 'substitution of signifier for signifier' (Lacan, 1957b, p. 512). Its 'formula' is 'one word for another' (p. 504).[32]
- *The chain of discourse*. It consists of 'the diachronic set of concretely pronounced discourses' (Lacan, 1956c, pp. 411–412). It appears as the succession of discourses, or words in discourse, or moments in time, which amount to the same thing. It includes the 'sliding' of 'signified entities' (1957–1958, 22.01.58, p. 196), but its principle is 'metonymy', which 'is based' on the 'connection' between 'signifiers' (1957b, p. 503). The 'connection' of one signifier ("pillar") to another ("construction") is 'nowhere other than in the signifier' (ibid.). Lacan stresses this '*word-to-word* nature of the connection' (ibid.). Although the sliding signified entities 'historically affect' the signifiers, it is the 'structure' of the signifiers which 'govern the pathways' of the signified (1956c, pp. 411–412).

The diachronic chain of discourse and the experience of reality	*The synchronic structure of language and its application*
Succession of signifying elements and sliding of signified entities	Differences between signifying elements
Metonymy: connection of one signifier to another ("pillar" – "construction")	Metaphor: substitution of signifier for signifier ("pillar"/"family")

Perpendicularity between metaphors in language and metonymy of discourse

Lacan retains the signified entities until 1958. Then, from 1958 to 1964, he reduces those signified entities to signifying elements. This reduction correlates logically with the transition from imaginary signification to symbolic signifierization. All this occurs during the most structuralist period in the evolution of Lacanian theory. During this period, even 'enjoyment' is 'signifierized' in a 'conceptual rewriting' that obtains 'symbolic terms' from terms included before in the 'category of imaginary' (Miller, 1999, p. 10).

After proposing the scheme of the parallels, Lacan (1958c) remarks that 'it is impossible to dispense with the function of the signifier', which 'is the only thing in the world that can underpin the coexistence—constituted by disorder (synchronically)—of elements among which the most indestructible order ever to be deployed subsist (diachronically)' (p. 135). This order is the order of the signifier. It is the condition for the coexistence of everything in the human world. It is thus a precondition for our experience of everything that coexists. This experience must be ordered according to the order of the signifier. Instead of the 'symbol attached' to a 'single experience', there is now the signifier as 'linguistic symbol' that orders coexisting 'experiences' into 'delimited classes of experience' (Sapir, 1921, pp. 12–17). As for the flow of experience, it is not an alternation of images anymore, but a connection between signifiers. The symbolic order of successive signifying elements absorbs the imaginary motion of sliding signified entities. There is thus a theoretical simplification that eliminates the imaginary from the analysis of the symbolic. Instead of the parallelism between the signifier and the imaginary signified organized by the signifier, there is now only the 'double register' of the symbolic 'signifier' (Lacan, 1958d, p. 96). There is 'the synchronic register of opposition between irreducible elements, and the diachronic register of substitution and combination' (ibid.). The whole experience of reality, as well as 'everything in interpersonal relations', is now 'structured' by the synchronic structure of 'language' and 'through' the diachronic chain of discourse (ibid.). It may be remarked that this diachronic chain is not precisely *parallel*, but rather *perpendicular* to the synchronic structure. This perpendicular relation between language and discourse is no longer covered by the imaginary screen of the parallelism between the signifier and the signified.

The parallelism between signifying elements and signified entities screens the perpendicular functioning of signifying elements. In this functioning, the discontinuous metaphors operate through continuous metonymy, or, to be more specific, the synchronic structure of linguistic oppositions and identifications operates through the perpendicular diachronic chain of discursive substitutions and combinations. For instance, Francisco Javier will have succeeded in his *identification* with a "consistent revolutionary" through a *substitution* of "familiar obligation" for "faithfulness from conviction", and then a *combination* of this "faithfulness" with "consistent revolutionaries". After these processes, language will have diachronically transformed Francisco Javier into a "consistent revolutionary" in the synchronic structure. Similarly, another language will have *opposed* the "revolution" to "Mexico", in a metaphorical trope (Mexico = the Establishment = a peaceful colonial city with its counter-revolutionary institutions), by the metonymical strategies of *substituting* "violence" for "revolution" and *combining* "violence" with "damage to Mexico". This is how the temporality of discourse can be used by language to redefine the positions of all persons and things in the timeless signifying structure of society.

Diachronic chain of discourse	*Synchronic structure of language*
Sequence of substitutions and combinations	System of oppositions
Metonymy (displacement)	Metaphor (condensation)

When undertaking a Lacanian Discourse Analysis, we must assume that the synchronic structure of language operates through the diachronic chain of discourse. Accordingly, we must analyze the system of linguistic oppositions through the sequence of substitutions and combinations. By the same token, the examination of metonymical 'displacements' in discourse should allow us to approach metaphorical 'condensations' in language (Lacan, 1958b, p. 166). The assessment of the movement from "pillar" to "construction", for example, should facilitate the analysis of the condensed conception of the "pillar" as a "family". Similarly, the structural significance of the opposition between "dissolution of the couple" and "identification in the perception of the world", inside this unintelligible perceptible world (i.e., the unconscious world), cannot be appreciated without considering the sequence of substitutions and combinations that go from "identification" to "dissolution" through "individual sexual love" and "faithfulness from conviction".

The substitutions and combinations may be regarded as continuous metonymical discontinuities, displacements or events of sliding, which offset each other and thus compose the continuity of the discursive chain. According to Lacan (1960–1961), this chain 'marks the subject' and 'establishes in him the metonymy', that is, the 'possibility of permanent sliding of signifiers under the continuity of the signifier chain' (01.03.61, p. 202). Instead of the sliding of signified entities under the succession of signifying elements, characteristic of the 1950s, there is now, in the 1960s, a sliding of signifiers under the signifying chain. In this sliding, the opposed signifiers of the structure can be combined between them and substituted one for another. In this way, the diachronic metonymies of discourse create new metaphors in the synchronic structure of language.

Thanks to the metonymies in the signifying chain, the signifying structure is reorganized at each moment. At each link of the discursive chain, the structure of language is enriched with new metaphors. These new metaphors are useful, but also dangerous. They may put the structure in danger. They may ultimately neutralize the necessary structural oppositions between symbolic values. We can even conceive of the hypothetical situation, described by Lacan (1960–1961), in which 'all the elements associated with the signifying chain' can be finally 'taken as equivalent to one another' (01.03.61, pp. 202–203). This can be illustrated by considering, in Francisco Javier's discourse, the trend towards the equivalence between the "pillar", the "monogamous family", the "couple", "marriage", and "individual sexual love". Rather than a "proletarian ideology", these equivalences involve the bourgeois ideology that dangerously weakens and impoverishes the signifying social structure by reducing first "individual sexual love" to the "couple", then the "couple" to "marriage", and finally "marriage" to the "monogamous family" (so that *my* "individual sexual love" becomes *our* "monogamous family"). In this reductive 'chain of equivalences' that Laclau (2000a) assigns to the functioning of ideology, we can be faced with a situation in which 'we must neglect the characteristics of each link to maintain what the chain of equivalences tries to express' (p. 120). To maintain Francisco Javier's *consistency*, for example, we must neglect the structural oppositions between individuality and monogamy, couple and family, etc.

Without a definite and definitive symbolic value, words can become totally equivalent. At the same time, being empty or devoid of a meaning that is merely imaginary, words can *float*. As the 'phenomenal form' of a word's 'emptiness', this 'floating character' implies that words turn out to be interchangeable (Laclau, 2000a, p. 121). This is only natural. On the one hand, words do not have any imaginary reality that would be proper to them and that would thus prevent their interchange. On the other hand, they do not have any symbolic value that would be independent from their position in the chain. Without this intrinsic value, a word can take any value, including the value of another word. For example, a 'circumstantial element', such as "love" in Francisco Javier's discourse, 'may take the representative value' of 'the object towards which the subject makes his way' (Lacan, 1960–1961, 01.03.61, p. 202). When it takes the value of this 'impossible object' that Laclau (2000a) identifies as the 'fullness of community' (p. 117), "love" *is* "faithfulness from conviction", as well as the "conviction" itself, but also the "consistency" of the "revolutionaries", and even the "revolution", the "new society", or "the pillar" as a "monogamous family". Unfortunately, these lovely words are nothing but words, empty words, *loveless words*, unconscious signifiers without a real conscious signification. The reality of the *fullness of community* is just an imaginary reality. Its value is purely symbolic. The only real thing here is the materialization of this value in the literal form of language, discourse, and words.

The retroactive enforcement of the laws of language

We already know that the real of the symbolic is the only real thing accessible to Lacanian Discourse Analysis. This empty real takes the three literal signifying forms of the synchronic structure of language, the diachronic chain of discourse, and an isolated element, a signifier, which can be anything in the world, since anything can function as a word or lexeme, as a morpheme or a phoneme. In a sense, these isolated *signifying elements* and their *signifying chain* belong to the *signifying structure* of language, which is simultaneously deployed as a discourse and composed of signifiers. Besides being the most elementary analyzable items in discourse, these signifiers are the material constituent elements of the real structure.

The signifiers make up 'a set of material elements linked by a structure' (Lacan, 1953b, p. 148). This 'structure of the signifier' is 'articulated' just 'as is commonly said of language' (1957b, p. 498). This articulation, as the distinguishing feature of the signifying structure, 'means that its units are subject to the twofold condition of being reduced to ultimate differential elements and of combining the latter according to the laws of a closed order' (ibid.). Here the laws are as fundamental as the signifying elements. A language is 'a field' that is 'structured' by 'laws' (1956c, p. 428). The laws are the actualization of the structure. We can even define the structure as an *enforcement of laws*. This enforcement can be described, in turn, as a retroactive application of the structure to a raw material, which is thus overdetermined, and thereby signifierized, or transformed into a set of signifiers. This synchronic process necessarily underlies the making of each moment or word in discourse. Even if each discourse is subject to specific rules, these diachronic rules of the signifying chain must be intrinsically related to the synchronic laws of a signifying structure.

Signifying chain of a discourse	*Signifying structure of a language*
Diachronic rules of metonymical displacement by substitution or combination	Synchronic laws of opposition and metaphorical condensation

To correctly analyze the signifying chain of a discourse, with its diachronic rules of metonymical displacement by substitution or combination, Lacanian Discourse Analysis must also analyze the signifying structure of a language, with its synchronic laws of opposition and metaphorical condensation, which are retroactively enforced in order to make each signifier of discourse. Without this enforcement, there would simply be no discourse to be analyzed. The analyzable signifiers of discourse are nothing but the result of the retroactive and recurrent enforcement of the laws of language.

The 'slightest appearance of a graph' involves 'orthography' (Lacan, 1956–1957, 20.03.57, p. 236). Likewise 'the most elementary appearance of the signifier' implies the enforcement of the laws of language (ibid.). These laws come into force 'with the signifier', *a priori*, unconsciously, 'internally, independently from any experience' (ibid.). Now, besides the necessary enforcement of the laws of a language (*langage*), there is always the obligatory application of the rules of a discourse (*discours*), as well as the unavoidable obedience to the conventions of a tongue (*langue*). These three compulsory symbolic systems concern the three levels of a tongue community, a discourse pronounced in specific circumstances, and a social or individual language that structures the unconscious, as we shall see thoroughly in chapter six.[33] When we analyze a concrete statement, we should expect to come across the three levels, as well as their respective compulsory systems, which are closely interwoven. In Francisco Javier's discourse, for instance, there should be *language laws, conventions of tongue* and *rules of discourse* that forbid certain combinations between signifiers, while allowing the combination of "consistent" with "revolutionaries" and "monogamous" with "family". First, in the Spanish tongue, as in English, the adjective ("consistent" or "monogamous") can only be combined with a substantive ("revolutionary" or "family"). Furthermore, in the language of Francisco Javier, there may be a law that forbids the combination of "revolutionaries" with "inconsistent" when using the verb "to be" in the first person plural, present tense, conditional mood, and negative form ("we would not be consistent revolutionaries if our conceptions ..."). Finally, in the specific discourse that we are using as an example, there is probably a rule that prevents the combination of the adjective "polygamous" with the substantive "family" that has the value of "pillar for the construction of the new society".

Obligatory application of the rules of a discourse *(discours)* pronounced in specific circumstances
Necessary enforcement of the laws of a language (*langage*) that structures the unconscious
Unavoidable obedience to the conventions of a tongue (*langue*) in a tongue community

Notes

1. In other words, 'signification' is impossible since 'it is only indeed possible against a background framework of rules and presuppositions that, as it were, co-determines my meaning' (Hook, 2008, p. 57). This being so, signification is *only indeed possible* when it is no longer a signification, but a *co-determination* by the signifying *background framework of rules and presuppositions.*
2. By assuming overdetermination, we accept that 'one interpretation does not preclude others' (Parker, 2005a, p. 171). In the case of Francisco Javier, the interpretation of the "pillar" as a *support* does not preclude its interpretation in relation to "faithfulness", "monogamous family", "man's total fulfilment", and "individual sexual love".
3. Here language includes 'people's practical reasoning' and 'settled institutional practices' for 'soliciting' and 'producing a *cognition*' (Antaki, 2006, pp. 13–14). As language functions with the social material of symbolic differences and identities, it makes it possible to 'divert the spotlight off the private mind' and to 'bring into view' that which 'conjures and sustains it in the public sphere' (p. 15).
4. As Parker (2003) notes, 'to treat *meaning* as self-sufficient and independent of the symbolic would be to render it, in Lacanian terms, as an imaginary order of experience' (p. 100). This idea is completely consistent with Lacan's early work. Provisionally, we may agree with it. However, we will radicalize it in a while, in a more structuralist position, by assuming that meaning is always *an imaginary order of experience.* The reason is precisely that meaning can only be treated *as self-sufficient and independent of the symbolic.* From this point of view, we can no longer regard the transition from cognitive psychology to Lacanian psychoanalysis as 'a shift from questions of mechanism to questions of meaning' (p. 99).
5. From our Lacanian point of view, this unsignifiable character of the real thing explains a 'multiplicity' in which 'there are, simply, too

many ways of speaking about things, and to do them justice one would have to use all these different ways, all at once' (Frosh, 2007, p. 641). Thus, to signify the real thing, one would have to use all the signifiers at once. This being impossible, the thing cannot be signified and the signifiers jostle to signify it.

6. In Lacan, as we shall see later, what really has a use value is not the language, but the subject, who is *used* by language, and *functions* as a 'language employee' (Lacan, 1969–1970, 21.01.70, p. 74). It would seem here that Lacan 'inverts' the '*instrumentalization*' of language (Cléro, 2008, p. 172). Instead of a language *instrumentalized* by the subject, there would be a subject *instrumentalized* by a language.
7. Instead of 'meaning based on denotation', we assume here a 'structural approach' in which 'a word is conceived to have a meaning by virtue of its relationships to other words' (Harré, Clarke & De Carlo, 1985, pp. 101–102). Fortunately, nowadays most constructionist social psychologists should be familiar with this structural approach of Lacanian Discourse Analysis.
8. This does not amount to saying that meaning results *only* from this configuration. It is true that 'meaning doesn't result only from language, unless we believe that cognition doesn't exist without language' (Camus, 1999, p. 277). Although we should actually believe that *human* cognition does not exist without the symbolic order of language, we should simultaneously recognize that human cognition is not only its symbolic value, but also its imaginary reality. Accordingly, meaning results from this reality of cognition and not only from the order of language.
9. As the assimilation to the signifying structure, signifierization embraces all the processes that usually come under the psychosocial heading of 'categorization' (e.g., Tajfel, 1982). Since categories are nothing more than signifiers implying structural relations between signifiers, categorization is just a form of signifierization that reduces things and people to *signifying categories* such as "black", "red", "revolutionary", etc. Together with other discourse analysts, a Lacanian must regard these categories as 'nouns' that are 'moulded in discourse' (Potter & Wetherell, 1987, p. 137).
10. It is the premeditated illusion of those who 'abstractly take a proposition as an intentional unit, corresponding to the meaning of a sentence in linguistic theory, and to the conceptual representation of a sentence in a cognitive model of language comprehension' (Van Dijk & Kintsch, 1983, pp. 112–113). In this way, the proposition opens the 'space of the rewording/paraphrase' which constitutes what Pêcheux (1975b) calls 'linguistic imaginary' (pp. 1962–1963).

11. In the justification of a social-psychological *semiotic discourse analysis* (Camus, 1999), this has been correctly described as a 'retroactive construction of meaning' (p. 282).
12. This is recognized by Camus (1999) when she remarks that words 'persuade the other that this particular reality constructed *in* and *by* discourse, is the reality, or eventually a reality, existing outside words' (p. 276). This is profoundly true as long as we see that 'reality', as 'meaning', is not the same for the speaker and for the listener (p. 277). For reality to be the same for the 'perceptions' of both interlocutors, it must be a 'signifying reality', but in this case it is not 'meaning' anymore and it becomes something indistinguishable from 'discourse' (ibid.).
13. As Billig (1998) notices, 'if adults impose meaning through conversational interaction, then this includes psychological meaning' (p. 18). After a cognitive content analysis, which had focused on imaginary psychological meaning, rhetorical and traditional discourse analyses studied symbolic conversational interaction, which imposes psychological meaning. As for Lacanian Discourse Analysis, it must *also* study the real structural signifierization that sustains conversational interaction.
14. Lacanian Discourse Analysis 'emphasizes form over content' (Parker, 2005a, p. 167). In this sense, it is consistent with its foundation in psychoanalysis, which 'is concerned primarily with questions of *form* rather than *content*' (Parker, 2008, p. 150). As a *psychoanalytical analysis of form* that prioritizes the signifying container over the signified content, our analysis is in complete contrast to a *psychosocial analysis of content* that is 'interested precisely (and exclusively) in the signified, by definition' (Muchielli, 1974, pp. 30–33).
15. Accordingly, we should avoid 'thinking that *attitudes* and *representations* are contents that exist before the speech act, which would translate them in a transparent form' (D'Unrug, 1974, p. 229). Rather than a simple translation, the form 'has to be seen as an act or process of elaboration' (ibid.).
16. What we imagine can only become *predictable* by a *simulacrum* of an exact science which is not ours. It can only be *objectified* by a *betrayal* of the real subject of our analysis. It can only be *generalized* through an *absolutization* of a relative imaginary which is necessarily related to the specific individual who analyzes discourse. Those three vices of 'absolutization', 'betrayal' and 'simulacrum' are judged with good reason as a 'form of Evil' by the Lacanian ethic that Parker (2005b) extracts from Badiou and recommends to psychology (pp. 240–241).

17. This distinction is crucial. However, the Thing and the object concern the same real whose 'insignifiability' indicates its unimaginable 'existence' somewhere in the 'mental', while its unsignifying character indicates its 'unsymbolizable' existence somewhere in the 'material world' (Hook, 2003, p. 22).
18. This is how a Lacanian would assume 'in a profound sense' the constructionist idea that 'accounts *construct* reality' (Potter & Wetherell, 1987, p. 34). However, unlike the theoretical perspective of much discourse analysis in social psychology, a Lacanian Discourse Analysis does not treat this 'constructive activity' as a 'creation of a *world out there*' (p. 181). This *world out there* is a discursive world. It is discourse itself. By using our enunciating workforce, it constructs itself and it does not need *another discourse* to be constructed. What would supposedly need a discourse to be constructed is not this *world out there*, but my inner world. Nevertheless, this conscious world is just a reified portion of a discursive *world out there* which is constantly constructing, although not always 'consciously constructing', as Potter and Wetherell have remarked (p. 34). We will see in chapter six that, actually, the discursive *world out there* corresponds to *the* unconscious as Other's discourse.
19. Unlike traditional discourse analysis (Potter & Wetherell, 1987), Lacanian Discourse Analysis, though 'radically non-cognitive', does not force us to concentrate 'exclusively on discourse itself' (p. 178). In Lacanian 'discursive constructionism', we focus certainly on the symbolic field of 'people's practices', but that does not rule out the possibility of taking into account the imaginary sphere studied by 'cognitive constructionisms that consider the way images of the world are mentally put together through processes of information processing' (Potter, 2004, p. 610). This imaginary sphere is nevertheless entirely subordinated to the symbolic field of discursive constructionism.
20. Therefore Lacanian 'discursive constructionism' involves a 'social constructionism' (Potter, 2004, p. 610). In the Lacanian constructionism, the 'social relationships' and the 'social perceptions' (ibid.) are determined by signifying relations and positions within the structure of discourse. In actual fact, as we shall see later, a social relationship can be analyzed as a signifying relation between structural positions occupied by different individuals. Likewise, a social perception can be analytically reduced to a position from the point of view of another position that is shared by different individuals. In Lacanian Discourse Analysis, all of these positions are nothing more than signifiers composing the analyzed discourse.

21. In this way, from the perspective of 'Lacanian theory', the 'symbolic allows human subjectivity to form, creating the conditions for communication and hence for some kind of deeper recognition of subjecthood' (Frosh, Phoenix & Pattman, 2003, p. 40).
22. Lacanian communication thus has nothing to do with 'communication' defined as an 'exchange of meanings' (Anzieu & Martin, 1968, p. 193), a 'sharing of representations' (Rimé, 1984, p. 446) or 'a process of *intersignification*' (Le Blanc & Almudever, 2000, p. 291). Lacanian communication is rather a process of *inter-signifierization* in the 'inter-signifying relation' that we call 'inter-subjective relation' (Lacan, 1970–1971, 13.01.71, p. 10). What is communicated is a structural overdetermination, and not a signification, a meaning, or a representation. All this is 'incommunicable' (Sapir, 1921, p. 12). It cannot be either shared or exchanged. It cannot move from one's mind. When a meaning travels from one mind to another, it simply becomes another meaning. When a representation seems to be shared between a couple of people, there are, in reality, a couple of similar representations.
23. It does not *inform* us about the 'assigned properties' of a 'reference object' (Newcomb, Turner & Converse, 1965, p. 252). It is not 'content' referred to an object, but rather a simple 'informing action' or 'operation' of information (Anzieu & Martin, 1968, p. 189).
24. In my opinion, when social psychologists assume the 'worthwhile ideal' of the 'transparency of communication', *they simply do not* 'need a more radical approach to grasp how our understanding is always structured by the symbolic order' (cf. Parker, 2003, p. 106). This need of a *more radical approach* does not affect those psychologists who can satisfy all their needs 'on the axis of the *imaginary*' (ibid.). By the way, the imaginary will always be more satisfying than the symbolic.
25. Lacan's 'fundamental insight' has nothing to do with the idea of 'bringing psychoanalysis and semiotics together' (cf. Juignet, 2003). Lacan's insight, on the contrary, is his decision to keep the signifier away from the 'semiotic universe' of the sign, the signification and the signified (ibid.).
26. Therefore it is not comparable to a conscious or pre-conscious psychosocial 'communication contract' as the one proposed by Bromberg (2004). In relation to this contract, the symbolic pact functions as the implicit structure that precedes and determines the contractual clauses, namely the 'selection' of a 'plausible context' for interpretation (p. 104), the 'institution' of this 'context' as 'interpretative frame' (p. 107) and the contribution of a 'default interpretative framework' (p. 106).

27. Language constructs the imaginary reality, granted, but that does not mean that it exists as a 'tool' used by our 'mind' to construct that 'reality' (cf. Ghiglione, 2003, p. 498).
28. It follows that we cannot put Lacan's language in any of the four 'models' distinguished by Habermas (1981), in which language is always a way of doing something in order to achieve something else, whether to 'influence' in 'one's interest' in the 'teleological model', to 'communicate cultural values' in the 'normative model', to 'appear on the scene' in the 'dramatic model', or to 'intercomprehend' in the 'communicational model' (pp. 110–112). The first three models would consider only one function of language, while the fourth one would 'take into consideration all the functions' (ibid.). By contrast, the Lacanian model does not consider any function apart from the signifying function. So language is merely a way of signifying to signify.
29. Unlike Propositional Discourse Analysis (Ghiglione et al., 1985), Lacanian Discourse Analysis must not look for anything such as the 'nodal referents' that would refer to an extra-discursive real or reality (p. 36). As 'discursive objects with structuring power' (ibid.), those referents assimilate its reference to the signifying structure of discourse. Once assimilated, the reference forms part of discourse. The "proletarian ideology" of Francisco Javier, for example, forms part of his discourse. Its 'expressive value' is its symbolic value in discourse and not its 'reference value' in relation to something real outside discourse (cf. Ghiglione et al., 1985, p. 38).
30. This Lacanian idea of the form as content presupposes a real structural container of the symbolic form. This form can be then regarded as content. We find a similar idea in the cognitive differentiation between the 'verbal exchange', the 'linguistic content of that exchange', and the 'information structure of discourse', that is 'richer than its content alone' (Roberts, 1999, p. 231). This differentiation perfectly describes the Lacanian distinction between the real container of the symbolic, the symbolic form or content, and the purely imaginary content, which is naturally *richer* than the symbolic content alone, which cannot be enriched by the rich imagination of cognitive psychologists. We will again encounter this triple distinction in chapter four (between the enunciation, the enunciated statement, and that which is stated), in chapter seven (between the absence, the representative, and the representation) and in chapter nine (between the literal being, the signifying being, and the signified being).

31. Pêcheux (1975a) notes that 'syntactical rules are constantly overloaded, covered and partially erased, what means that semantic theory is not purely and simply exterior to linguistic theory, which cannot be regarded as a theory about a logical homogeneous systematic matter' (p. 3). Accordingly, we must be prepared to encounter imaginary impurities in the analyzed discourse, as well as symbolic emanations, prolongations, or propagations outside *printed discourse.*
32. Lacan reduces the metaphor to the symbolic level of words and language. So, he would agree with Billig (2006b), who treats metaphor as a 'use of the linguistic phrase' in contrast to an 'internal state of mind' (p. 19). As Billig notes, 'it seems implausible to expect metaphors to be linked to precisely defined inner experiences' (ibid.). However, in a Lacanian Discourse Analysis in which we are not compelled to disregard the imaginary, we may *expect metaphors to be linked to vaguely defined inner experiences.* We may also acknowledge Francisco Javier to 'experience a particular inner state' when he 'uses a metaphor' such as "pillar" (ibid.). Although there is no evidence that this *inner state* is identical to mine, I have evidence which demonstrates 'the existence' of *my* 'internal state of mind' (ibid.). This evidence is precisely *my internal state of mind.* This state of mind may just be imaginary, and worse than useless to discourse analysis. It is nevertheless the case that it exists.
33. The tongue conventions include 'grammar, syntax and vocabulary (or *la langue* of formal linguistic theory)', while discourse and language embrace 'moral precepts' and 'social codes' that Billig (1998) connects soundly to 'repression' and 'unconscious' (pp. 16–17). The unconscious actually results from a 'language-in-interaction' that 'creates moral imperatives' (Billig, 1997, p. 156). Now, according to Billig, these imperatives 'repress' and thus cause a 'dialogic unconscious' (pp. 155–156). By contrast, according to Lacan, the unconscious is already the language-in-interaction, or *the discourse of language* (as discourse of the Other), that creates those moral imperatives. In a sense, Lacan's unconscious creates the imperatives that create Billig's unconscious.

CHAPTER THREE

Full speech and empty speech

Bearing in mind the primary distinction between the symbolic and the imaginary, this chapter turns to a secondary distinction between *full speech* and *empty speech*. When applied to discourse analysis, this Lacanian distinction will help us to differentiate between two kinds of structural aspects of discourse. On the one hand, there is the structured emptiness of descriptive speech, a word without consequences that is nothing more than a receptacle for an imaginary objective reality. On the other hand, there is the structuring truthfulness of decisive speech full of truth, full of its true consequences, full of the consequential, consistent subject that will exist by the mere fact of the enunciation of the word.

The structuring power as the fullness and truthfulness of full speech

Speech may be regarded as a concrete implementation of language laws, conventions of tongue, and rules of discourse. Accordingly, the speaker cannot freely decide what he speaks. It is, rather, up to speech to decide everything regarding itself and the speaker. In the 'relation of man to speech' as the 'base' of Lacanian psychoanalysis

(1958b, p. 165), it is speech itself that 'develops' its 'structure' and 'imposes' it 'on the subject' (Lacan, 1957–1958, 22.01.58, p. 179). This is true, provided that speech is *full*, full speech containing and structuring the subject, and not *empty*, empty speech 'floating above the subject' (ibid.).

Established between 1953 and 1958, the Lacanian distinction between *full* and *empty* speech is a distinction between a *structuring* and a *floating* speech. If the empty speech floats, it is precisely because it lacks the *structuring weight* of full speech. In Lacan's early work, this weight is a power to 'perform' the subject (1953–1954, 17.03.54, p. 174). In Lacan's later work, the performed subject is literally 'spoken' by his 'full speech' (1970–1971, 10.03.71, p. 78). For instance, Francisco Javier is *literally spoken*, as a "consistent revolutionary", by his own consistent speech, which performs his "revolutionary consistency" by assigning to him the "conceptions of marriage and the couple" that are "based on love, respect and faithfulness". Thus, in general, speech is not only full of its structuring power, but it is also full of the effect of this power, that is, the *spoken speaker*, who is moulded by his own speech. From a psychological angle, the speaker can be spoken and even moulded by his own speech for the reason that he is not only 'the one who speaks', but also 'the one who listens' to his own speech (Lacan, 1953b, p. 137). By listening to himself, the speaker may be transformed into someone else, a listener, who will not be identical to the speaker. Put differently, what the speaker hears from himself *will have changed* him. Speech can thus be full of a listener who *will have existed* as a result of what is spoken by himself. Supposing that I am Francisco Javier, for example, I *will have been part of* "consistent revolutionaries" (as a listener) by explaining (as a speaker) that "we would not be consistent revolutionaries if our conceptions of marriage and the couple were not based on love, respect and faithfulness".

By speaking to himself, the subject is transformed into someone else. Through his 'full speech which performs', he 'finds himself, afterwards, other than he was before' (Lacan, 1953–1954, 17.03.54, p. 174). He appears to himself, afterwards, as a new subject who will have been transformed by his own speech. This *new subject* will have literally *existed* by virtue of his speech. He will have been the effect of this speech. Therefore his speech precedes him. The structuring power of speech precedes its structured outcome. When the power is exerted through speech, the subject is scarcely beginning to exist. When he fully exists in his full speech, the power has already been exerted.

Logically, the structuring power is exerted before the appearance of the one who will have appeared because of this power. When the listener appears, the power of speech has already been exerted. In a sense it is no longer, so its effect cannot be conscious of it. The causal power of speech is logically unconscious for its consequential listener.[1] This is why the listener offers no resistance to it. He cannot resist the power because the power was already exerted before him and he does not even know it. So he cannot speak about it. He is not an active speaker anymore. At this moment, he is just a passive listener. He cannot yet speak about the power of speech, and when he finally does speak about it, he is not under its spell anymore, because he is no longer the listener caused by it, but now a speaker that has escaped from it.[2]

Since the listener follows from the power of speech, he cannot also be the one who exerted this power, who is always *Other* than him. This Other articulates the speech of the listener. Accordingly, this speech is a *discourse of the Other*, or a discourse of a language, as we shall see in chapter six. For the time being, we must remember only that the listener is not the one who articulates his own speech. Nevertheless it is his own speech. He *expressed* it. Yet he did not *articulate* it. He is not the author. He is rather the *truth* of speech. He is thus the truthfulness as the fullness of full speech. This truthfulness is the 'truth of the subject' that is 'realized' by full speech (Lacan, 1953–1954, 03.02.54, p. 83). It is, for instance, the inconsistent truth of the "consistent revolutionary" that will have been realized by saying exactly that which must be said in order to be a "consistent revolutionary" according to what is said.

By realizing the inconsistent truth of the "consistent revolutionary", Francisco Javier's full speech retroactively assigns a historic revolutionary symbolic value to his "conception of marriage" and to other conformist moments of discourse. These moments are thus promoted to the 'dignity of history' (Lacan, 1950, p. 129). They become historic moments of the consistent revolution undertaken by Francisco Javier. Since this revolutionary "would not be consistent" if his "conceptions of marriage and the couple were not based on love, respect and faithfulness", then it is *necessary* for the consistency of the revolution to base "marriage and the couple" on "love, respect and faithfulness". These three conjugal eventualities become, paradoxically, "familiar obligations" of the consistent revolutionary. Francisco Javier's full speech transforms them, in this way, into historical requirements that will have to be satisfied in order to achieve a consistent revolution. Thus 'the effect of full speech is to reorder past contingencies by conferring on them the sense of necessities to come' (Lacan, 1953a, p. 254). These necessities are, so to speak, the *life's necessities* of the subject who will have existed thanks to his full speech. They arise from the laws of language and rules of discourse that must be obeyed by the speaker in order to become a specific listener. These laws and rules are, in fact, enforced through the necessities of speech. This supposes continuity between the laws and rules, the ensuing necessities of speech, and their structuring power, in which lie the fullness and truthfulness of full speech.

The fullness and truthfulness of full speech lie in its structuring power. Exerted through the intrinsic necessities of speech, which enforce the laws of language and the rules of discourse, this power constitutes the truth of the subject who will have existed by virtue of his full speech. In Francisco Javier's discourse, the structuring power can be illustrated by the structured *consistent inconsistency* of the "consistent revolutionary" who will have existed retroactively by virtue of his conformist revolutionary speech. As the *truth of the subject*, this *consistent inconsistency* constitutes *the* necessity of other necessities as "love, respect and faithfulness". In general, the truth of the subject amounts to the necessity of the subject who will have existed retroactively as a consequence of this necessity. Obviously, this *necessity to come,* as the signifying fullness and truthfulness of speech, is not yet an actual reality already signified by speech.[3] To be sure, the truth of speech, from the Lacanian viewpoint, is not a mental concordance with an objective reality, but a verbal revelation of a subjective truth. In other words, the discursive truth is not an *adequatio rei et intellectus*, but an *aletheia* of the subject. The truth does not lie in the retrospective cognitive signification of a sign, but in the retroactive discursive signifierization of the subject who will have appeared as a specific signifier in his speech and because of his speech.

If there is truth in Francisco Javier's discourse, then this truth lies in the signifierization of the "consistent revolutionary" who will have existed because of his discourse. In the interim, this discourse cannot signify its subject, the "consistent revolutionary", for the reason that *he does not yet exist*. As we know, *he will have existed* as a result of his discourse. Meanwhile, he fills his discourse as clay fills a mould. Just like clay, the "consistent revolutionary" is a promise that will have been kept by his full speech. This speech is literally *full of promise*. And *a promise is a promise*. The promise will have been kept by discourse. However, at the moment of discourse analysis, it has not yet been completely kept. Discourse is always a work in progress. The "consistent revolutionary" can exist only by a *permanent revolution* that takes place within the discourse that we analyze. In this discourse, the subject is never fixed as a signified, but he is in a constant state of flux.

For Lacanian Discourse Analysis, the subject is a sort of molten material in the changing form of its discursive mould. In this matrix of full speech, the subjective fullness constitutes a psychic fluid without a definitive and definite form. The form is always unstable and provisional. It is never a fixed general psychic form. Actually there is no such form that could be reproduced by a psychological model.[4]

There is no general psychic form. There is only the matchless form of each actual discourse that will have formed its own potential unique subject. This psychic form is a signifying structure full of itself, full of its signifierized subject, full of its structuring power, full of its rules and laws. In a sense, it is a form full of its own form. This specific form, in general, is nothing but matter, the only matter, the linguistic matter, as the form of all forms. This form is the only material fullness of full speech. It is the only content of discourse. This 'content' is 'language' (Lacan, 1968–1969, 11.12.68, p. 89).

In a Lacanian perspective, language is the only true content of discourse. All other contents (mental, cognitive and even semantic) are just imaginary. They are not inside discourse, but they come from the imagination of the analyst. Unfortunately, they cannot get into the analyzed discourse. They can barely be reflected in the false depth of the analytical mirror. Behind this mirror, speech is only full of language. Now, as speech is language, then speech is only full of itself. Its fullness is its own literal consistency. It is the revolutionary *consistent inconsistency* in the discourse of Francisco Javier. This *in-consistency* lies in the signifying structure of laws and rules, in its necessities and structuring power. Here is the fullness of speech, its consistent inconsistency, or its real structural emptiness.[5]

The structuring powerlessness as emptiness of empty speech

Speech is full of the emptiness of what is not, but has to be and will have been. As lack and desire, this emptiness of the past and the present involves a fullness of the future. The emptiness is a structured and structuring fullness of needs and necessities, obligations and expectations. The real emptiness of the structure contains a symbolic structural fullness. This fullness refers to an oracular truth and not to a memorable reality. What is 'at stake' here 'is not reality, but truth' (Lacan, 1953a, p. 254). This truth is not realistic, but prophetic. Its symbolic value is not evocative or descriptive, but imperative and predictive.

From a Lacanian viewpoint, the truth does not relate to the meaning or signification of what has happened, but to the sense in which it will have happened. This 'sense' can certainly be 'noticeable' in the 'uniqueness of the signification developed by discourse' (Lacan, 1953b, pp. 149–150). However, in Lacan, the *signification* is not the same thing as the *sense*. The imaginary reality of the former must not be confused with the symbolic value of the latter. Now, full speech is 'full of sense', while 'empty speech has only a signification' (1976–1977, 15.03.77). This signification of empty speech is reversible and retrospective, while the sense of full speech relates to the irreversible retroactive signifierization according to the necessities of the signifying structure. By the way, it is precisely this structure that overdetermines reality in the 'reversibility' of its retrospective signification (1953c, p. 19). From this, one may conclude that the signification of empty speech is nothing but a derived consequence, or tangential effect, of the signifierization that full speech achieved somewhere else.

Unlike empty speech, full speech does not contain only the signification imagined by the one who understands the spoken signifiers. Besides the imaginary reality of this objective cognition that can be inserted in any discourse, full discourse entails the truth of a real subjective recognition. Actually, 'full speech is speech which aims at, which forms, the truth such as it becomes established in the recognition of one person by another' (Lacan, 1953–1954, 17.03.54, p. 174).

In this recognition, as discussed above, 'one of the subjects', the first one, 'finds himself, afterwards, other than he was before' (ibid.). Our recognition of him does not only entail his recognition of himself, but also his transformation and his separation from himself. In a sense, his full speech creates another subject. It reveals an Other different from the One that was before. Francisco Javier's full speech, for example, anticipates a revolutionary who will have differed from the one who existed before his engagement in the answer to our question about "familiar obligations". Unlike the previous revolutionary, whose revolution was not a sexual revolution and had nothing to do with marriage and the couple, the one who answered our question "would not be consistent" if his "conceptions of marriage and the couple were not based on love, respect and faithfulness". To exist, this new "consistent revolutionary" must demonstrate his inconsistent truth by basing his "conceptions of marriage and the couple" on "love, respect and faithfulness". This demonstration of the truth of the subject is at the same time, both for him and for us, an immediate recognition of the subject in his consistent inconsistency. This direct subjective recognition, which is characteristic of Lacanian Discourse Analysis, has nothing to do with the indirect inference of an objective cognition supposed by cognitive content analysis. The former is a demonstration of a symbolic truth by the one who generates discourse, while the latter is a presumption of an imaginary reality by the one who analyzes discourse.

Empty speech	*Full speech*
Only full of signification	Also full of sense
Presumption of an imaginary reality by the one who analyzes discourse	Demonstration of a symbolic truth by the one who generates discourse
Inference of an objective cognition by cognitive content analysis	Subjective recognition in Lacanian Discourse Analysis

Cognitive content analysis takes advantage of any emptiness of speech and fills it with an imaginary mental reality. On the other hand, Lacanian Discourse Analysis derives its benefit from the analyzable fullness of speech. This fullness enriches our analysis just as the emptiness of speech makes possible the enrichment of cognitive analysis. This emptiness, as structuring powerlessness, represents the best opportunity for a psychologist to exert his power, or the structuring power of his discourse, and insert his own mental structures into the analyzed discourse without being disturbed by it. This is why full speech may deliberately be emptied by the psychologist who trivializes or oversimplifies it, and pays no attention to its specific fullness, or replaces it with a general psychological model.

Whether innate or emptied, empty speech suffers from its emptiness or structuring powerlessness, which facilitates its unrestrained filling, with mental structures, by cognitive content analysis. On the contrary, full speech is full of its own structuring power, which must be either violated or obeyed. Obeying this power, Lacanian Discourse Analysis fathoms the evident verbal structure of the analyzed discourse instead of filling it with the hypothetical mental structure of a psychological theory. Unlike the mental structure, the verbal structure does not concern the cognition of the analyst, but instead the analyzed discourse and its intrinsic subject. The truth of this subject is revealed immediately through the verbal structure of full speech. This immediate revelation makes possible the recognition of the subject. Thus it contrasts with the mediation of empty speech, whose emptiness can be described as the imaginary space in a two-sided mirror that comes between the interlocutors, contains their mental structures, reflects their respective cognitions, and impedes their mutual recognition. Here, in empty speech, 'if speech functions as mediation, it is on account of its revelation not having been accomplished' (Lacan, 1953–1954, 03.02.54, pp. 82–83). This *immediate revelation* is distinctive of full speech, while *veiling mediation* is the proper function of empty speech.

The truth of the subject and the structure of wisdom

Every kind of speech 'constitutes a mediation' (Lacan, 1953c, pp. 35–36), of course, but empty speech would constitute, by definition, nothing but this mediation. At least in theory, empty speech would only be a mediating speech that mediates between two speakers who do not have anything revealing to say. Thus, without any kind of revelation, an empty discourse would supposedly express just the mediation as is. It would communicate no more than communication. It would communicate merely itself, its mediating substance, its pure *face value.*

The only value of an empty discourse would theoretically be its *face value*. Yet, in practice, this value is never the only value of discourse. Lacan observes that 'however empty discourse may seem, it is so only if taken at face value' (Lacan, 1953a, p. 250). Now, besides this face value, an empty discourse always has its symbolic *exchange value*. In view of this, Lacan may compare empty speech to a worn 'currency' (ibid.). This image (of Mallarmé's) illustrates both the connecting capacity and revealing incapacity of empty speech. On the one hand, the 'figures in the obverse and the reverse' of the 'currency' have been 'worn away' (ibid.), which shows that empty speech lacks the revealing capacity of full speech. On the other hand, the worn currency 'passes from hand to hand', which demonstrates that empty speech keeps not only its mediating formal substance but also its connecting structural capacity as a symbolic 'exchange value' (ibid.).

The connecting capacity of speech operates in a shared structural sphere of language, or *wisdom*, which amounts here to the same thing. As a net of connections, this sphere deploys a signifying social structure that exerts its structuring power over the speaking individual subject. But this *truth of the subject* can only be revealed through full speech. *Unlike full speech, empty speech cannot reveal to us the truth of the subject under the power of the signifying structure of wisdom. Nevertheless, it connects us to the position of the subject in this structure.* This connection is logically made up of wisdom (*savoir*), inherent in the signifying social structure of language, which has nothing to do with the truth (*vérité*) of the subject under the structuring power of wisdom.

Empty speech	*Full speech*
Connection with the position of the subject in the structure of wisdom	Revelation of the truth of the subject under the structuring power of wisdom

In order to establish a connection of wisdom, empty speech obstructs the revelation of the truth. This truth is lost in wisdom. The subject 'loses himself in the machinations of the system of language, in the labyrinth of referential systems made available to him by the state of cultural affairs to which he is more or less an interested party' (Lacan, 1953–1954, 03.02.54, p. 83). In this way, 'the subject becomes involved here in an ever greater dispossession of himself as a being' (1953a, p. 247). By wandering in our shared wisdom, he wanders from the subject of his own truth. This can be seen in the empty speech that is used only for connecting positions in the shared spheres of conventional psychological journals, sectarian psychoanalytical associations, doctrinaire communist parties and imperialist capitalist common sense. When approaching empty discourses massively produced in these spheres, Lacanian Discourse Analysis will have a great deal of difficulty in identifying the truth of the subject lost in the shared wisdom. Francisco Javier's truth, for example, seems to be completely absent in the middle of his long discourses about the Marxist-Leninism of his party. As *Eperrist wisdom*, these discourses are of outstanding importance, but they are not a good place to identify the truth of the subject. To find this truth out, it is better to analyze those fragments in which Francisco Javier speaks about family, Amerindians, questions of gender, or the topicality of Marxism. Likewise, to find truth among psychologists or psychoanalysts, the best thing would be to look for it far from the consensual core of their respective wisdom, that is, at the borders where different types of wisdom clash between them. Full discourses are generally produced in those margins, in which a kind of shared wisdom comes into contact with other kinds of wisdom and is torn by this contact. Along with this bordering failure of the connecting structural function, there is unavoidably a revelation of the truth of the subject that suffers from the structuring power of wisdom. There is also the recognition of this subject who is ignored in the core of wisdom.

The true subject and the imaginary object called ego

In the core of wisdom, instead of a revelation and a recognition, there is the ignorance of the subject, as well as the 'dispossession of himself as a being' (Lacan, 1953a, p. 247). To compensate for this real dispossession, empty speech contains, for the subject, the imaginary being of his objective ego (*moi*) and retrospective self (*soi*).[6] Now, this being is characterized, defectively, by 'sincere portraits which leave its idea no less incoherent, rectifications that do not succeed in isolating its essence, narcissistic embraces that become like a puff of air in animating it' (1953a, p. 248). In view of all these tropes of empty speech, the subject 'ends up recognizing' that his 'being' inside empty speech 'has never been anything more than his own construction in the imaginary' (ibid.).

Empty speech is full of an imaginary object, an ego, which passes itself off as the true subject who will have existed by virtue of his full speech. Naturally the object could never be identical to the subject. Here, as Bakhtin (1938) remarks, 'the absolute identity', which identifies the subject with 'the ego about which he speaks', is 'as impossible as hanging oneself up by his own hair' (p. 396). Apart from the Baron of Münchhausen, who rose into the air by pulling himself up by his hair, there is no one who can overcome this real impossibility. Yet, we can always disregard this, and believe in the mirror of the imaginary, in which the object often seems to be identical to the subject.[7]

Despite the seeming identity between the subject and his ego, this objective ego is not the subject. When 'empty speech' refers to the ego, 'the subject seems to speak in vain about someone who, even if he were such a dead ringer for him that you may confuse them, will never join him in the assumption of his desire' (Lacan, 1953a, p. 252). Although the ego can be a desired imaginary object, it obviously cannot be a desiring real subject. Nor can it *have* a cognition, even if it *is* a cognition. Likewise, we can now speak against the ego, but fortunately the ego cannot speak against us. There is, nevertheless, 'the ego's language' in empty speech, that Lacan (1956c) describes in terms of 'intuitive illumination, recollective command, retorting aggressiveness of verbal echo', as well as 'automatic scraps of everyday discourse: rote-learning and delusional refrain' (p. 426). So this ego's language exists. However, it is not expressed by the ego, which is expressed, but cannot express anything.

Empty speech	*Full speech*
Language of consciousness: speaks about a retrospectively perceived ego	Unconscious language: speaks the subject who will have been retroactively created by this speech

Expressed by the subject, the ego's language constitutes the language of his consciousness. In empty speech, there is only this language, which speaks about a retrospectively imagined ego. Instead, in full speech, there is an unconscious language, or *the* language, which *speaks the subject* who will have been retroactively created by this speech. As we know, this subject is Other than the One who was before speech. Besides that, he is indistinguishable from the unconscious language that speaks him, since he is *what is spoken* and not the object *about which one speaks*. Therefore the subject, as speaking and spoken Other, *is* unconscious language. For Lacan, as we shall see in chapter six, this language is the unconscious itself. Now, this language fully speaks through us and our world, which is then composed of the signifiers whose structure contains and retroactively creates us with everything we perceive. This signifying structure of the perceived world is that which creates and contains, for instance, Francisco Javier and his "perception of the world". Overdetermined and signifierized, the perceived world is nothing but its unintelligible structure of perceptible signifiers, its *unconscious structure*, which is full of the future-oriented structuring power that 'governs our being' (Freud, 1912, p. 159). The perceptible signifiers can thus be compared, as constituent elements of the world, to the Leibnizian unconscious 'little perceptions' in which 'the present is full of the future' (Leibniz, 1704, pp. 42–43).

Notes

1. Likewise, the 'conditions of existence' of the 'reader-effect' must be 'hidden from this effect', which Pêcheux and Fuchs (1975) consider 'constitutive of subjectivity' (p. 8).
2. As Billig (2006) notices, 'power is typically reproduced within interaction without the participants explicitly discussing it', and when the participants 'bring up the topic, they are likely to be challenging patterns of power, rather than routinely reproducing them' (p. 21).
3. Assuming that 'the signifier is empty' and 'the sign is full' (Barthes, 1956, p. 198), a semiologist should not discern the particular fullness of Lacanian full speech. This fullness has nothing to do with the signified fullness of the sign, which is just imaginary, because of the 'impossibility for a sign' to 'occur in the fullness of a present' (Derrida, 1967, p. 102). Presupposing this impossibility, the Lacanian 'full speech' is *not* full of the signified ideal reality that would justify the accusation of 'logocentrism' against Lacan (cf. Derrida, 1972, p. 118).

4. If Lacanian Discourse Analysis assumed a 'psychological model', then 'the battle between psychology and psychoanalysis' would be won 'by psychology' (Parker, 2008, p. 157). In that case, our analysis would look for a fixed and general psychological model contained in discourse instead of analyzing the changing discursive form that incessantly moulds a psychic fluid which is always unique and peculiar to the analyzed discourse. In so doing, Lacanian Discourse Analysis would become a psychological analysis of content. As is, it would betray psychoanalysis, which 'is concerned primarily with questions of *form* rather than *content*' (p. 150). And what is more and worse: besides yielding to the temptation to 'decipher underlying content' (p. 152), our analysis would disregard the specificity of each discourse and would always decipher the same general underlying content composed of enjoyment, desire and other kinds of 'affect' (p. 157).
5. Full of its structural emptiness, the full speech can be full of the subject, his truth, his life, his breath in the vowels that are 'gnawed' by the consonants of the structure (Derrida, 1967, p. 322). Without this fullness, empty speech is 'pure consonant, pure articulation', and becomes, prematurely, a sort of 'dead language' (pp. 443–444).
6. We can assimilate this imaginary identity to the *self* of cognitive psychologists. Take for example, in social psychology, the *self* of Martinot (1997), with its 'cognitive component', as the 'concept of self', and its 'internal face', as the 'memories of self' (pp. 39–42). The objective and retrospective character of these entities is evident and does not need any comment.
7. This illusion arises precisely from what is called '*Münchhausen effect*' by Pêcheux (1975b). To avoid this 'imaginary effect' in discourse analysis, 'we must not regard the subject of discourse as the source of discourse' (p. 142). Our Lacanian Discourse Analysis, together with the Althusserian-Lacanian Discourse Analysis proposed by Pêcheux, must rather take language as the only source of a subject who cannot be the 'cause of himself' (p. 141).

CHAPTER FOUR

Enunciation and enunciated

Concentrating on the realm of full speech, this chapter concerns itself with how Lacan redefines the two levels, originally defined by Jakobson, of the *enunciation* (the process of stating something) and the *enunciated* or the *statement* (what is stated). A reflection on the first of those levels enables us to tackle the problem of the real in discourse analysis. In so doing, I discuss why study of enunciation necessitates an examination of the real that cannot be reduced, either to a discourse analysis of the statement, or to a content analysis of the imaginary reality signified by the statement. In order to locate *the real of the symbolic* that is at stake in *the enunciation of the enunciated*, I reassess several ideas of Austin and Jakobson. By means of this reassessment, I explain why Lacan decided to temporally contextualize the real subject of the enunciation, in a latent future perfect tense, as a subject that *will have existed* by the fact of the enunciation.

The signifierizing enunciating act and the signifying enunciated fact

When speaking, the subject of full speech is not yet created, but he will have been created by his speech. Even if he is spoken by now, that does not mean that he is plainly enunciated. He is not explicitly told, but rather implicitly foretold. He is thus implicated in the telling of his foretelling. His discourse heralds him. But even if he appears to us as a promise that already fills his discourse, he is not a piece of this enunciated discourse. He is just the truth of his discourse, but this truth is not enunciated by this discourse. The truth of his structural subjection cannot be objectively enunciated. His real signifierization cannot be expressed as a symbolic signifier.

The causal overdetermination and constitution of the "consistent revolutionary" cannot be confused with the consequential "consistent revolutionary". The subject's articulation is not articulated. This articulation is not enunciated wisdom, but the truth of this wisdom. It is the truth of the subject who will have existed by virtue of his enunciation of wisdom. This truth is also the retroactive investment and positioning of the subject, through his enunciation, in the signifying social structure of wisdom. It is thus the structuring power that constitutes and confirms, retroactively, the truthfulness and fullness of speech.[1]

As structuring power, the truth of the subject is his retroactive situation, overdetermination, signifierization, positioning and investment in the signifying structure. In a sense, this truth amounts to the real subject himself, to his life, to his speaking and spoken history. His truth is actually his structural constitution as a real subject, or, to put it more correctly, his subjectivation through his subjection to the structure. Now, this truth *is enunciation*, but it *is not enunciated*. There is here a crucial difference between two things:

- *The enunciation*. It is *the act of enunciating or stating something*. It involves the signifierization of the subject who expresses a discourse. It functions as an assimilation of this expressing subject to the enunciating structure of language that articulates the enunciated chain of discourse. At stake here is the individual truth (*vérité*) of the subject, which lies in the real foundation of the symbolic, the structure of the signifier, the fullness and truthfulness of full speech.
- *What is enunciated*. It is the *enunciated fact*, the *statement* or the *stated thing*. It involves the unfolding of the signifierized events that are enunciated. Thus it corresponds to the enunciated chain of discourse, which is expressed by the subject and articulated by the structure of language. At stake here is the symbolic signifying stuff of general

wisdom (*savoir*), which precedes and determines all knowledge (*connaissance*) of the imaginary objective reality of the signified.

Enunciated fact	*Enunciating act*
Objectivity, reality, general wisdom	Subjectivity, the real, the individual truth
The symbolic of the imaginary: retrospective signification	The real of the symbolic: retroactive signifierization

Borrowed from Jakobson, this conceptual distinction 'between the levels of the enunciation and of the enunciated' (Lacan, 1959–1960, 16.12.59, p. 79) predominates in the most structuralist period of Lacanian theoretical evolution (1958–1964). At this moment, the conceptual distinction takes the place of the differentiation between full speech and empty speech (1953–1958). From this previous differentiation, the new distinction recovers the parallel oppositions between subjectivity and objectivity, the real and reality, truth and wisdom. The new distinction also recuperates two conceptual polarities: symbolic-imaginary and signifier-signified. However, after the structuralist shift from signification to signifierization, the enunciation and the enunciated can operate as two symbolic signifying levels. *In depth, in the real of the symbolic, the enunciating act enables a retroactive signifierization. On the surface, in the symbolic of the imaginary, the enunciated fact makes possible a retrospective signification. This signification depends on signifierization just as the enunciated fact depends on the act of enunciation.*[2]

The objective distinction between the *enunciated fact* (symbolic wisdom or imaginary reality) and the *enunciating act* (the truth of wisdom) also implies a subjective distinction between the *symbolic subject of the enunciated fact* (the grammatical subject) and the *real subject of the enunciating act* (the enunciator).[3] This real subject is an individual in the flesh, while the symbolic subject is nothing more than a signifier. Apparently, they are independent of one another. Yet they both arise from the same identification of the real one with the symbolic one. So, in reality, they are dependent on one another. Actually, the identification of an individual to a signifier, through his enunciating act, entails his alienation in language, that is to say, his signifierization and subjectivation through his subjection to the structure, which generates both him as a real subject and his signifier as a symbolic subject. Thus, all things considered, the enunciation entails a creation of both the symbolic enunciated subject and the real enunciating subject.[4]

In a Lacanian perspective, the real subject arises from the enunciating act. He exists through this act. The protagonist of this act is consubstantial with the act. The speaker is the truth of his speech act. He is the truthfulness of his full speech. By revealing the real subject of the enunciation, full speech thus immediately reveals its truthfulness, which is the truth of a particular subject, such as the one identified with a "revolutionary", who will have been through the enunciation of his speech. Now, besides this real subject identified with the signifier, there is the signifier or the symbolic subject, the "revolutionary", whose existence is also determined by the enunciation and identification of the real subject with it. However, unlike the real subject, this symbolic subject is not the unique truth of the enunciation, but it is part of a shared wisdom. This is why many people can identify with a symbolic "revolutionary" in Marxist general wisdom. On the contrary, there is only one person who can incarnate the individual truth of a real subject, like Francisco Javier, with his particular way of telling the "revolutionary". In other words, the *told* "revolutionary" can be applied to everybody, but the *telling* will not be the same for everybody. The telling can be serious or humorous, risky or safe, proud or ashamed, and countless other things combined one way or another. As an individual truth, the telling would only be characteristic of one individual and only by a combination of circumstances. On the contrary, what is told, as general wisdom, can be told of various individuals in diverse circumstances.

What is told obviously depends on what one can tell, must tell or wants to tell under certain circumstances. But all this is not entirely translated into what is told. All this can only be expressed by the telling, and it concerns only the telling *or* its subject, the real subject of precise structural circumstances, of incomparable necessities, of a distinctive structuring power, of specific laws and rules characteristic of only one individual position in the world. The telling refers precisely to this one and only position held by the real subject of *an* unconscious, of *a* language, of *a* particular expression of the signifying social structure. What is told or not told logically depends on this unique structural telling position, or, to be more specific, on the unparalleled way in which this enunciating position is overdetermined by the structure.[5]

Lacanian Discourse Analysis presupposes, behind the analyzed discourse, a real subject who tells exactly what has to be told in his unique telling position. In this structural position, the subject does not decide anything, but tells what has been decided somewhere else by the structure. In so doing, the enunciating individual subject does the work of the signifying social structure. Since this structure includes the economic system of society, we may regard the subject as a 'proletarian', or a pure enunciating workforce, which is there to do the work of the unconscious (Lacan, 1968–1969, 12.02.69, pp. 172–173; 1969–1970, 17.12.69, pp. 33–35; 1970–1971, 21.05.71, p. 203; 1974b, p. 187). To do this work of the signifying structure, the worker is indispensable. There would not be a telling without a real teller. Unlike what is told (which can even be told by the cognitive abilities of a software tool), the telling involves a real subject in the flesh (an actual person who cannot be replicated by any kind of virtual simulation).

What is told involves only a 'grammatical subject' as the 'place where something' is symbolically 'represented' (Lacan, 1968–1969, 11.12.68, p. 83), while the telling involves the real presence of a 'living subject' whose 'subsistence' depends on his telling 'workforce' (Marx, 1867, II, VI, p. 133). This force is the prerequisite for the real subject to exist in the human world, or in the structure, which is the only place where he can exist. As Lacan (1968–1969) postulates, 'there is only a subject of a telling', and 'the subject is the effect of this telling' (04.12.68, p. 66). The subject arises from his telling. As for this telling, it arises from the signifying structure, which needs to make a real subject in order to do its work. So the telling requires a structure, which, in turn, requires the subjection and subjectivation of an individual. Francisco Javier's consistent revolution, for example, needs a language, which, in turn, needs the engagement of Francisco Javier as a "consistent revolutionary". This subject will have thus existed by being subjected to the language of his telling. This telling 'calls' the subject 'to existence' (Lacan, 1972a, pp. 449–450). Thus, through this telling, the signifying social structure creates the real subject by summoning him to appear.[6]

By creating a real subject, the signifying structure generates the individual telling truth that substantiates its own general told wisdom. It generates, for instance, a concrete revolution, such as that of Francisco Javier, which confirms the general conventional theory that asserts "the importance and significance of marriage as a starting point for the establishment of family and thereby for the constitution of society". But the confirmation of this theory relates only to the revolutionary, called Francisco Javier, whose promise is filling his speech. On the contrary, the confirmed theory can be told by him as well as by another Eperrist. In actual fact, the theory can also be told by a counter-revolutionary, in an empty speech; or by me, here; or by somebody else, elsewhere.

The enunciated fact may be told by quite a few individuals. It can represent them and be communicated between them. Contrarily, the enunciating act is incommunicable and inalienable, as it concerns only one individual subject of the structure. Unlike the slogan 'proletarians of every country, unite!', which can be inherited and enunciated by workers of every country, its ad hoc enunciation by Francisco Javier supposes a truth that concerns only him in his particularity and in particular circumstances. The particularity thus characterizes the truth of the enunciating act, while the universality gives its full symbolic value to the wisdom of the enunciated fact.

The enunciating act generates a particular truth of the universal wisdom, while the enunciated fact simply regenerates this wisdom, which makes it possible to imagine a reality. For this wisdom to be regenerated, the enunciated fact functions as a mechanism that is immanent to the symbolic system of the real structure. It is a sort of device that shall simply restore and reinforce this latent existing system of wisdom. As for the enunciating act, it must transcend the system. Otherwise, the structure cannot be particularized, as a particular language or unconscious, for the structural position which is already kept for the subject. This particularization of wisdom underlies any generation of the truth. It thus underlies any constitution of the subject by a subjection to the structure. In sum, when an individual is subjected to the signifying social structure, the enunciating act will transcend and particularize this structure for him, while the enunciated fact will simply reproduce the universal immanence of the structure.[7]

Analyzing the concrete psychology of an enunciating subject

On the enunciated side, there is the 'sense' of the universal 'true' wisdom (Lacan, 1975–1976, 09.03.76, p. 117), which is also the symbolic value of an 'imaginary' reality, as 'that which makes sense' (13.04.76, p. 131). On the enunciating side, there is the particular 'truth' of the subject, or the 'true real' (10.02.76, p. 85), which 'doesn't make sense' (09.03.76, p. 117). Even if this nonsensical true real corresponds to the fullness and truthfulness of full speech, it is not *content* in the strict sense of the word, and it should not be confused with the imaginary signification that makes sense.[8] Far from it, the true real is the literal container of all conceivable content. It is the structure of everything in the human world. First and foremost, it constitutes the real matrix of all symbolic forms. As for these forms, they are thus contained by the real, but they also contain the imaginary. In other words, the symbolic form of discourse is both the content of the real enunciating structure, and the enunciated container of the imaginary content. The structural position of the "consistent revolutionary", for example, represents at the same time: internally, the mould in which the signified revolutionary takes its imaginary shape; and externally, a symbolic form of discourse determined by the structure of a language in which a "consistent revolutionary" bases his "conceptions of marriage and the couple" on "love, respect and faithfulness".

Enunciated fact	*Enunciating act*
True wisdom of reality	Real truth of wisdom
Form of discourse: symbolic container of the imaginary content	Structural matrix: real container of the symbolic content

Lacanian Discourse Analysis must be levelled, primarily, at both the enunciating structural matrix, or the articulating real container, and its articulated symbolic content, as the enunciated form of discourse and the container of the imaginary content. In the analysis of this articulated content, we must begin by examining the signifying chain of discourse, the succession of symbolic events, before eventually proceeding to the imaginary signified reality. In the analysis of the articulating container, we must, in parallel, analyze the literality of the signifier, the real material structure of the symbolic form, the body of the soul, or the *hypokeimenon* of the *entelechies*. When analyzing this enunciating body, we must regard each person in the flesh as a support of the structure. We must approach thus the relation between the corporeal individual subject and his literal position in the structural social matrix, as real emptiness and space of his lacks, needs or desires, as well as his anguishes, drives or enjoyments.[9] All of this should make it possible to describe the subjecting of individuals, or the positioning of subjects in the structure, and not only their structural positions. In this description we should deal with the real act of overdetermination, structuration and signifierization, and not only with the symbolic system of the overdetermining signifying structure. In this way, the description of the real of the symbolic should give an explanation of the symbolic. The analysis of the enunciating act of positioning the subject in the structure should elucidate the enunciated structural position of this subject.[10]

Besides helping to elucidate the symbolic, the real enunciation should help in some way to clarify the imaginary. In fact, by explaining the enunciated fact, which creates the 'image of objective reality', the enunciating act also indirectly explains the 'subjective creation' of this 'image' (cf. Schaff, 1964, pp. 225–227). The reason for that is the 'creative function' of language, which has been so authoritatively considered by Humboldt (1834, §7, p. 163). Fulfilled through the 'acted' reality, this function concerns the enunciating level of the 'acting' truth (§14, p. 202). At this level, language is not 'an instrument intended for the representation of a known truth', but a way 'to discover an unsuspected truth' (1820, §20, p. 88). Such a truth reveals, 'in language', a structuring 'autonomous power' and a 'divine liberty' to create reality (1834. §3, p. 147).

With regard to the divine creating liberty or creative function of the enunciating act of language, we must acknowledge that 'in the beginning was the Word' (John, 1: 1). In Lacanian Discourse Analysis, we must accept, to be more specific, that *in the beginning was the telling of the Word* or *the enunciating act that enunciates the enunciated fact*. The Lacanian synthesis of John (*Word*) and Faust (*act*) thus poses a 'beginning' in which the 'action of the Word' is 'essential to the Word and renews its creation every day' (Lacan, 1953b, p. 135). Through this renewed enunciating act of creation, the imaginary reality is created, while 'the real' is 'demonstrated' by the 'act reached in the symbolic' (1970b, p. 592).

In the symbolic system, the real act of enunciation is also an act of retroactive demonstration of the real subject. From this enunciating act, the enunciated fact of the symbolic subject and its predicative world determines the entire imaginary reality of the *ego* and the *other* in the mirror. This determined mental reality of the signified self is prioritized, as we know, by cognitive content analysis (Lacan, 1957–1958, 25.06.58, p. 486). On the other side, traditional discourse analysis focuses on the determining enunciated fact of the signifying discursive chain. As for Lacanian Discourse Analysis, it must also examine the fundamental enunciating act of signifierization and structural overdetermination. In so doing, our analysis aims at illuminating the subjection of the individual to the structure, as well as the structure itself, its structuring power and its real emptiness, that is, the real matrix of the symbolic form, the literal foundation of the signifying determination, the articulating structural reason of the articulated discursive functioning, *the why of the how*.

In Lacanian Discourse Analysis, the *why of the how* refers to the enunciating structure whose real emptiness is negatively composed of logical identities and differences, literal positions and oppositions, as well as gaps, but also lacks, anguishes, desires, motivations, drives, repetitions, and other factors that are evidently inseparable from the symbolic.[11] As the real of the symbolic, these factors function retroactively as the cause of their own cause. Thus, paradoxically, they underpin what gives rise to them. Let us take the case of "love" in Francisco Javier's discourse. As that on which the "conceptions of marriage and the couple" are "based", this "love" might indicate a real thing that would support the same signifying "conceptions of marriage and the couple" which might stimulate it. Those discursive "conceptions" *are* the same language that generates the thing indicated by the word "love", of course, but that does not mean that a discursive psychology of those "conceptions" would be enough to explain the "conceptions" as well as their "base". Once generated by the told "conceptions", what is indicated by the word "love" exists retroactively as a real telling thing that explains the told "conceptions". This thing directly concerns the individual subjected to the structure, that is, the concrete literal incarnation of this structure, which constitutes, logically, the real "base" of any symbolic signifying "conception". If that is the way it is, the real thing called "love" deserves, beyond discursive psychology, a concrete psychology of the enunciating subject as an incarnation of the structure.

Through the concrete psychology that characterizes the enunciating subject of an enunciated statement, Lacanian Discourse Analysis should reveal the incarnate real structure of the symbolic form in the analyzed discourse. The analysis should expose, in this way, the retroactive signifierization of the signifier, the telling truth of the told wisdom, the corporeal thrust of the discursive movement. So, the analysis does not confine itself to strategic discursive operations, but it is also interested in the structural and structuring gesture that animates these operations. This gesture is analyzed as the corporeal enunciating act that generates the enunciated discursive fact.[12] It is the movement that articulates the analyzed discourse. So it is crucial for our analysis. Its *muscular force* is also crucial. It is the unremittingly applied workforce of a proletarianized subject who makes, in discourse, the continuous work of the structure, of language, of an unconscious.

Parallelism between enunciated general wisdom and enunciating individual truth

As the *executed work* and the *execution of the work* (or the *application of the workforce*), the enunciated fact and the enunciating act function as two superposed levels in a second scheme of parallels (for the first one, see chapter two). Instead of the parallelism between the signifying structure and the sliding signified of the first scheme (from 1956 to spring 1958), the new scheme (from summer 1958) establishes a parallelism between the two signifying chains of the enunciation and the enunciated. The two new chains present 'opposed structurations' (Lacan, 1958–1959, 03.12.58). As for their opposing 'relation', it embraces 'the whole grammar' (ibid.).[13]

Let us now proceed to examine separately and thoroughly the two Lacanian parallel and opposed signifying chains of the enunciating act and the enunciated fact:

Parallels (from 1958)

------------------- Enunciation

------------------- Enunciated

- Above, there is the enunciating act of the enunciated fact, or the 'signifying articulation' of the articulated discourse (Lacan, 1957–1958, 25.06.58, p. 486). This articulation of discourse is 'a moment of existence' of the subject (1972a, p. 450). It is 'the place in which the subject is implicit in pure discourse', which can be illustrated by the 'imperative' or the 'fire alarm' (1958c, p. 141). In these cases, the subject, who gives the command or burns and shouts, is implicit in the command and his shout. He is not explicitly enunciated when he cries "Fire!" or when he commands Francisco Javier to "Be consistent!". However, the enunciating subject is there, as he cries and gives orders. So he must not be forgotten either by the fireman, or by the revolutionary, or by the analyst of discourse. Unlike the reliable fireman and the consistent revolutionary, who must simply respond to the call, the scrupulous analyst of discourse will be faced here with a huge problem. As the 'truth' of the enunciated wisdom in the analyzed discourse, the enunciating subject can only express himself through 'enigma', 'wisdom without wisdom', and the 'half-told' or 'hints' (Lacan, 1969–1970, 17.12.69, p. 39). It may even be the case that he expresses himself through the telling silence of the non-told. Contrary to the enunciated fact, the enunciating act can thus be a 'silence' which 'does not amount to the absence of its subject' (Todorov, 1977, p. 363). Actually, whether in silence or in speech, an individual cannot speak about the enunciating truthfulness of his speech. The *telling truth* of the enunciation cannot be told or enunciated. As an incarnation of the articulating structure, the real subject cannot be present *in* that which is articulated. He can only appear in the gaps of his discourse. His telling truth can only be revealed in the fissures of his told wisdom, that is, in the silences, breaks, holes, leaps, ellipses, and all kinds of discursive deficiencies, which must not be disregarded by Lacanian Discourse Analysis.[14] Demonstrating the accomplishment of repression, those absences present the subject of the unconscious, a subject whose presence permeates his own absence, his fading, or the erasure of his telling by what is told. This erasure amounts to the enunciated fact of its enunciating act. The act erases itself. Thus, it erases the subject, who 'disappears and fades away' because of his enunciation, which entails, intrinsically, his 'repression' (Lacan, 1958–1959, 03.12.58).[15]

- Below the articulating enunciation, there is the enunciated chain, or the articulated statement, in which the real enunciating subject is denoted by 'shifters' (Jakobson, 1957, p. 178): proper nouns ("Francisco Javier"), common nouns ("revolutionary") and personal pronouns ("I" or "we"). These signifiers function as *clutches* that engage the subject in the signifying machinery. They refer to the points in which the individual is subjected to the structure. They are 'particles and inflections fixing his presence as the subject of discourse' (Lacan, 1958c, p. 141). Contrary to the real enunciating subject, this symbolic enunciated subject of discourse is explicit and explicitly present as a signifier. As is, as a word, he constitutes the symbolic representative of the imaginary representation of the absent real presence of the subject. So, as a signifying representative of a signified representation, the enunciated signifier involves the imaginary reality of the signified. In the mirror of discourse, the enunciated fact returns 'as a signified to the subject' (Lacan, 1957–1958, 25.06.58, p. 486). As far as the subject is concerned, he is reflected as a signified thing, a conscious 'ego', an object of consciousness (ibid.). Instead of the subject of the unconscious and his retroactive determination by the 'structure of enunciation', there is now the object of consciousness and its retrospective determination, its 'remembering' actualization, its updating by the enunciated chain (1958c, p. 148). In this updating, the latent essential tense can only be the 'present of chronology' (p. 141), that is, the Augustinian time of the consciousness, the 'present of the present', the 'present of the past' and 'of the future', the present as the essence of consciousness, as that which 'is present' (Augustine, 400, XI, pp. 267–270). This present is nevertheless only present as long as it is passing and thus becoming past, the past participle of what is already enunciat*ed*, then end*ed*, complet*ed*, accomplish*ed*, *presented*, so stabilized and ready for an analytical use, and misuse.[16]

As time passes, at each stabilization of the present, an enunciated general wisdom is totalized in discourse. In parallel, in each one of these totalizations, there are imperfections, flaws and destabilizations, which reveal the enunciating individual truth of discourse. This revelation discloses the real emptiness of the signifying unconscious structure, while the parallel totalization closes the imaginary fullness of a signified conscious reality.

The parallelism can be illustrated by differentiating the two levels in Francisco Javier's discourse. At the enunciated level, from a stabilized "revolutionary point of view", what is told is included in the totalization of "proletarian ideology, culture and values" (*general wisdom*), which certainly "contributes to man's development and total fulfilment" (*imaginary fullness*). In parallel, at the enunciating level, there is a destabilizing relation between our question about "familiar obligations" and the answer in terms of "marriage" and "monogamous family", which cannot be truly regarded, from a "revolutionary point of view", as a distinguishing feature of the "proletarian ideology, culture and values" (*flaw in totalization*), but rather as something else that should concern Francisco Javier and the quite particular "consistent revolutionary" that will have been retroactively created by his discourse (*enunciating individual truth of discourse*).

The future perfect tense in the perlocutionary act of the unconscious

The revolution forms the revolutionary. The enunciating act creates its enunciating actor. Thus, as '*Mythos*', the retroactive working of the enunciation reverses the psychological temporality of the enunciated '*Epos*' (Dunker, 2008, p. 85). Contrary to this ordinary temporality that governs articulated 'accounts' and 'stories', the 'circular' time of the articulating structure functions in such a way that 'something coming before may come after that which comes after' (ibid.). This inverted 'historical' time permits the 'revelation' of the 'truth', while the psychological epic temporality allows only the 'recitation' of an 'indirect account' (Lacan, 1953a, pp. 252–256). In this account, the recitation is centred on the 'present tense' and follows the signifiers in the enunciated signifying chain (ibid.). Its timing obeys the epic temporality of the latent present, as the essence of consciousness, in which past things are present causes that must precede their present effects, which are future things. Conversely, in the retroactive logic of the enunciation, there is the timelessness of the unconscious and its tragic historicity in which effects precede their causes.[17] The completed fate looks after its fatal completion. Similarly, speech makes its speaker. History makes those who make it.

Through the making of history, or the enunciation of discourse, the signifying social structure retroactively creates each one of its subjects. These subjects will have been thus created by their acts of enunciation. They will have been creations of their creations and outcomes of their outcomes. So, to be present, they must wait for their future. But this future is *never yet* present. In this future, the subjects are *never yet* present. By definition, as subjects of the unconscious, they cannot be present for consciousness. Therefore, as always absent enunciating subjects, they cannot function according to the conjugations that express the psychological temporality of the always present enunciated subjects.

Unlike the enunciated fact, the enunciating act is never tacitly conjugated in a latent present tense of the indicative mood. Nevertheless, it can be expressed in this present tense, as evidenced by explicitly performative assertions such as: "That's enough, I oblige myself to marry my comrade"; or, "Well, I authorize myself to cause a revolution". These assertions join the enunciated fact (obligation of marriage or authorization of revolution) and the enunciating act (the truth of the consistent revolutionary who obliges or authorizes himself). Apart from these assertive-performative statements, there is only the prescriptive enunciated fact which can openly express its enunciating act in the present tense. Now, in this case, the mood of the fact is not indicative, but imperative. Let us suppose that Francisco Javier ordered himself to: "be consistent!" or "be faithful from conviction!". Here again, these commands constitute, simultaneously, the enunciated facts (the commands to be consistent or faithful from conviction) and the enunciating act (the same commands).

In addition to the prescriptive and assertive-performative statements, there is the greater part of assertive enunciated facts, namely, the 'essentially representative or descriptive' ones, which we usually analyze in discourse (Recanati, 1981, pp. 180–185). Normally, as far as I can judge, those enunciated facts do not present an explicit expression of their enunciating acts. Therefore, we must discover these acts through our analysis. In order to facilitate this hard task, we must at least know the latent verbal tense of what we are looking for. We already know that this verbal tense of the enunciating act cannot be the present, since what is at stake here is *never yet* present. Accordingly, at first sight, we can gather that the tense must be the future, in the sense that the subject *will be* created by his enunciation. However, if that were the case, the subject would only be present after his enunciation, which is absurd, because the enunciator should have logically existed *already* before the end of his enunciation. Actually, the enunciating existence of the subject is proved by the enunciating act itself. So, paradoxically, the real subject should exist *before the future* and not only *after the present*. His place is an interstice between the present and the future. This narrow place can only be expressed by the *future perfect* tense, which is used to describe an event that *will have happened* in the future. This event is future in relation to the present and past in relation to the future. In this impossible temporality, the real enunciating subject is now of the future, as he does not exist yet, but later he will be of the past, because he *will have existed* already. Understandably, this subject will be unconscious, as he will never be present to consciousness, either in the present, when he is not yet present, or in the future, when he will not be present anymore, because he will have already been present.

The enunciating subject *will have existed* by his enunciation. Then, after his enunciation, he *must have existed* already, since his enunciating act will have already been completed. There is here a structural necessity, or a logical obligation, which can justify any other obligation (moral, legal, methodical, etc.,) in the signifying social structure. The laws and rules of this structure actually get their force from this logical obligation.[18] It is also this obligation that should explain all those 'linguistic forms' that 'impose a defined direction to our mind and submit it to a certain force' (Humboldt, 1821, p. 129).

Under the logical obligation of the enunciating act, Francisco Javier will have been in a condition to be a "consistent revolutionary" provided that his "conceptions of marriage and the couple" are "based on love, respect and faithfulness". As his conceptions are really based on those values, Francisco Javier *can be* a "consistent revolutionary". Furthermore, he *must have been* a "consistent revolutionary", since he "would not" have been one "if…", *which implies that he must have been one*. This implication (the sufficient condition to be a "consistent revolutionary") reveals the logical obligation of the enunciation, but it can only be detected at the end of the phrase, once we have known the values of "love, respect and faithfulness" (the necessary condition to be a "consistent revolutionary"). Therefore, the "consistent revolutionary" must have been only from this *point of view*, the *final point*, which functions retroactively as the *anchoring* and *starting point* for the existence of the "consistent revolutionary".[19]

In Lacanian Discourse Analysis, the minimal analyzable discursive unit corresponds to an enunciated fact which is settled and limited, from a *final point of view*, by the retroactive movement of the enunciating act. This unit can be defined as 'the unit of the signifying chain' (expressed in the formula S1–S2), which 'finds its achievement at the point that cuts the intention in the determining future perfect tense' (Lacan, 1968–1969, 27.11.68, p. 50). For the analyzable enunciated chain to be achieved, it has to 'meet' the 'retroactive' enunciating chain (p. 51). This is only possible in full speech, in which a specific speech does not get completely lost in general shared wisdom, but *withdraws into itself to fill itself with itself*, with its own subject, its individual truth or its enunciating act. Without this real filling, the enunciated fact would continue forever, which can be seen in all those discourses that are never-ending precisely because of their vast insatiable emptiness.

A discourse comes to an end when it is a true discourse that withdraws into itself. Now, to withdraw into itself, the true discourse must also turn against itself. To be *true*, in the Lacanian sense of the word, a discourse must be contradictory. As a flaw of wisdom that reveals the truth of discourse, the enunciated contradiction (S1–S2) implies the enunciating division of a subject whose existence depends on this division ($). Caused by the contradiction, this division causes, in turn, the existence of the real subject and the accomplishment of his enunciating act, as well as the truthfulness and finishing of his enunciated fact. In Francisco Javier's discourse, for instance, without a contradiction between the consistency and the inconsistency, there would neither be a consistency to be realized nor an enunciation to be accomplished. Without the interval between the rather bourgeois "moral conquest of our time" and the "proletarian ideology" of the "new society", there would not be enough time to cause a revolution. There would not be time for the retroactivity of the revolutionary enunciating act. There would not be the time of its future perfect tense. Devoid of this 'circular' time of the revolution, the empty enunciated fact is a simple epic 'story' (Dunker, 2008, p. 85). It is a *story* that cannot become *history*. It is a tautological account that cannot be really conjugated. Its latent present tense corresponds to the imaginary time of consciousness.

Behind this mirror of signified reality, the signifying empty fact seems to be in the infinitive.[20]

Diametrically opposed to the imaginary present tense of enunciated facts, there is the latent future perfect tense of most enunciating acts. This tense describes a future that passes while always remaining future, that is, the *timeless time of the unconscious*, of what could never be present to consciousness. It is the impossible retroactive instant embedded in full speech, in its 'authentic symbols', which are always 'regressive-progressive', as was perspicaciously observed by Ricœur (1965, p. 478).

When a Lacanian assumes that the enunciating act of a full speech will have been performed in the future perfect tense, he does not take the enunciating act as a simple act of enunciating the enunciated fact. If that were the case, the empty enunciated fact would also presuppose an enunciating act, since the fact would have been enunciated by the act. In this case, the act corresponds, in the Speech Act Theory of Austin (1955), to the 'locutionary act of saying something' (VIII, pp. 94–108), which is inseparable from all enunciated facts. Obviously, the Lacanian enunciating act is not only this locutionary act, but also an 'illocutionary' and 'perlocutionary act' (ibid.). On the one hand, the enunciating illocutionary act, which is 'performed in saying something' (ibid.), can be well illustrated by prescriptive and assertive-performative enunciated facts, such as "be consistent!" or "I authorize myself to cause a revolution", which are performed (which *command* or *authorize*) *in* being told (*in* pronouncing the command or the authorization), and which necessarily involve a full speech or an 'authentic discourse' (XI, pp. 133–147). On the other hand, there is the enunciating perlocutionary act, which can be observed in all full enunciated facts, including prescriptive and assertive-performative ones, but also descriptive ones, whose latent tense will then be the future perfect. In any case, the perlocutionary act seems to *result from* the enunciation. However, in reality, it *is* the enunciation. It is the enunciating accomplishment of the enunciation. It is the commanding effect of the command (the obedience), or the authorizing effect of the authorization (the authorized fact), but also the creating or *causing* effect of the description (the materialized thing). It is, for instance, the commanded or authorized or caused *consistent revolution*. At the origin of this revolution, the 'perlocutionary act' is 'achieved by saying something', effectively commanding or authorizing or causing the revolution, but also 'persuading, deterring, and even, say, surprising or misleading' (IX, p. 109). In these examples, the act will have deceived, prevented, surprised or persuaded a listener who may be the speaking subject himself. In so doing, the perlocutionary act *will have created* retroactively (in the future perfect tense) a persuading-persuaded or deceiving-deceived subject (e.g., the "consistent" or "inconsistent revolutionary" who will have listened to his own discourse).

Unlike the illocutionary act of describing or prescribing, the perlocutionary act of deceiving or persuading, or causing something or imposing a prescription, is not predominantly explicit.[21] But this does not diminish its performative structuring power. The implicitness of the act, on the contrary, ensures its effectiveness as an act. Therefore, what directly causes its factual implicitness should also indirectly determine its actual effectiveness. What impedes the act to be a 'told' fact should be precisely what transforms it into a telling 'act' (Butler, 1997, p. 121). What is it? It is the signifying social structure. This structure explains the structural repression as well as the structuring power of the repressed.

Repressed and empowered by the signifying structure, the locutionary enunciating act becomes the perlocutionary act of the unconscious. Unlike the enunciated fact, this act cannot be either present to the consciousness, or conjugated in a latent present tense, but can only be deployed in the retroactive time of the unconscious, and described by the future perfect tense, as that which will have been performed by the enunciating act of a real subject who will have existed by this performance. As we discussed above, this locutionary-perlocutionary act can enunciate any kind of statements, even assertive-descriptive ones. Therefore, it must not be reduced to the locutionary-illocutionary explicit enunciation of prescriptive and assertive-performative statements. This enunciation has not necessarily been repressed and thus empowered by the structure. Consequently, it can be present to consciousness and even conjugated in the present tense of the indicative or imperative mood. The same holds true in respect of the locutionary enunciations of empty descriptive statements, which are used to describe reality and are conjugated in a present tense that hides their latent infinitive.

Enunciating act	*Enunciated fact*
Locutionary (latent infinitive)	Mainly descriptive, in empty speech
Locutionary-illocutionary (present, indicative or imperative)	Prescriptive or assertive-performative, in full speech
Unconscious, locutionary-perlocutionary (latent future perfect)	Mainly assertive-descriptive, in full speech

Doubt in the cartesian cogito, the truth of the liar's paradox, and the enunciating real subject behind the enunciated symbolic subject

In full speech, the 'act of enunciating (enunciation) remains forgotten behind the enunciated' (Lacan, 1972a, pp. 449–450). The perlocutionary articulating act of language vanishes behind the articulated fact of discourse. Thus the structural "familiar obligation" disappears behind "faithfulness from conviction". The telling necessity of the counter-revolutionary signifying social structure withdraws behind the told revolutionary consistency.

The real subject hides in his enunciating act, that is, behind its enunciated fact. To reach him, we can go by the shortest route and ask ourselves what he will have become in the course of his enunciation. For a definite discourse, the answer will be found just around the corner, at that anchoring point which simultaneously represents the final point of the enunciated sequential temporality and the starting point of the enunciating retroactive movement. Nevertheless, strictly speaking, this point is an analytical heuristic abstraction. The enunciation of a real subject is concretely coextensive to his existence. This is why a Lacanian Discourse Analysis may tend towards a Biographical Analysis. After all, the analyzed discourse is always a disconnected and fragmentary passage that is abstracted from a concrete biography. Its enunciation is always a lifelong enunciation. Therefore, its starting point coincides with death, not simply the organic first death, but the symbolic 'second death' (*Apocalypse*, 2: 11; 20: 6; 20: 14; 21: 8), the final full stop of the enunciated life, the silence of the exhausted enunciation, the fall into definitive symbolic oblivion, the symbolic death of the real subject, his disappearance in the enunciating 'chain of what he is' (Lacan, 1959–1960, 22.06.60, p. 341). The problem is that this 'limit of the second death' is 'indefinitely' delayed (ibid.). The point of intersection between the enunciating and enunciated parallels takes place in the vanishing point of a symbolic infinite. This infinite can be illustrated by the immortality of the classical authors, whose full speech is always *telling*, because it is a full speech that is still full of its telling subject. So, we have not yet reached the starting point of its telling act. And before this point, nothing is yet definitive.

Every year, 'Socrates, Descartes and Marx' tell us their 'truth', which is 'always new' (Lacan, 1946, p. 192). Each time, this *new truth* changes our interpretation of their wisdom. It objectively changes everything in their discourses. For this reason, the analysis of these discourses must be started again every year. That applies to all full discursive material that we encounter in discourse analysis. An analysis of a full speech is always provisional, since its enunciating subject is still alive, and still enunciating and changing himself retroactively by virtue of his enunciation. This must be formally acknowledged in the perspective of Lacanian Discourse Analysis. In this perspective, the results of our analyses are always provisional conclusions.[22] They are refutable, or *falsifiable*. Therefore, they are also informative, and *scientific*, in the Popperian sense of the term.

Discourse analysis is always provisional because the analyzed 'enunciated' discourse is 'inseparable' from an 'enunciating position' that is always here with us, in the signifying social structure, changing constantly with this structure (Lacan, 1966b, p. 205). This is also why an enunciating subject, such as Francisco Javier, is still *alive*, and quite lively, as he cannot stay in one place, but must be in perpetual motion, always on the move, at least as long as we analyze his discourse. In this discourse, the subject is always a living subject of the signifying social structure. So, he is changing incessantly according to the changes in the structure, which entail *his changes of position*, and not only *changes of his position*.

Unlike a fixed occurrence of the enunciated "revolutionary", the enunciating revolutionary is always moving *in* the structure and not only *with* the structure. Similarly, *I* am a living subject who will have been moving through this book, even after my organic death, and who is not boringly fixed to the non-living 'I' that I wrote, a moment ago, in the phrase 'I am a living subject'. Thus we can again distinguish the written or enunciated 'I of the statement' and the writing or enunciating 'I of the enunciation' (Lacan, 1964, 22.04.64, p. 156). The former is a signifier that may become the symbolic inanimate subject of an abstract discursive psychology, while the latter is a real animate subject whose psychology must be radically concrete.

In two archetypal discursive situations, we can easily make the distinction between the moving *I* of the enunciating act and the inert *I* of the enunciated fact:

- In the paradoxical statement '*I am lying*', it goes without saying that 'the *I* of the enunciation is not the same as the *I* of the statement, that is to say, the shifter which, in the statement, designates him' (Lacan, 1964, 22.04.64, p. 156). This enunciated *I* is 'lying', while the enunciating *I* is 'deceiving' (ibid.). Therefore they must not be confused. When I say 'I am lying', I can only deceive as long as I am 'not lying' (ibid.). I can only deceive by 'telling the truth', by admitting that the enunciated 'I' is lying and by distinguishing myself from this lying 'I' of my statement 'I am lying' (ibid.). But this implies that I am lying when I say that I am lying. However, if I am lying, then I am telling the truth. Likewise, in general, *I* enunciate 'the truth by means of an enunciated lie' (Lacan, 1972b, p. 499). So, despite this lie, the enunciating I 'is not a liar' (ibid.). He is not lying precisely because the enunciated I 'is lying' (Lacan, 1964, 22.04.64, p. 156).
- In the Cartesian statement '*I think, therefore I am*', we can make with Lacan, and despite Descartes, a distinction between two different subjects. On the one hand, there is the explicitly enunciated *I* of 'the statement', the symbolic 'subject of the *I think*' (Lacan, 1964, 05.02.64, p. 53), which underpins the *ego*, the 'image' that *I* 'draw' by thinking (Wittgenstein, 1969, IX, §113, p. 215), or the imaginary representation of the 'extensive thing' or the 'assembling of members that we call the human body' (Descartes, 1640, II, pp. 83–85). On the other hand, there is the implicit *I* of 'the enunciation', the real 'subject of the *I doubt*' (Lacan, 1964, 05.02.64, p. 53), the 'thing that doubts' (Descartes, 1640, II, p. 85), or the doubtful enunciating subject ($) who 'splits' (Lacan, 1965a, p. 199) between

his identification with the enunciated *I* who thinks (S1) and his alienation in what he is or thinks (S2), or, to be more specific, in what language is and thinks at the place of the doubting subject.[23] As the workforce of language, this real doubting subject is a proletarianized philosopher named Descartes who does the work of the unconscious (the work of enunciating, speaking, thinking, meditating on metaphysics, writing the meditations). Apparently this subject thinks that *he thinks* and therefore he concludes that *he is*. These thoughts are accurate, granted, but they are not, strictly speaking, the thoughts of the subject. They are, rather, the thoughts of *the Other*, of a language, or a signifying social structure that thinks at the place of the individual subject, who functions here just as the enunciating workforce of language, or the operator of the linguistic machine. When Descartes thinks that *he is*, it is rather a language (as a thinking system or a symbolic system of thought) that *is* in his mind and thinks that *he is*. It is also this language that tricks the philosopher into knowing for certain that he thinks and is. This 'certainty' would thus be 'acquired on the basis of a trickery' (Cottet, 1987, p. 20). The Cogito would be the ruse of the pervading *genius of language* that *informs* the philosopher, and imposes a being on him by *misinforming* him (hence the pertinence of the Augustinian *si enim fallor, sum*; if I am misinformed, I am). On that assumption, the genius of language is the 'cunning genius' that manages to 'deceive' Descartes (1640, I, p. 75), in the end, by *being* and *thinking* instead of him. More precisely, while the *cunning genius of language* is deceiving the philosopher, there is one signifier that *is* instead of him (S1: enunciated *I*) and other signifiers that *think* instead of him (S2: enunciated statement). As for him, he is *split* ($: enunciating *I*) between these signifiers that compose the unconscious (S1–S2). So, in Lacan (1965a), the Cartesian Cogito 'does not underpin consciousness', but this 'splitting' in which lies 'the unconscious' (p. 199).

Enunciated *I*	Enunciating *I*
"*I* am lying" (lie)	*I* am deceiving by telling the truth (≠ lie)
"*I* think, therefore *I* am" (certainty)	*I* doubt (≠ certainty)

The Cartesian Cogito and the Liar's Paradox operate implicitly in every statement, so far as every statement implements a language that *is and thinks*, that *lies and admits its lie*. Francisco Javier, for instance, gives us an inkling of the Cogito that we can formulate in the words: "I enunciate a consistent revolutionary discourse, therefore I am a consistent revolutionary". As for the Liar's Paradox, we catch a glimpse of it in the implicit confession: "I am a consistent revolutionary who preaches marriage". In both cases, we can clearly see the difference between the symbolic enunciated subject (the "I" of the statement "I am a consistent revolutionary") and the real enunciating subject (the one who enunciates that he is a "consistent revolutionary"). Now, in reality, the former is *nothing*, or *nothing but a signifier* that lies by claiming to be *someone* as a "consistent revolutionary", while the latter involves the truth of the real Eperrist, or the *impossibility* for him to be a real consistent revolutionary through the deceitful wisdom of a language that simply uses him, and exploits his enunciating workforce, by making him believe that he is a real consistent revolutionary when he preaches "marriage" for the "new society". Here we can appreciate the relation between the enunciated 'nothing' and the 'real' as the 'impossibility' that is 'at the origin of every enunciation' (Lacan, 1961–1962, 07.03.62). This relation underlies the Cartesian Cogito as well as the Liar's Paradox. In both discursive situations, the enunciated subject is really *nothing*. When the liar enunciates his lie ("I am lying"), he is lying because he is not lying, so his lie comes to nothing, and so his *lying being* also comes to nothing. Similarly, when Descartes enunciates his certainty ("I am"), he is certain because he is doubting, so his certainty comes to nothing, and therefore his *certain being* comes to nothing also. All of this leads us to the real impossibility of enunciation, that is to say, the impossibility for the liar *to be* or *to be the one who lies*, which is also the impossibility for Descartes *to be* or *to be the one who is certain of being*.

By doubting, Descartes cannot be someone who is simply certain of being. In the same way, by admitting that he lies, the liar cannot be someone who is simply a liar. Both Descartes and the liar must be someone else, a doubting and sincere *Other*, a language, or a pure symbolic system that deceives them by making them believe that they really are a sincere liar and a doubting philosopher. At the same time, by demonstrating their impossibility to be only *the one who lies* or *the one who is certain of being*, this *Other* reveals the incarnate *truth* or *doubt* of a divided real subject who does not persist in a lie or in a forced certainty. Likewise, by demonstrating the impossibility for Francisco Javier to be a "consistent revolutionary", his discourse reveals the revolutionary consistency of someone who does not artificially persevere to the last with a forced consistency that would thus result in a fossilized revolution, such as that of the most rigid and dogmatic revolutionaries, whose consistent revolution is quite the opposite of a consistent revolution.[24]

In Lacanian Discourse Analysis, the transcendent truth of the enunciating subject can be revealed, in the analyzed enunciated discourse, through the logical demonstration of the impossible existence of this real subject at the immanent level of symbolic wisdom. This impossibility lies in the division of the enunciating subject ($) between two mutually exclusive possibilities (S1–S2), namely, the enunciated subject (S1) and its predicate (S2), the *One* and the *Other*, a signifier and a language, the liar and his sincerity, the certain Cogito and the Cartesian doubt, the "consistent revolutionary" and his "conceptions of marriage and the couple", the "new man" and "our time". On the surface of the enunciated discourse, this division will appear to us as a gaping impossibility, or a real gap in the symbolic possibilities. This opening proves to be constitutive of the enunciating subject, who can even be described as a pure division, or fracture in discourse.[25] The real subject *opens himself up* on the symbolic surface of discourse. His truth consists of a fissure in the consistency of wisdom. It consists of the *consistent inconsistency* of Francisco Javier in the *inconsistent consistency* of his revolution. In this instance, the truth *is* the gap between the "revolutionary" and his "conceptions". *In general, between what I am and what I think, there is a doubt that represents the truth of the Cartesian Cogito. It is the same truth that appears, in the Liar's Paradox, between the liar and his lie. Here, between the enunciated symbolic subject and its predicate, the interstice gives substance to an enunciating real subject who reveals the truthfulness of speech in the structural emptiness of language.* In this deceiving consistency of wisdom, Lacanian Discourse Analysis must look for the only truth and true consistency of the analyzed discourse.

Notes

1. Here is the outline of the problem that will be treated in this chapter. Posing this problem in all its complexity, Frosh, Phoenix and Pattman (2003) note that the 'investment' of 'people' in 'subject positions is not necessarily captured by the articulation of the discourses themselves; rather, it may hinge on unspoken and at times unspeakable events, experiences and processes, all of them cultural, but also deeply embedded in subjectivity' (p. 42). As will be seen, Lacanian Discourse Analysis must replace these events in the spoken and speakable sphere of the enunciation. In this sphere, we *are* these events which *speak themselves* when we speak. That does not mean that they can be told or enunciated. Even if we *speak them*, we cannot *speak about them*. The fact remains that they are speaking and spoken through enunciation. If they are embedded in subjectivity, this subjectivity is embedded in enunciation. In fact, subjectivity arises retroactively from enunciation. Therefore, we must assume, together with Pêcheux (1975a, 1975b), an idea of enunciation in which the subject 'is not at the origin of the enunciated sense' (Pêcheux, 1975a, pp. 3–4), but it is its 'retroactive effect' (1975b, p. 139).
2. In the semiotic perspective that Camus (1999) wants to 'introduce into social psychology' (p. 277), there is a 'retroactive construction of signification' which 'concerns' the enunciation or the 'act value of the enunciated' (p. 282). In our Lacanian perspective, all this can be accepted, provided that the *construction of signification* is not confused with the *signification* itself, but rather conceived as an unconscious signifierization, which would retroactively determine the conscious signification. Alas, this conception is hardly reconcilable with a semiotic perspective.
3. Here is the Lacanian version of the four elements originally distinguished by Jakobson (1957): the 'related event' or 'process of the enunciated', the 'discursive action' or 'process of the enunciation', the 'protagonist of the enunciated process', and the 'protagonist of the process of the enunciation' (p. 181).
4. Together with the Althusserian-Lacanian Analysis of Pêcheux and Fuchs (1975), our Lacanian Discourse Analysis regards 'enunciation' as a 'subjection' and a 'constitution of the subject' (p. 15). We can also assume the Althusserian explanation of this constitution as a 'retroactive effect' of the '*interpellation*' (Pêcheux, 1975b, pp. 138–139), that is, the movement that 'calls out the individual to become a subject of discourse' through his 'identification' with this subject (p. 240).

5. Even if Pêcheux and Fuchs (1975) disregard this unparalleled character of each individual overdetermination, they do not fail to observe that 'processes of enunciation consist of a set of determinations' which 'allow what is told and reject what is not told' (p. 20).
6. Pêcheux (1975b) already regards enunciation, in his Althusserian-Lacanian perspective, as the 'interpellation' of the subject who is 'called to existence' (p. 138). Similarly, in our Lacanian perspective, the enunciation is considered the gesture of the signifying social structure which calls for a subject to exist in order to do its work, that is, the work of the unconscious. In this way, together with Pêcheux, we analyze the enunciation as a subjective 'effect' of the 'structural determination' and 'positioning of the subject' in the structure (p. 157).
7. In the terms of Billig (1987), the enunciating act needs the 'particularization' with its 'capacity for transcendence', for 'rule-creation, rule-breaking and rule-bending', while the enunciated fact implies 'categorization' and 'rule-following' (p. 130). Explaining the 'natural propensity for prejudice' (p. 132) in Allport, this categorization can be explained, in turn, by the natural propensity of the symbolic system to reproduce itself through the enunciated facts. Obviously, this propensity is challenged by the 'natural tendency to form particularizations and to make special cases' (ibid.). However, for the particularizations to be produced, the categorizations must be reproduced. Francisco Javier, for example, must be a "revolutionary" among other "revolutionaries" (as an enunciated subject) in order to be unique among them (as an enunciating subject).
8. Accordingly, the Lacanian Discourse Analysis of this true real should not be confused with the cognitive content analysis of the imaginary reality. Our analysis, together with the precursory analysis proposed by d'Unrug (1974), assumes that 'formal indicators' of the enunciated fact 'refer to analyzable processes', at the level of the enunciating act, and not to 'contents which are attributed rather than observed' (p. 231).
9. This analysis of the enunciation corresponds, in Frosh, Phoenix and Pattman (2003), to the 'move required if one wants to understand the specificity of each subject's personal investment in discursive positions, a move which goes *beyond* or *beneath* discourse to explore the needs which are being met, the *enjoyment* created, by the positions which are taken up' (p. 52). In the Kleinian theory of the 'defended subject' proposed by Hollway and Jefferson (2000), this move leads us always to a 'need to defend oneself against feelings of anxiety', as 'crucial motivation for investment in particular

discourses' (p. 59). The discourse about the "monogamous family" would then be explained, for instance, by Francisco Javier's anxiety when facing our question about "familiar obligations". This seems to be plausible, especially when we consider the tension between "obligation" and "conviction", as well as the reference to the "dissolution of the couple".

10. So 'a psychoanalytic frame of analysis can provide plausible reasons for the adoption of specific identity positions' (Frosh, Phoenix & Pattman, 2003, p. 42). From this point of view, 'there may be important reasons why each one of us ends up where we are, and these reasons are the legitimate target of psychological inquiry' (p. 52). These reasons are also the legitimate target of Lacanian Discourse Analysis, as long as they are connected, through enunciation, to the enunciating structure.
11. Such factors may explain 'why speakers *choose* to inhabit particular subject positions over others (motivation, personal investment) and why certain *choices* persist over time and place (continuity, repetition)' (Gough, 2004, p. 247). In discursive psychology, those questions are 'sidestepped in favor of concentrating on participants' practices' (ibid.). In this way, discursive psychology disregards the *why* in order to concentrate on the *how*. Similar to Gough, I think 'discourse analysts within social psychology need to do more to examine subjectivity' and subjective factors which explain 'why individuals take on certain positions and reject others' (p. 265). Now, avoiding a relapse into the purely imaginary 'subjectivism' of the psychological mirror, we must situate those subjective factors in the enunciating structure (Pêcheux, 1975b, pp. 161–162). After all, these factors are not immanently 'subjective' in the sense that they would 'affect' an already constituted 'subject', but they are transcendental factors 'in which the subject is constituted' by the enunciating act of the structure (pp. 136–137).
12. Here is my Lacanian structuralist reinterpretation of the 'action orientation' that Potter (2003) gives to 'discursive psychology' and to 'discourse analysis' in general. In Lacanian Discourse Analysis, this *action orientation* must not orient us only to the activity inherent in discourse, but also to the structural impulse that determines this activity. Unlike other kinds of discourse analysis, ours must scrutinize the *why* and not only the *how* of the action. Together with the Lacanian-Althusserian Discourse Analysis of Pêcheux (1975b), ours must go beyond any 'utilitarian and pragmatist theory' in which 'language is first used by me to act on others' (p. 233). Language acts on others, granted, but that does not mean that I use it for that

reason. In any case, in spite of myself, language acts on me as much as on the others.

13. Notwithstanding this inclusion of grammar, the two parallel and opposed Lacanian chains of the enunciation and the enunciated must not be confused with the perpendicular and correlative structures that Chomsky called 'surface structures' and 'deep structures' or 'initial phrase markers' (1975, pp. 81–82). In the Lacanian perspective, there is no 'transformational component' which 'converts' the enunciation, 'step by step', into the enunciated 'sentence' (ibid.). Unlike the Chomskyan 'initial phrase markers' that 'initiate' this conversion, the Lacanian enunciation is just *the action of* the 'deep structures' that initiate *sentences* and 'determine semantic interpretation' (ibid.). Confused in the first *standard theory* of Chomsky, these two factors, *transformational* and *semantic*, correspond respectively to the explicit Chomskyan transformational grammar and to the implicit Lacanian structural semantic theory on enunciation. This theory can be compared, in the Althusserian-Lacanian Discourse Analysis of Pêcheux and Fuchs (1975), to the 'formal semantic' theory that 'reaches inside language the point of construction of the subject-effect' (p. 18). Now, unlike this theory, ours cannot reduce this 'subject-effect' to the 'subjective illusion of speech' (p. 79). Behind this imaginary effect, we must look for the real retroactive effect in the fullness and truthfulness of speech.
14. As Parker (2005a) notes, 'it is this that makes Lacanian Discourse Analysis radically different from forms of *conversation analysis* that aim to carefully redescribe only what is present' (p. 171).
15. Repression is thus accurately located by Billig (1998) in the enunciating 'activity of speaking' (p. 42). In his opinion, however, repression would depend on 'cultural, moral precepts' (p. 16), which would originate in a 'language' that 'provides the crucial rhetorical devices for the operation of repression' (p. 12). Then, in Billig (2006), language 'provides the means' which make it possible to achieve 'repression' (p. 22). Instead, in Lacan, language entails, intrinsically and immediately, not only the virtual 'necessity for repression' (ibid.), but also the actual reality of a repression that cannot be differentiated from language. The enunciated fact of language implies the repressive enunciating act. The signifying structure presupposes the real emptiness of the structure. This structure of the symbolic needs to hollow out the real. The symbolic representative called the "consistent revolutionary" implies the real absence of Francisco Javier. Speech sounds only in an empty space. Words take place only in the silence of repression. Now, by taking place

in this silence, words take the shape of it. So they acquire the form of repression. They provide the devices for repression, as Billig observes, because they have in themselves the conformation of those devices. Words have the structure of the silent empty spaces that resound with them. They thus have the real signifying structure inherent in the silence of the unconscious. This silence structures all rhetorical figures of speech, all discourse, all dialogue. Hence the importance of silence in a 'Lacanian Discourse Analysis' in which 'the unconscious is what functions as absences in the text' (Parker, 2005a, p. 171).

16. In contrast to the 'process' of the 'enunciation', the enunciated fact appears as a 'finished product' that can be 'immobilized' and 'divided into segments' by discourse analysis (D'Unrug, 1974, p. 67). In this way, the analyzed discourse, just as any other enunciated wisdom, can be used as well as misused. This depends on our intentions. Unlike the hints of truth, the fragments of wisdom can easily be manipulated.
17. With its available resources, current social psychology is incapable of grasping this logic of enunciation. Ian Parker (2003) sees here the main reason for the 'misunderstanding' that underpins the 'apparent connection' between 'Lacanian views of discourse' and 'dominant tendencies in recent discursive psychology' (p. 107). Actually, with its 'commonsensical notions of cause and effect reconfigured through *stake* and *function*' (ibid.), discursive psychology could never go beyond the enunciated level of the signifying chain and its *epic* succession of present causes and present effects. Limited to this psychological temporality, discursive psychology is just a sign of 'an era in which everything has become *Epos*' (Dunker, 2008, p. 85).
18. Pêcheux (1975b), for instance, refers to the 'future perfect of the law that states: *the one who will have caused damage...*', which 'generates the subject of law' (p. 143). This subject is 'duplicated', as the author remarks, by the one who is 'called-constituted' by 'statements of fact such as *a French soldier doesn't move back*, which actually means *if you are a true French soldier, what you are cannot move back*' (ibid.). Likewise, in the statement "a revolutionary communicates the values of love, respect and faithfulness", we can interpret: "if you are a consistent revolutionary, you must communicate the values of love, respect and faithfulness".
19. This is why Lacanian Discourse Analysis 'will search out' those 'anchoring points that serve as the *conclusion* of sentences or other stretches of text, anchoring points that only then, at the concluding

moment, posit their own original starting point' (Parker, 2005a, p. 170). At this starting point, there is a sudden structural integration of the sufficient and necessary conditions of the enunciating act. Such an integration is the truth of any kind of discursive totalization of knowledge. It is also the truth of a cognitive 'semantic integration' that accomplishes and closes the fullness of an imaginary signified reality (cf. Kintsch & Van Dijk, 1978).

20. Although the infinitive 'indicates its relation to the *sense* or the *event* in its internal time' (Deleuze, 1969, p. 215), this internal time is generalized and separated from the subject of a particular event. For instance, instead of statements such as "I order you to cut off his head", or "I am innocent of the blood of this just person" (Matthew, 27: 24), an infinitive can only express "to order someone to cut off a head", or "to be innocent of the blood of a just person". This general time is not the individual time of a precise enunciation and it does not involve, whether in English, in Spanish or in French (contrary to Portuguese), any relation to the enunciating subject. This is why history does not need perforce a particular revolutionary, such as Robespierre, *to cause a revolution* or *to order someone to cut off a head*. As demonstrated by Marx, the revolutionary fact, in the infinitive, can be empty of particular revolutionary actors. It is the 'scripture' that must be 'fulfilled' (John, 19: 28). This does not mean, however, that particular actors are innocent of the blood of just persons.

21. Potter and Wetherell (1987) already observed that 'in ordinary talk participants often do not make the act their speech is performing explicit' (p. 29). When 'people are persuading, accusing, requesting, etc., they do not always do so explicitly' (p. 32). As will be seen, a Lacanian would only rectify here that it is the *Other* (the language or the signifying structure), instead of *people*, which persuades, accuses, requests, etc., not always explicitly. Hence the existence of the unconscious, as discourse of this Other.

22. In this regard, Parker (2005a) judiciously notes that 'the reading of a text will always be provisional, for the meaning is determined not only by the last signifiers to appear but also by signifiers that may appear even later (to reconfigure what will come to serve as the key points that serve as anchors of representation)' (p. 170).

23. By pointing out this movement in which 'Lacan displaces the Cartesian cogito', Parker (2003) emphasizes that this 'challenges the presumption of cognitive psychology that an understanding of the nature of human thinking is also an insight into what is a human being' (p. 100). From a Lacanian point of view, in fact, *human thinking* is merely what *language is and thinks* at the symbolic signifying place

of the real subject. As for the understanding of this discourse of the Other, it amounts to an insight into the image drawn by thinking, that is, the imaginary signified being of the *ego*.

24. We must remember here that the term 'revolution' was originally used to describe the orbital movement of planets, in 'celestial mechanics', in which the *consistent revolution* can only persist until the 'return to the departure point' (Lacan, 1969–1970, 21.01.70, p. 62). Similarly, human revolutions can only persist until their reactionary stabilization. On that, Miller (2003) observes, from a Lacanian viewpoint, that 'the more it changes, the more it is the same thing' (p. 118).
25. We can wonder here, with Žižek (1999b), if this 'gap/opening/void' can 'still be called *subject*'. Just like Žižek, we can answer with 'an emphatic yes', since 'the subject is at once the ontological gap' and 'the gesture of subjectivization that closes, or heals up the wound of that gap (in Lacanese: the gesture of the Master which establishes a new harmony)' (ibid.). In other words, the subject is at once the enunciating real subject ($) and the enunciated symbolic subject (S1) in an 'irreducible circularity' in which 'the power' of the enunciated subject 'does not fight an external, resisting force', but 'an obstacle that is absolutely inherent', which 'ultimately *is*' the enunciating 'subject itself' (ibid.). The "consistent revolutionary" (S1) of the Popular Revolution Army (EPR), for example, does not only fight the "consistent reactionary" of the rightist National Action Party (PAN) or the "inconsistent revolutionary" of the Institutional Revolutionary Party (PRI), but also his own subjective enunciating division ($) between the revolution (S1) and the reaction (S2), the consistency (S1) and the inconsistency (S2), etc. Behind the hood of the "consistent revolutionary" (S1), such division *is* the enunciating subject himself.

CHAPTER FIVE

The subject as a signifier to another signifier

Having contextualized the real subject of the enunciation, I undertake, in this chapter, to locate the symbolic subject of the statement in the context of this statement. In this context of discourse, I show how the symbolic subject, that with which the real subject is symbolically identified, intervenes as a signifier for another signifier. I then make a distinction between this *subject of the signifier* and the *subject of knowledge,* the psychological subject that is repudiated by Lacan and still accepted in social psychology. Taking Lacan's side, I appeal to Kleist, Humboldt, Sapir, and also Stalin and Wittgenstein, through an innovative interpretation of their ideas, to justify my choice of the subject of the signifier to be the subject prioritized by discourse analysis. Finally, I review relevant contributions by Kant, Benveniste, Bakhtin and Derrida in order to specify the transcendental situation of such a subject, before the elaboration of any kind of particular social or historical knowledge, in both the spatial environment of language and the temporal dimension of the signifying chain.

The individual support of the social structure

In relation to full speech, the real subject does not appear only as an effect, but also as a cause. As such, he is a speaking 'thing' that supports 'speech' (Lacan, 1956c, pp. 406–408). This thing is the *letter*, a *literal body*, an *extensive thing* that materializes that which is enunciated, the signifiers, or the 'thoughts' of Descartes (1640, II, pp. 83–87).

Unlike the Cartesian 'thinking thing', the Lacanian speaking thing *is* an 'extensive thing', that is to say, a 'body' which can be 'perceived by touching, seeing, hearing, tasting, smelling' (Descartes, 1640, II, pp. 81–85). To incarnate speech, the speaking thing must be this perceptible body. It must be material in order to materialize a discourse whose letters have to be visible or audible, but also touchable and capable of being tasted or smelled. As a matter of course, the Lacanian Analysis of this discourse must be a materialist analytical approach to a perceptible discursive materiality. Its psychology must be a 'concrete psychology' such as the one that Politzer (1947) 'binds to a materialist tradition' (II, III, p. 100). This is the only psychology that can properly use a Lacanian Discourse Analysis. Its materialist stance is diametrically opposed to the idealist standpoint of neo-Cartesian or pseudo-Cartesian cognitive psychologies. The thing of concrete psychology must not be a *non-extensive thinking thing*, but an *extensive speaking thing* (which does not only mean the neuronal stuff of the brain, of course).

To embody 'thought', the speaking thing has to be a 'body' that is 'carved' by the 'structure' (Lacan, 1973a, p. 512). It has to be corporeal to materialize the signifiers corporeally, bodily, not only through hysterical or psychosomatic symptoms, but also by means of each gesture, each movement, each articulated voice, or piece of writing. All these *words* incarnate thoughts through a perceptible and unintelligible body.[1] Crossed by the words, this unconscious body expresses discourse. It is also violently or sensuously expressed in discourse, especially by the discursive effect of the 'drive' (*pulsion*), as the 'conjunction between logic and body', the symbolic and the real, the speech and the speaking thing (Lacan, 1968–1969, 12.03.69, p. 229).

As a speaking thing, the enunciating subject is 'the support of the signifier' (Lacan, 1960–1961, 01.03.61, p. 201). He is the incarnate word, the real of the symbolic, the substratum of discourse, or the fertile soil of the cultural environment. As a 'human being', he can be called the 'humus of language' (1969–1970, 14.01.70, p. 57).

Like humus, he nourishes the same organism that nourishes him. He gives his substance to the signifier that signifierizes him.

The individual real subject is not only signifierized and overdetermined by the signifying social structure, but he must be also a corporeal support that bears the weight of this structure, constitutes its material substratum, nourishes its symbolic system and functions muscularly as its enunciating workforce. In Marxian terms, the 'individual' must be the 'support' of the same 'relations that create him socially' (Marx, 1867, p. 37). The real enunciating subject must support the same symbolic system that generates him. It is a necessity, but also an impossibility. This is why, one day, Lacan (1968–1969) decided to regard the real subject, 'in relation to the signifier', not as an impossible 'support', but as the 'anticipation', which is only 'supposed' or 'induced' (11.12.68, p. 90).

The supporting subject turns out to be impossible as he should exist already, before his existence, in order to support the signifier that induces him to exist. The impossibility of the real subject thus lies in the necessity of his existence before the beginning of his existence. The subject should be before himself. He should be in order to be.[2] Francisco Javier, for example, should already be a particular consistent revolutionary in order to enunciate the discourse that will have created him as this particular consistent revolutionary. Likewise, as involuntarily argued by religious people, *man* should exist already in order to create man 'in his image' (*Genesis*, 1: 26). But human nature cannot be something real before it becomes what it is in the cultural environment of the symbolic system. So the real subject, with his human nature, is impossible precisely because he is real. His impossibility thus lies in his consequential real nature, which should be previous to its cultural cause.[3]

The culture of human nature needs at the beginning what can only come at the end, namely, human nature as the humus or the cultural medium in which human nature can be cultivated. All the same, this nature can be cultivated, perhaps because it cultivates itself. To be sure, the analogy between *humus* and *human* does not imply that the human subject, as the material support of the signifier, occupies a passive position. By supporting the signifier, the real human subject is actively enunciating that which is supported by him. The subject is the producer of that which produces him. As the humus of language, he is a 'living being' that lives on its own signifying decomposition, and that becomes, through this decomposition, the 'agent' and not only the 'support of the signifier' (Lacan, 1960–1961, 12.04.61, p. 273).

As the agent and support of the signifier, the subject produces himself through the signifying social structure that overdetermines and signifierizes his being.[4] This being is not just a spoken being, but also a 'speaking being' who takes over the 'incidence of the signifier' and thus integrates by himself 'into the apparatus' of language (Lacan, 1969–1970, 14.01.70, p. 57). In this way, through an enunciating act, the subject actively assumes his own signifierization by the structure. As the real of the symbolic, the enunciating subject supports what determines him. He takes charge of his own structural overdetermination. So he should also take responsibility for what he will have become retroactively by virtue of his enunciation.

Unlike the enunciated subject, the enunciating subject is responsible for what he is. He cannot disclaim his responsibility. Although the structure determines him, he cannot share his responsibility with the structure, which is not somebody who can be responsible for something, but something which is responsibly enunciated by a responsible subject. By enunciating, this subject should assume honestly and courageously all the colossal responsibility of the structure. He should not avoid his family commitments, social debts, cultural faults, historical obligations, etc. In his discourse, for instance, perhaps he will have been guilty for the fact of being "white", "Christian", "European", or an "heir of an exploiter". Lacanian Discourse Analysis cannot and must not release the enunciating subject from all this guilt.

The living matter of the signifying structure

The subject is retroactively responsible for that which follows from the transmutation of his formless *living* or *grey matter* into his characteristic individual form, a subjective form, as a manufactured product of his full speech. Now, if the subject is responsible, his responsibility is inherent in his subjective form. One is not responsible as the raw material of the structure. One is only responsible as a subject, or element, or part of the structure. The responsibility goes along with the structural position. As a structural position, the subject *is* the structure, and his responsibility is, in a sense, the responsibility of the structure. Through the *structured subject*, the structure is no longer an irresponsible *something*, but turns into *someone* who may assume a responsibility.

By enunciating a full speech, my living matter is automatically signifierized, or seized by the signifying social structure, and thus becomes a structural position, a human living part of the structure, a subject of rules and laws, of obligations and responsibilities. The subject arises here from the structural mould, which gives a signifying form to his living matter. As we know, this mould is the only real matrix of the human subject. It is the only real foundation of everything that concerns him. In view of this, Lacan (1959) defines the structure as 'the network of the signifier in which the subject must already be caught up in order to be able to constitute himself there as self, as part of a lineage, as existing, as the representative of a sex, and even as dead' (p. 182).

Before being anything that he can be, the individual subject has to be a subject, who can only be so by being subjected to the signifying social structure. Now, as discussed above, this structure initially needs to be supported by the subject, who should then exist impossibly sooner than he is subjected. The impossibility of this existence of the telling real subject does not change the fact that he shall necessarily exist and cannot be symbolically told. His real enunciation is a necessary condition of the structure, but his impossibility prevents the structure from enunciating him.

Because of being impossible, the real enunciating subject can only be expressed by the telling absences in what is told. In the symbolic facade of the signifying chain, the openings are clues to the real subject and the real structure. They are silences *articulated* by this structure of the unconscious. By analyzing those silences, Lacanian Discourse Analysis may approach the unconscious of the subject.[5] More precisely, the silences allow us to move towards the truth of the subject as enunciating workforce in the analyzed discourse, that is to say, his enunciating act as a gesture articulated by the structure in the work of the unconscious. On the enunciated surface, this gesture must be approached through the gaps, holes or fractures, precisely because of its impossibility and resulting incommunicability. Because of this, the enunciating 'speech act' does not function as 'communication', but rather as a 'foundation' of the subject in his 'annunciation' through the irregularities of his enunciated fact (Lacan, 1953b, p. 136).

The real subject is founded on his enunciating act. By definition, as an enunciating subject, he is *always enunciating*. Now, to be *always still enunciating*, he cannot be *never yet enunciated*, or communicated. This is why he lies in the silences of discourse. This is also why the enunciated symbolic surface shall twist, become corrupted, deteriorate, tear and even dissolve to make way for its enunciating real subject (e.g., James Joyce). We can then understand that 'Lacan's science of the real draws its *subject* in the lines, points, intersections and overlaps that appear in language as mysteries, confusions, mistakes, miscommunications' (Ragland-Sullivan, 1992, p. 62).

With the aim of locating the real subject, Lacanian Discourse Analysis takes into consideration the lacks, flaws, slips, abnormalities, aberrations and contradictions on the symbolic surface of the analyzed discourse.[6] In order to be on the right track of the enunciating subject named Francisco Javier, for example, we must take notice of details such as the correlated incongruity and strangeness of the two elements "monogamous family" and "individual sexual love as the foundation of the monogamous family". We must also pay attention to the apparent unsuitability of the answer to our question, the lack of reference to "familiar obligations", or the connected mention of "faithfulness from conviction". In that case, the tension between "obligation" and "conviction" may be revealing the logical junction between the symbolic necessity and the real impossibility of the enunciating subject, or, to be more precise, between his irresponsible position (overdetermined by the structure) and his enunciating responsibility (as the real support of the structure). In Lacanian psychoanalytical theory, this junction also demonstrates the point of sameness of law ("obligation") and desire ("conviction"), discursive rules and sexual drives, signifying structure and literal or corporeal support.

Desire and law, body and structure

'Seized by the words of his mouth' (Proverbs, 6: 3), Francisco Javier will not have been a "consistent revolutionary" if he does not *want to* be faithful in "marriage and the couple". Therefore, to be a "consistent revolutionary", he will have been paradoxically *obliged* ("familiar obligation") to be really *convinced* of being faithful (personal "faithfulness from conviction"). In this way, 'seized by his own lips' which are already 'seized by the words of his mouth' (Proverbs, 6: 2–3), Francisco Javier will have been *corporally convinced of his structural symbolic obligations.*

Seized by a body which is already seized by the signifying social structure, the real subject will have desired what he will have been compelled to desire according to the laws of the structure. The enunciating responsible subject is thus indistinguishable from the overdetermined irresponsible subject. Whether free or forced, he is the same real subject. He is the same whether he is supporting the external structure, or being internally determined by this structure. For Lacan, the external power of this signifying social structure is the inmost motivation of the individual enunciating subject. Behind the mirror of the mental imaginary interiority (*intus*), the signifying exteriority of the perceptible unconscious (*foris*) thus paradoxically forms the real trans-individual motivational interiority of the subject (the Augustinian *intimum cordis*). The external signifying structure (the structure of relations between the positions of persons and things) is not in due course internalized, but from the beginning constitutes the only real interiority of the subject.[7] Leaving aside a mental interiority that is just imaginary, the subject is internally nothing more than his externally signifying and supporting structural position. This position functions internally as the whole signifying social structure particularized for only one individual subject. As we shall see in the next chapter, this structural particularization articulates the unique unconscious matrix that constitutes each subject and his consciousness.

The subject is constituted in a 'material' and 'social structure' that cannot be reduced to 'consciousness' (cf. Althusser, 1976, p. 246). Through the 'work of the unconscious', this 'structure' formulates that which characterizes each individual subject, namely, the 'encoding' of *a* 'language' (Lacan, 1973b, p. 558). As the unconscious of a particular subject, this encoding creates a particular subjective structured form. In this way, it confirms the structuring power of the real signifying structure. From this 'real-of-the-structure', the 'subject of the unconscious' appears as an effect that 'clutches at the body' (1973a, pp. 536–537). As an effect of the embodied 'structure', the subject is a real thing that arises from 'the real that comes to light in language' (1972a, p. 476). Now, in this real of the body, the subject is not completely alone. In the real structure made flesh, it is not only 'the subject', but 'the subjects, seized in their inter-subjectivity', who 'shape their being' according to their unconscious matrixes, structural positions, or corporeal 'moments' in the 'signifying chain' (Lacan, 1956a, p. 30). By coordinating these 'moments' occupied by the 'subjects', the signifying structure 'determines' at each 'moment' their social contacts, exchanges and interactions, as well as their individual 'acts, destiny, refusals, blindness, success, and fate' (ibid.).

As a 'support of the signifier', the supporting subject is 'determined' by the supported signifier at each link of the signifying chain (Lacan, 1960–1961, 01.03.61, p. 201). At each moment, through this 'determination', the subject receives a sudden complex 'overdetermination' from the signifying structure (12.04.61, p. 273). But the extreme suddenness and unthinkable complexity of this overdetermination are incompatible with consciousness. Therefore, even from a psychological angle, the subject shall be 'unconscious' of the structural 'overdetermination' (ibid.). Moreover, he shall be unconscious of the overdetermining structure, which governs his time, or the succession of signifying moments. At each one of these moments, the subject cannot be conscious of a structure that *does not give him any time to be conscious of it*. In fact, the subject has only the negative retroactive time expressed by the future perfect tense. Once he will have been retroactively overdetermined by the structure, all the moments of the signifying chain will have already been exhausted. In the intersection point between the enunciating act and the enunciated chain, the subject will have instantaneously spent all his time. All his moments will have lasted for less than one moment. So, there is not enough time for something to be really present for consciousness. The subject cannot linger in order to become aware of the immediate structuring power of the structural mediation.[8] In this immediacy, which does not leave any pause or break for consciousness, the subject shall be unconscious of the instant 'major determination' that he 'receives from the itinerary of a signifier' (Lacan, 1956a, p. 12).

At each moment of the enunciated chain, the enunciating subject will be unconscious of the way the structure is organized, in a flash, for his momentary structural position. Without the positive time of the enunciated fact, the real subject will be unconscious of what will have carried him away in the negative time of the enunciating act. In this *always already exhausted time* expressed by the future perfect tense, the subject shall be unconscious. Actually, for him to be obliged by the structuring power, he shall be unconscious of the instantaneous exercise of this power. Similarly, in Francisco Javier, the structural "obligation" shall vanish behind the thickness and opacity of the obligatory "conviction". The structural determination of the enunciating act shall thus disappear behind the fact of the enunciated signifier. In this fact, the 'act' will have only the 'efficacy' that is 'stolen' by the 'signifier' (Lacan, 1960–1961, 12.04.61, pp. 273–274). The convincing "obligation" will be only an obligatory "conviction". More precisely, the "familiar obligation" of the "revolutionary" (in the signifying social structure) becomes his "faithfulness from conviction" (in "individual sexual love as the foundation of the monogamous family"). The enunciating "revolutionary activities" become the enunciated values of the "consistent revolutionary" (e.g., "love, respect and faithfulness"). The enunciating truth gets muddled with the enunciated wisdom.

Without time to cope with his enunciating act, Francisco Javier gets muddled by the enunciated fact. He gets into a muddle because he 'doesn't know yet what he is going to say when he opens his mouth' (Kleist, 1806, p. 10). Just as he, all men are over and over again in the situation of the 'man who gets into a muddle' because he 'thinks' without 'realizing that he speaks before thinking' (Lacan, 1980, p. 317). The muddle results from the precedence of unconscious perceptible speech over conscious intelligible thought, or, in other words, the fact that 'thought comes by speaking' (Kleist, 1806, p. 8). This is also a reason for why we stumble when we speak. In this case, we stumble as our thoughts, which must be preceded by our speech, try nevertheless to precede it. In this way, the imaginary understanding of the symbolic enunciated fact aims vainly and absurdly to pave the way for the real enunciating act. Then the act stumbles over the fact. Otherwise, in well-expressed discursive situations, the act gets into the muddle of the fact. In any case, the truth of the enunciating act deals with the wisdom of the enunciated fact. At the same time, speech manages the thought of the speaker.

The subject as the exploited speaking workforce and thinking workplace of language

The thinker, even when mute, is always a speaker. When he thinks, he speaks to himself. We cannot conceive thought without taking speech into consideration. Actually, the relationship between both human faculties is so close that we cannot easily make a distinction between them.[9] In a sense, 'thought and speech are the same' (Plato, *Sophist*, 263d-e). Both are language. It would seem that the only difference between the two faculties lies in their particular accessibility. To be sure, speech is a directly or immediately accessible emergence of language, while thought is language that can only be indirectly accessible through the mediation of speech.[10] Nevertheless, as will be seen, 'there is no metalanguage', so speech is composed of the same language that composes thought (Lacan, 1960a, p. 293). All things considered, the reality of thought is nothing but a language that is immediately accessible in the form of speech. Accordingly, as Marx (1846) notes, 'language is the immediate reality of thought' (p. 1324). We must simply understand here, with the plainness and confidence of Stalin (1950b), that 'language manifests the reality of thought', that 'thoughts are born and exist only on the basis of the material of language', and that there are no 'nude thoughts', devoid of their 'natural language matter' (p. 181). As Wittgenstein (1949) observes at the time of Stalin, 'thought' is not an 'incorporeal process' which can be 'removed' from 'speech' (§339, p. 161).

In Lacan, as in Stalin and Wittgenstein, thought can only take place in language.[11] The explanation is that thought is not only inseparable and even indistinguishable from language, but also that it is generated by language. In the 'discourse' of language (or the *discourse of the Other*), Lacanian Discourse Analysis must then look for the 'cause' of 'thought' (Lacan, 1968–1969, 13.11.68, p. 13). This cause is language.

In a Lacanian Discourse Analysis, we analyze the discourse of a language which thinks and speaks instead of the subject, the so-called speaker *or* thinker, *who is just the exploited speaking workforce and thinking workplace of this language*. Thus, in our Lacanian perspective, *my* organ of thought is not *my* brain, but *a* language that is also *my* organ of speech, which is basically out of myself, even if it crosses and controls my body and my brain. This idea is not really new. Almost two centuries ago, Humboldt (1821) already described 'languages' as 'the organs of the ways of thinking' (p. 121). Like Wittgenstein, Humboldt is certain that thought cannot be removed from the *linguistic organ* that 'makes it possible' (p. 125). Without the functioning of the organ, there would not be any thought. Likewise, in our perspective, language is the *indispensable condition* of thought and not only its *dispensable expression*. Actually, we do not have a language to express what we think, but we think because there is a language that thinks in our place.[12]

In the Lacanian Cogito, I imagine that I think, but it is language that thinks in my place and imagines that I think, therefore language *is*. Without this language, we would not be able to think. In this regard, we must agree with Sapir (1921) when he declares that 'the feeling entertained by so many that they can think, or even reason, without language is an illusion' (p. 15). We must also take him seriously when he observes that 'speech' is 'the only road we know of that leads' to 'the domain of thought' (p. 16). This is so because 'language' is the only 'material' and 'immediate reality' of 'thought' (Marx, 1846, pp. 1061, 1324). Even if we distinguish the 'ideas' of thought and their material 'formulations' in language, we should acknowledge, much like Kleist (1806), that both 'go hand in hand' (p. 15). Similarly, even if we naively regard the separation between 'thought and language' as a division between 'knowledge' and the 'use of language' for 'communication', we should recognize, like Schaff (1964), that both are 'indivisible elements of a unit' and that 'their unity is so organic and their interdependence so close, that both elements cannot appear independently in a pure form' (p. 194). Now, in a Lacanian perspective, we put *language* itself (and not *the use of language*) apart from *communication* (of Schaff) or the *formulation of ideas* (of Kleist). In this way, we can analyze the materiality of language in its *pure form*, or regardless of the ideality of thought. Our analysis thus makes possible an accurate account of a language that exists independently from thought.

Despite Schaff, the materiality of language does exist *independently in a pure form*, or independently from the ideality of thought, as evidenced by those incomprehensible writings found in Chiapas or on Easter Island, but also elsewhere, and even everywhere, since no writing can really be comprehensible, all comprehension being imaginary. But on the other hand, thought cannot be separated from language. Even an unspeakable thought is dependent on the unthinkable materiality of language. Incidentally, this dependence on the unconscious is precisely the reason why thought proves to be, in a sense, *always unspeakable*. If thought wants in vain to be spoken, its unspeakable character demonstrates that speech is not in the hands of thought. On the contrary, thoughts are in the hands of speech. They are shaped and arranged, pushed and interrupted by language. The ideality of thought is thus determined by the unthinkable materiality of language.[13]

The unconscious materiality of the language that thinks in the place of the subject

The determination of thought by language is an essential idea in one of the less anti-Lacanian philosophies of language that I know of, namely, that of Wilhelm von Humboldt (1820, 1821, 1822, 1834). This philosophy actually focuses on 'the incidence of language in thought' and the 'properties of language that underpin thought' (1821, p. 123). In this regard, the most radical Humboldtian assumption is that 'language creates a definite thought, puts its mark on it and gives a form to it' (1822, p. 149). Then, 'through' this 'form', language 'pushes for the creation of new thoughts and new connections between thoughts' (p. 155). This *linguistic creation of thoughts* demonstrates, in the eyes of Humboldt, that 'language meets an interior need of mankind' (1834, §4, p. 151). As a kind of romantic Lacanian, this philosopher believes that language 'does not simply fulfil an exterior need of social communication', but represents 'the necessary condition' for 'mankind to materialize its spiritual forces' (ibid.). This is the reason why 'language governs the thought of the singular individual, even in his solitary existence and independently from his communication with others' (p. 194).

Whether in dialogic or monologic situations, thought is governed by language, composed by signifiers, developed by discourse. If we infer a thought from a discourse that we analyze, the so-called *thought* will just be a development of the analyzed discourse. It will be a discursive explanation or prolongation, a paraphrase of an accessible phrase.[14] Now, in an accurate discourse analysis, the analyzed phrase determines its analytical paraphrase. Thus, in general, the phrase is the signifierizing data that determines the signifierized expressible thought, as well as every imaginary signified thought.

The inaccessible ideality of thought is generally determined by the accessible materiality of language. The *accessibility* and the *determining capacity* of language represent, in Lacanian Discourse Analysis, two decisive reasons for prioritizing language at the expense of thought. We can formulate these two reasons as follows:

- *Language is internally the only determining or significant original data.* In this regard, Sapir (1921) observes that 'language, as a structure, is on its inner face the mould of thought' (p. 22). We shall see later that we can translate this into Lacanese: *the unconscious, as a structure, is on its inner face the mould of consciousness.* This inner face corresponds logically to the 'inner form of language' that contains thought and consciousness in Humboldt (1834, §21, p. 231).
- *Language is externally the only accessible or available material for analysis.* In this regard, Wittgenstein (1921) observes that 'language', as a perceptible 'exterior form', is on its outer face the 'garment' that 'disguises thought' (4.002, p. 71). We shall see later that we can translate this into Lacanese: *the unconscious, as a perceptible form, is in its outer face the garment that disguises the intelligible content of consciousness.* This garment, though exterior and perceptible, would then be strangely unconscious. For what reason? Wittgenstein gives us the answer: 'We cannot infer the form of the disguised thought from the exterior form of its garment, as this form does not aim for the recognition of the form of the body' (ibid.).

The perceptible form of language does not aim for the recognition of the intelligible form of thought, but rather for the *formation* or creation of this form. This is why Sapir (1921) stresses the fact that language, in relation to 'thought', is 'a mould' and *not* 'a garment' (p. 15). The only problem with this idea is that it misses the outer face of language. To solve this serious problem, we should proceed dialectically, through a synthesis of Wittgenstein and Sapir, and compare language to those providential moulding garments, such as the old corset and the new Wonderbra, that give handsome forms to our sadly formless bodies. Just as our bodies, our souls are formless. Their form is not their form, but the form of language. Now, internally, this external and accessible form of language is also the moulding structure of the moulded soul. Even if this perceptible structure of the analyzed discourse is unintelligible or unconscious, it is the only structure of the intelligible or conscious content.

The 'corporeal and crude' material of discourse is the only formal structure of the spiritual or 'ethereal substance' of the soul, of thought and cognition (Kleist, 1811, p. 32). In this manner, as Marx (1846) notes, 'spirit is under the curse of being sullied by matter' that 'takes the form of language' (p. 1061). This matter corresponds, in our Lacanian materialism, to the 'symbolic' as the 'preformed matter' of 'the unconscious' (Lacan, 1972c, p. 548). It corresponds also, as signifierized matter, to the 'signifier' defined as 'matter transcended in language' (Lacan, 1966b, p. 209).

The Lacanian signifier constitutes the external materiality of language. By focusing on this external materiality and neglecting the internal ideality of the signification, Lacan embraces a sort of symbolic materialism and turns his back on idealism, which he relegates to the sphere of the imaginary.[15] Contrary to idealism, Lacanian materialism, just as any other genuine materialism, 'regards' unconscious 'matter' as 'primary data', and 'consciousness' as 'secondary data' (Lenin, 1908, I, §1, p. 44). However, unlike Marxist-Leninist materialism, our symbolic materialism cannot treat 'sensation' as an imaginary 'copy, photography, reproduction, projection of things as in a mirror' (cf. Lenin, 1908, IV, §6, pp. 241–242). From our radical materialist viewpoint, sensation must be considered a material thing among other material things. Just like any other human thing in our symbolic universe, our 'sensation' is a material 'symbol' (cf. Lenin, 1908, IV, §6, p. 241), a literal 'sign' (Helmholtz 1878, p. 255), or, more precisely, an external *signifier* or 'a sort of hieroglyph' that 'is not similar' to 'the fact' it represents (Plekhanov, 1892, p. 437).

Adopting the symbolic materialism of Lacan, Lacanian Discourse Analysis must concentrate on the materiality and externality of the symbolic form of discourse. It must also acknowledge the imaginary character of the internal ideal content of mind and discourse. To be compatible with this method, our social psychology must be a 'concrete psychology' (Politzer, 1928, 1947). It must be a 'materialist psychology' that recognizes the 'mythological character of inner life' (1947, II, III, p. 100). It must be a 'psychology without inner life', but also 'without the slightest trace of physiology or biology' (1928, V, II, pp. 228–229). Instead of these isolated fields of purely analytical knowledge, our concrete psychology must be also dialectical. Its materialism must be a *dialectical materialism* in which the symbolized or signifierized *physis* and *bios* are inseparable from the materialized and externalized *psyche*.

In his symbolic materialism, Lacan always keeps in mind the dialectical movement of symbolization and materialization, signifierization and externalization. Thus, in a sense, his materialism is dialectical and not only symbolic. What we can identify here as *Lacanian dialectical materialism* brings us closer to Marxism-Leninism. Now, unlike Lacanians, Marxists-Leninists regard language only as *a* part of the basis and *a* specific matter among other matters. Lacanians instead take the signifying structure of language as *the* matter and *the* basis or the infrastructure of the human world. The fact remains that, in the eyes of Lacan (1966b), Marxism stands, 'concerning language, quite above logician Neo-positivism' (p. 208). This is because Marxism recognizes both the *material* and *infrastructural* character of language (pp. 208–209). Stalin (1950a, 1950b) is categorical on these two points. First he postulates resolutely that 'language is the matter of thought' (1950b, p. 181). Then he claims again and again: 'it is false' that language is a 'superstructure' (1950a, p. 147), it 'differs from the superstructure' (p. 149), it 'differs as a matter of principle' (p. 151), the 'confusion between language and superstructure is a grave mistake' (p. 154)—and we should consider here the gravity of what Stalin regards as a *grave mistake*!

Together with *good* Marxists and *true* Lacanians, Sapir (1921) observes rightly that language is situated on 'a lower plane' than 'the conceptual plane' (p. 15). He also remarks that 'thought arises' here 'as a refined interpretation' of the 'lower plane' of 'language' (ibid.). Likewise, in Lacanian materialism, the unconscious signifiers compose the material basis or infrastructure that underpins every superstructure of conscious thought or cognition.[16] Language is the basis on which 'depends every determination of the subject' and his 'thought' (Lacan, 1969–1970, 20.05.70, p. 178). In this way, it is not only 'the thought' of the subject, but also the thinking 'subject' that Lacan 'subordinates' to the base of language (1961, p. 181). So, the Cartesian thing that thinks rests also on the language that speaks. In actual fact, the thinking thing of Descartes is nothing but its material base or infrastructure of language, that is, the 'matter transcended in language' (Lacan, 1966b, p. 209) as the 'preformed matter of the unconscious' (Lacan, 1972c, p. 548). This unconscious matter incarnates the body of the subject as a *Thing*, an extensive thing, which consciously thinks. It is the Freudian *id* or the Lacanian *ça*. It is *that*. And *that thinks, therefore it is.*

Lacan advances the idea of a material trans-individual articulation of language that thinks in the place of the individual subject.[17] This idea must be treasured in Lacanian Discourse Analysis. Contrary to cognitive psychologists who visualize an individual 'mind' which 'uses language as a vehicle of thought', Lacanians must analyze 'a language which thinks through the dynamics of its trans-individual articulation' (Schepens, 2002). In this way, by treating language as the trans-individual material base of the alleged individual thought, Lacanian Discourse Analysis proves to be suitable for a discursive and concrete social psychology. When Francisco Javier thinks about "family", for example, a Lacanian assumes that it is a language which thinks *in* him, or rather *through* him, but also *outside* him, in a particular cultural and social environment, as evidenced by the "significance of marriage for revolutionaries, as a starting point for the establishment of family and thereby for the constitution of society". It must be granted that an oddly enough traditional and revolutionary Mexican society, based on marriage and family, should already be constituted in order to think and speak about the "significance of marriage for revolutionaries". Francisco Javier is just the thinking workplace and speaking workforce of this society.

To explain the conscious ideal thought of an individual subject, a concrete psychology must analyze the unconscious materiality of a language which trans-individually thinks in his place. Logically, to analyze this materiality, the psychology must be social and discursive.[18] Its psychic matter must be discursive. As for its psychological subject, it must be the signifying social structure of language, which includes all our structural positions in it. Strictly speaking, these positions are not ours, but they are the positions of the structure. In these positions, our thought belongs to the signifying structure, which materializes through a nervous system and not only through an economic system. Our psychology is the psychology of this Other. This Other is *he who* thinks instead of us. Therefore *he* is instead of us (*he* and not *it*, because the Other takes from us all of our humanity and personality).

When the Other thinks in my place, I should ask myself, with Foucault (1966), if 'I can still say that *I am* this language that *I speak* and in which my thoughts enter and find all of their capacities' (p. 335). The answer is *no*. I am not this language whose 'sedimentations could never be entirely grasped' by me (ibid.). Yet *I* still speak and *I* still think when this language speaks or thinks in my place. Therefore the *I* is language. *I is Other* (*Je est un Autre*). Here is the 'failure to recognize myself' as the origin of the 'unconscious' (p. 337). The unconscious refers here to our absence in the language that thinks our thoughts.

The ontogenetic precedence of language and the phylogenetic precedence of humankind

However material it is, language is not a 'secretion of thought' (Lacan, 1953b, p. 135). It is rather 'the mould of thought' (Sapir, 1921, p. 22). Its 'materiality' plays a 'constituent role' for 'thought' (1953b, pp. 135–136). Its structure is the 'framework' in which 'thought' is 'constituted' supposedly 'beyond' (1967c, p. 341).

Instead of the naïve representation of a social context where individuals communicate their thoughts by means of language, Lacanian Discourse Analysis must assume the representation of a language as a signifying social structure which trans-individually constitutes its subjects as well as their thoughts.[19] Seized by this structure, the animal becomes a human subject. He is converted into *someone* by speaking, because he is humanized by the structure of language. In a virtuous circle, he is a human subject as he is subject to 'the laws of language', but he is subjected to these laws as he is 'indebted' to them, and he is 'indebted' to them precisely because his 'human' subjectivity depends on them (Melman, 2007, pp. 52–54). In the end, his human *subjectivation* is nothing but his *subjection* to the signifying structure of society. This subjection, as the 'assimilation to the signifier', has 'the function of *subjectivating*' (Lacan, 1958–1959, 13.05.59). Accordingly, the *signifierization* also involves a *subjectivation* and not only a *materialization* and an *externalization*. While the 'signification' brings about an imaginary 'objectivation' of the enunciated or constructed reality (Berger & Luckmann, 1966, p. 35), the signifierization entails a real subjectivation of the enunciating workforce which is proletarianized and exploited for the construction of reality.

In Lacan (1960–1961), the subject is 'constituted' by the signifier (01.03.61, p. 201). This constitution presupposes a logical anteriority of the signifier in relation to the subject. Understandably, 'for the coming of the subject, the signifier is required as a syntax previous to the subject' (Lacan, 1961, p. 182). What is subjected must follow what subjects it. The structure should precede the subject of the structure. Language should be already here to create its enunciating workforce. Humanized and symbolized by speech, 'man speaks' because of 'the symbol' which 'has made him man' (Lacan, 1953a, p. 274).

The human humus nourishes the tree of language thanks to the creation of the humus by the rotten, dead leaves of the tree. So the tree should precede the humus. But simultaneously, as discussed above, the humus should precede the tree. On that assumption, Lacan (1973c) defines language as 'what the human humus invents for its everlastingness from generation to generation' (p. 311). Now, from this definition, we can easily avoid a circular reasoning and understand the feedback between the language and the human being. *From a phylogenetic point of view, there is the logical precedence of humankind, which creates and preserves a language in order to exploit it as a work system, a subjecting system that makes it possible for humankind to exist and subsist. Conversely, from an ontogenetic point of view, there is the logical precedence of a language, which creates and preserves a human being to exploit him as a workforce, an enunciating force that makes it possible for language to exist and subsist.*[20] The fact of the matter is that the two points of view refer to the same phenomenon. The exploitation of each individual by language involves the exploitation of language by humanity. In the 'employment of language', each employer becomes an 'employee' (Lacan, 1969–1970, 21.01.70, p. 74). He is instrumentalized by his 'instrumentalization of language' (Cléro, 2008, p. 172). He is exploited because he belongs to a system that is exploited by humankind. Thus, in the ontogenetic experience, language 'imposes the phylogenetic experience of humankind' on a human being (cf. Schaff, 1964, p. 204). But this human being cannot enjoy *his* experience of humankind. He is 'a language employee and not an enjoyment user' (Josselin, 2006, p. 52). Hence, his discontent in civilization.

In the ontogenesis of the language employee, we may discern two successive moments. First, *a priori*, there is the signifying structure of language, in which the subject already has a position reserved for him. Then, *a posteriori*, there is the signifying chain of discourse, by which the subject will have retroactively existed. In Lacanian Discourse Analysis, we must deal simultaneously with these two moments in which the subject appears, respectively, as a virtual workforce (e.g., "familiar obligations") and as an actual work of an enunciating act (e.g., "faithfulness from conviction"). In the gap between the two moments, we must analyze the 'link' that Lacan (1953b) establishes between 'the material of language' (in contrast with 'the instrument of language'), as a 'geometrical place' in which 'everything is already there', and the 'action of speech' (in contrast to 'the function of speech'), which 'underpins' and 'constitutes the subject' (pp. 147–154).[21]

In speech as well as in language, the signifier precedes the ontogenesis of the subject. This precedence is either *chronological* (because of the phylogenetic foundation of the signifying structure of language) or *psychological* (because of the retroactive functioning of language in the signifying chain of speech). In any case, the genesis of the signifier takes place before the ontogenesis of the subject, which is only natural, since the subject is constituted by the signifier (both synchronically by its structure and diachronically by its chain).

Conscious identification and unconscious alienation

In the evolution of the Lacanian theory, the ontogenetic constitution of the subject by the signifier has been considered in two different ways, each corresponding to one of the two successive periods mentioned in previous chapters. First, until 1958, the subject is constituted by a signifier which 'engenders' a 'signification' that 'seizes the subject, branding him as a signified' (Lacan, 1958b, p. 166). Then, from 1958, the emergence of the subject as an 'effect of the signifier' does not 'respond at all to the signified', but 'to a signifier' defined as 'what represents a subject for another signifier' (1969, p. 390).

In Lacanian reinforced structuralism, the subject is no longer signified and constituted by its signification, but rather he is constituted by the fact of being represented by a signifier for another signifier. Actually, the subjection or constitution of the subject resides in this relationship between the signifier that represents him and the signifier to which he is represented. As the 'personification' of this 'relationship' (Marx, 1867, I, §2, p. 77), the subject is not a *signified* according to the strictest definition of the term. If he is a signified (which does not go without saying), he is not the signified of a signifier, but 'the signified of the signifying relation between two signifiers' (Lacan, 1967d, p. 580). If we persist in regarding Francisco Javier as a signified, for example, we must at least acknowledge that he is not the signified of his "revolutionary point of view", but rather the signified of the relationship between two "points of view", that of the "revolutionary" and that of "our time" and its "moral conquest". Now, first of all, this relationship consists of a difference between both viewpoints and their respective positions in the signifying chain and structure. Perhaps we may say here, in Gramscian terms, that Francisco Javier is signified by the difference between the domination of his "revolutionary point of view" and the hegemony of the *conquering morality* or "our time". Whether here or elsewhere, the difference *in* discourse refers to the subject *of* discourse. Here is a new reason why Lacanian Discourse Analysis must take a great deal of interest in difference. This difference is decisive as it represents a necessary condition of any subjective relationship between signifiers.

The relationship between signifiers necessarily implies a difference between them. But, at the same time, this difference necessarily implies a contradiction. With Mao Zedong (1937), we can assume that 'in every difference there is already a contradiction and the difference itself constitutes a contradiction' (II, p. 60). This contradiction may also eventually entail a 'conflict' that Bakhtin (1934) already examined in discourse (pp. 125–135). In Francisco Javier's discourse, for example, the difference between the "revolutionary point of view" and the "moral conquest of our time" constitutes a contradiction, which entails antagonism, a rivalry, a fight, a battle and a battlefield. Now, this battlefield comprises a "point of view", a "time", a bourgeois ideology, but also a "proletarian ideology, culture and values". As for the battle, it does not only signify Francisco Javier, but also other individuals who relate to the same discourse. In this way, the subject is signified, and constituted, in a battle of words that takes place in a sociocultural battlefield.[22]

Signified by a battle of words, the subject finds himself divided between the contradictory signifiers that fight the battle. This 'primary division follows from the fact that one signifier represents the subject only for another signifier', which is the enemy, but also the 'repressed' holder of the being of the subject (Lacan, 1967e, pp. 277–278). The division ($) is then between the representative of the subject and his repressed enemy, that is to say, between the subjective identity (S1) and a predicative alterity (S2) of the being of the subject in discourse (S1–S2).

In the battle of words inherent in every discourse, the enunciating subject is divided between his conscious identification to the signifier that represents him, as the enunciated subject, and his unconscious alienation in the enemy signifier which is repressed, as the enunciated predicate. Francisco Javier would thus be divided between his conscious identification with the "revolutionary", as the grammatical subject of his discourse, and his unconscious alienation in "our time" and its "moral" environment, as a predicate that includes "marriage", "monogamous family", etc. The Eperrist would then be torn between his conscious, dominant "proletarian ideology", and the unconscious, hegemonic bourgeois language that holds his being. Besides being bourgeois, this language should be fundamentally conventional, institutional, conformist, conservative, reactionary, anti-revolutionary. As the Other of the revolutionary, language should be everything that Francisco Javier assigns to his adversaries, to the external environment, to the Mexican political and economic system. Repression entails, in general, this externalization of that which is repressed, as well as the division of the subject between his two contradictory parts, namely, his conscious identity and his unconscious alienation in that which has been externalized.[23] Now, in Lacan, this negative *division by repression and externalization* also entails a positive constitution of the subject. The Lacanian subject can only be positively constituted as a divided subject, or, more precisely, as a subject divided between his internal identification to a signifier and his external alienation in language. Thus, in actual fact, the division by the signifier *is* the constitution of the subject, his emergence as an effect of the signifier.

The subject as a signifier and not only as an effect of the signifier

One of the most important contributions of Lacan to our discipline is his demonstration that 'facts of human psychology cannot be conceived in the absence of the function of the subject defined as the effect of the signifier' (1964, 27.05.64, p. 231). This demonstration is logically based on the assumption that a 'subject arises as such from the effect of the signifier' (1961–1962, 06.12.61). It is a 'radical assumption' that puts the subject, as an 'effect of the signifier', in a 'secondary position' of 'dependence on the signifier', as the cause of the subject (1961–1962, 30.05.62).

As an effect of the signifier, the subject depends on its cause. First, he is only 'sustained' by the 'signifier' that 'keeps recurring' (Lacan, 1966c, p. 223). Then, by his identification with this recurrent enunciated subject (S1), the enunciating subject begins living in the alienating predicative environment of the signifying structure (S2). Here he lives on words. His 'life is a parasite of language' (Barthes, 1957, p. 90). Actually, the subject can only exist and subsist in the consecutive links of the signifying chain. These links are the successive instants of his life.

Luckily for us, the living instants of a real subject are linked together in analyzed discourse. Adopting the viewpoint of the concrete psychology of Politzer (1928, 1947), we can assume that each one of these discursive links expresses 'a segment' of life, a moment in 'the drama that represents one's life', which can only emerge as a 'gesture illuminated by a narrative' (1928, C, §11, pp. 247–248). In this narrative deployed by discourse, the link is a 'dramatic segment' of a 'material performance' (1947, I, VIII, p. 49). Its 'dramatic value' (ibid.) is nothing but its symbolic value. As for the 'dramatic meaning' of this value, it is that which is 'taken by psychology' and transformed into an objective mental or cognitive reality (ibid.). Now, in a Lacanian concrete psychology, such meaning shall not be transformed into this imaginary objective reality. It shall be neither reified nor objectified. Instead, it shall be reduced to its truth, to the real of the symbolic, to the gesture illuminated by the narrative, to the subjective enunciating act elucidated by the enunciated fact of discourse, by this 'objective data' or 'objective material that can be studied from the outside' (1928, II, I, p. 81).

Besides constituting a way to approach the subject and his subjective enunciating act, the objective material of the enunciated fact *constitutes* the subject. *The subject is not merely the truth contained in his full speech. Moreover, he incarnates this speech. He is structured and not just retroactively subjected to the structure. He is language and not just the inhabitant of language. He is the signifier and not only an effect of the signifier.*

From 1960 to 1961, Lacan focused on a subjective signifierization whereby the subject 'disappears as a subject beneath the signifier he becomes' (1960b, p. 315). In this signifierization, the signifier turns out to be 'identical to the subject' (1960–1961, 12.04.61, p. 273). The 'presence' of the 'subject' proves to be constitutionally 'a signifier rather than a body' (1961, p. 182). The Eperrists who were tortured or died for their revolution, for example, already proved to be signifiers ("consistent revolutionaries") rather than bodies. By sacrificing their bodies for the revolution, the comrades of Francisco Javier were totally signifierized by their discourse. The criminal Mexican Army is guilty of their pain and death, granted, but the tortured and dead "revolutionaries" were signifiers who *knew* the Mexican Army as well as the price to be paid in Mexico for the symbolic value of "revolutionary consistency". They were still "consistent revolutionaries". Together with Pascal (1662), they decided to 'risk' their mortal body for the living signifier (§233, pp. 113–117). They lost the body, but they gained the 'signifier' (Lacan, 1968–1969, 15.01.69, 22.01.69, 29.01.69, 05.02.69, 12.02.69, pp. 107–183). Consequently, they became what they are at present, that is, clean discourse, wholesome names, pure signifiers, "consistent revolutionaries". Their signifierization will have been just the prolongation of Francisco Javier's discourse, which, by the way, may cost him his life. But even before any kind of heroic death, Francisco Javier is already his discourse. This discourse by now deploys the signifying subjectivity of the "consistent revolutionary". Our hooded subject can then be regarded as identical to his signifierizing discourse, which can be correspondingly treated as identical to the signifierized subject.[24]

The subject can be regarded as a signifier, or as identical to the signifier, because his 'identification' as a 'subject' is necessarily an 'identification' with a 'signifier' (Lacan, 1961–1962, 06.12.61). As discussed above, the subjectivation is a signifierization. It is a signifierization as it entails a subjection to the signifying structure. To be subjective, our living matter should have a signifying form. It should be 'taken by the mechanism of the signifier' (20.12.61). It should 'slide' into the 'signifying chain' (1972–1973, 16.01.73, p. 65). Now, in the signifying chain, the enunciating subject cannot be reduced to an enunciated subject. The speaker cannot simply be spoken as the other signifiers. If he becomes a signifier, he should be a signifier different from all of the others, an ineffable signifier, a missing signifier. It is thus 'the elision of a signifier as such, the missing signifier in the chain', which makes possible 'the appearance of the subject' (1959–1960, 11.05.60, p. 264). The appearance of the subject amounts to the *dis*-appearance of the only signifier of the chain that could never appear among other signifiers. It is the *enunciating signifier*, that should be outside all the other enunciated ones, in order to enunciate all of them. In this manner, it is *the signifier of the signifiers*. It is a signifier 'identifiable with the game of the signifier' (1961–1962, 20.12.61).

In the chain as well as in the structure, the position of a subject is an enunciating position fundamentally different from all the other objective enunciated positions. And yet, the subject is a mere position in the structure. He is just a signifier. Even if he is a signifier different from all the other signifiers, he is still just a signifier and he should be just that to be a subject. For his living matter to be transformed into a subject, it should be subjected to the signifying social structure, which overdetermines, signifierizes and structures subjectivity.[25] But in this structure of signifiers, the subject should be nothing more than a signifier. As symbolization, his signifierization is not only a subjectivation, but also a *de*-realization, or annihilation of the real. Therefore, the real subject 'disappears as a subject', or as *something more than a signifier*, 'beneath the signifier he becomes' (Lacan, 1960b, p. 315).

In a sense, and oddly enough, the Lacanian real enunciating subject turns out to be just as symbolic as the symbolic enunciated subject. His enunciating or speaking aptitude is then nothing more than his signifying and signifierizing character. This is why the Lacanian real subject is the same thing as his truth. By telling his truth, he incarnates it. He is the letter, the literal, signifying presence of his truth, not only written in ink, but also in blood, in the flesh, as a gesture, a countenance, and a symptom. The truth is thus articulated by the tongue as well as by all the other natural and artificial muscles and organs of the body, through each movement, behaviour, decision, perception, cognition. As a truth, the signifying real subject is not only a speaking subject, but also a living subject, and even a perceiving subject, a reader or listener who is instantaneously signifierized by what he listens to or reads. In this way, by encountering a signifier, the subject is 'assimilated' by it and 'becomes a signifier in his turn' (Lacan, 1960–1961, 26.04.61, p. 307). Furthermore, he becomes *the signifier*, the truth of the signifier that he encounters, or, more precisely, the truth of the encounter with the signifier. In this sense, the analyst of a discourse *is* the truth of his analysis. For example, as a signifier, I am the truth of my analysis of Francisco Javier's discourse. This truth *is* a missing signifier, an enunciating invisible position in the structure, a place that cannot be easily spotted. However, we can approximately trace this place through my identification with a number of signifiers, such as "Lacanian" or "materialist". In Lacanian Discourse Analysis, we must not avoid this reflexive tracing of the analytical enunciating position within the signifying social structure.

The subjects of concrete, discursive and cognitive psychologies

Besides the missing condition, there is another negative feature, this time an intrinsic one, which distinguishes the implicit enunciating subject (*my truth*) from the explicit enunciated subject that represents him (such as "Lacanian" or "materialist"). This intrinsic negative feature is the division of the subject ($) between his identification to the signifier of the enunciated subject (S1) and his resulting alienation in language (S2). This division distinguishes him, as the divided subject of an actual truth (*vérité*), from the individual subject of factual wisdom (*savoir*), but also from another individual subject, namely, that of forged knowledge (*connaissance*). Accordingly, *we can make a distinction between three subjects who are prioritized in three different psychological positions: in Lacanian implicit concrete psychology, the divided real subject of actual enunciating truth; in discursive psychology, the individual symbolic subject of factual enunciated wisdom; in cognitive psychology, the individual imaginary subject of forged or imagined knowledge.*

Cognitive psychology	Individual imaginary subject of imagined knowledge (*connaissance*)
Discursive psychology	Individual symbolic subject of enunciated wisdom (*savoir*)
Concrete psychology	Divided real subject of enunciating truth (*vérité*)

Unlike the imaginary subject of cognition, our real subject of discourse does not have an individual 'unity' that would be 'warranted and crowned by consciousness' (Althusser, 1976, p. 237). He is not an ideal subject who would relate individually and consciously to an object, but a material subject who is divided between the signifiers in the signifying social structure of the unconscious. This material subject of the unconscious is covered by consciousness, while the ideal subject of consciousness is 'called into question' by the 'unconscious' (Lacan, 1967d, p. 579). Thanks to the unconscious and its 'symptomatic' expressions, the imaginary character of the subject of consciousness was satisfactorily demonstrated, a long time ago, when Marx and Freud 'denounced' the 'fundamental trickery of the theory of knowledge' (Lacan, 1970–1971, 16.06.71, pp. 164–165). All the same, the old and boring imaginary subject of knowledge is still *the* subject of cognitive psychology.[26] Actually, he is the prevailing subject of psychology. He is the 'psychological' subject par excellence (Lacan, 1967d, p. 579). The explanation might be that this subject is the only conceivable subject in a 'bourgeois ideology' which is 'implicit to psychology' (Althusser, 1976, p. 237). As the hegemonic symbolic system of the signifying social structure, this bourgeois ideology needs an individual subject who *knows* exactly what pleases him and what to do to obtain it, namely, *work and buy*, or, to be more specific, *open the purse and pay*. This imaginary knowledge ensures a demand that corresponds exactly to the supply. It is obviously not a stroke of luck, but rather the eternal virtue of the mirror, which covers the division and proletarianization of a real subject, the subject of the signifier, whose real desire will never be met by what is sold by the shopkeeper.

It is clear that 'the subject of the signifier and the subject of knowledge have nothing in common' (Lacan, 1969–1970, 14.01.70, p. 53). The former is correlative to *other* signifiers, such as a revolutionary in relation to "our time" or "the world". Instead, the latter is 'the subject correlative to the object' (1958–1959, 19.11.58), such as a psychologist in relation to an objective family known in the form of a pillar.[27] Unlike a subject of the signifier who irrefutably demonstrates himself through his enunciation of the signifier, the 'subject of knowledge' is only 'deducible' from his hypothetical relation to the object (1969–1970, 14.01.70, p. 53). He can only be conceived, in theory, through an abstraction of the already abstract 'relation of subject-object' (1957–1958, 25.06.58, p. 476). He is supposed from this conjectural 'relation to the world', which is actually nothing but 'the relation of his eye to the world' (pp. 476–477). Therefore, in reality, he can be reduced to 'an eye, a photoelectric cell', or a so-called 'consciousness' (1957–1958, 14.05.58, p. 394).

As a 'particularization' of 'human existence', the subject of knowledge does not refer to *homo sapiens* in general, but to the specific '*homo psychologicus*' (Lacan, 1953b, p. 142). Subjectified as a 'psychological subject', this human idea of the human thing may be understandably 'called into question' (1967d, p. 579). He is just 'ideal' and 'problematic' or problematically 'supposed' (1958–1959, 19.11.58). On the contrary, the *subject of the signifier* is not 'supposed', but necessarily embedded in the 'signifying implication' (1967d, p. 579). Implied thus by the spoken signifier, the speaking subject of the signifier 'imposes himself with complete necessity' (1958–1959, 19.11.58). He is the real subject who will have been 'born' *automatically, without human intervention*, 'just as the human individual is emerging in speech' (1957–1958, 25.06.58, p. 476).

The time of discourse and the space of language

For Lacan, the subject of knowledge is just supposed and problematic, while the subject of the signifier constitutes a real and necessary incarnate truth. As for the 'subject of wisdom', he refers merely to a perceptible signifier, that is to say, an evident and analyzable thing, a material 'subject of discourse', presented and 'animated' by 'discourse' (Lacan, 1970a, p. 433). This discourse actually materializes 'wisdom' that presents its symbolic enunciated subject (p. 408). At the same time, the wisdom 'surrounds' the 'real', which cannot really be 'known', but only 'demonstrated', in its necessity, as a real enunciating subject (ibid.).

As long as the real cannot be known, the knowledge relates only to an imaginary reality. But this reality belongs exclusively to the subject of knowledge. It is his own reality. He cannot communicate it through analyzable discourse. He cannot share his knowledge with us. He can only share his wisdom, which is already shared, at least in part, as it is inherent in the signifying social structure of language. In fact, when we analyze a discourse, we analyze 'wisdom', as that which has a 'structure of language' (Lacan, 1973a, p. 536). Unlike the knowledge of the subject, this wisdom of the structure, or *discourse of the Other*, can be reached to a certain extent through a Lacanian Discourse Analysis. And besides being partly accessible, this wisdom has the advantage of being fully determining. It is actually that which shapes any kind of knowledge. As the *discourse of the Other*, the wisdom of the structure logically decides the knowledge of the subject.[28]

Benveniste (1958b) shows strikingly how the 'linguistic structure' and its 'linguistic categories predispose the categories of thought' (p. 73). Assuming that 'language determines a subjectivity which in turn influences thought and sensation, knowledge and mental disposition' (Humboldt, 1821, p. 165), we should presume that linguistic categories, as signifying positions of the structure, predispose the categories of thought, but also the categories of knowledge and sensation. Put differently, in Kantian terms, we should radicalize Benveniste and take for granted that signifiers determine aesthetic spatio-temporal dimensions as well as analytical and dialectical logical categories. This should be our position in Lacanian Discourse Analysis. This was also apparently the position of Lacan. Actually, in the same year in which Benveniste showed the linguistic determination of thought, Lacan (1958c) had already decided that Kantian 'transcendental aesthetics', as well as the Aristotelian categories of Benveniste, 'have to be recast in our times, for linguistics has introduced into science its indisputable status, structure being defined by signifying articulation as such' (p. 126).

In Lacanian transcendental aesthetics, the *a priori* geometry of the spatial 'exterior intuition' of space (Kant, 1781, A, I, §2–3, pp. 55–61) shall be the synchronic signifying structure, as the place of language and exteriority of the unconscious. In this way, the so-called 'real space' shall be treated as the symbolic spacing, the 'purely verbal construction', carved, engraved or archi-written in the real, and 'spelled in three dimensions' (Lacan, 1975–1976, 10.02.76, p. 86). In the vertical dimension of the building inhabited by Francisco Javier, for example, there is a stacking, from bottom to top, of three symbolic architectural levels: an "individual sexual love", as a "foundation"; then, the "monogamous family", as a "fundamental pillar" on the "foundation"; and finally, "the new society", as a "construction" on the "fundamental pillar".

In relation to the newness of the "new society", Francisco Javier is not only situated in the vertical exterior spatial dimension, but also in the fourth Augustinian dimension, in the interior temporal one, in which "marriage" is the "starting point" for the "constitution of society". Therefore, to ascend to the constituted new society, the subject should first wait for the moment of marriage. In this case, from Francisco Javier's Marxist viewpoint, the moment of marriage functions eloquently as the aggravation of the contradiction between productive forces and productive relations. We should wait for this aggravation to make the revolution. Similarly, to start a revolution and thus ascend spatially or externally to the new society, our Eperrist should temporally or internally wait for a necessary marriage (whose necessity might arise, as it so happens, from an aggravation of the contradiction between productive forces of desire and productive sexual relations, or, more precisely, between enunciating forces and signifying relations). Here is the 'interior intuition' of the fourth temporal dimension, which makes it possible to conceive *a priori* expectation and revolution, 'duration' and 'change' (Kant, 1781, A, I, §4–6, pp. 61–65). Now, in our Lacanian transcendental aesthetics, this temporal intuition shall be determined by the diachronic chain of discourse. *The interior experience of time shall depend on the missing position of the enunciating subject in relation to the successive moments, or links of the enunciated chain of discourse. Correlatively, at each moment, the exterior experience of space shall depend on the same position of the same overdetermined subject in the overdetermining structure of language.*

In every analyzable discourse, the temporal-internal and spatial-external intuitions compose an indissoluble discursive-linguistic complex of time and space (discourse and language, domination and hegemony, revolution and reaction, internal "conviction" and external "obligation"). On the basis of the 'chronotope' of Bakhtin (1938), this complex can be defined as the 'essential spatio-temporal correlation' and the 'unification of space and time' as the 'fourth dimension of space' (p. 237). Of course, the correlation and the unification of time and space also presuppose a fundamental 'difference' (Derrida, 1967, p. 96) between the 'becoming-space of time and the becoming-time of space' (p. 101). In Derrida, this difference presupposes in turn a 'spacing (pause, blank, punctuation)', which reveals 'always the non-perceived, the non-present, the non-conscious' (p. 99). Thus, when we analyze a discourse, its ruptures, absences and silences should not be interpreted only as indications of the gap between space and time (or language and discourse), but also as the 'unconscious' (p. 101) of the transcendental signifying structure that opens the real and makes way for the spatio-temporal complex and for its perceptible, present and conscious phenomena.

In Kant, it is not only transcendental aesthetics that should be 'recast' (Lacan, 1958c, p. 126), but also, and particularly, transcendental analytics. With this aim in view, we can follow the 'purely formal categorical program' proposed by Melo (2000, pp. 382–469), in which categories are reduced to 'pure syncategorema', to 'logical-syntactical categories' (p. 380), to 'simple signifiers' (p. 443), to 'pure syntactic signs without signification' (p. 432). Without a conscious signification, those signifiers are unconscious. They are *the* unconscious. They compose 'the unconscious' as an 'ontological structure' (Resweber, 1998).

As for transcendental dialectics, there should be nothing to recast. All we have to do here is appreciate the purely discursive character of a 'reason' whose only 'immediate relation' is to the analytical signifiers of 'concepts' in the signifying chains of 'judgments' (cf. Kant, 1781, A, III, 2, p. 259). Those recast analytical entities shall have, in turn, a single 'immediate relation' to the reshaped aesthetic synchronic-diachronic signifying structure of 'intuition' (ibid.).

The subject symbolically represented to another signifier

In the Lacanian transcendental 'logic of the signifier', the signifier determines every 'intuition' of 'aesthetics' and every 'concept' of 'logic', every spatio-temporal 'perception' and every analytical or dialectical 'understanding' (cf. Kant, 1781, A, I, 2, pp. 76–84). Actually, in every 'pure' or 'empirical knowledge' (B, introduction, §1, pp. 31–32), the only real 'knowledge' is the traumatic experience of the truth, 'the symptom' or the gap of wisdom, when a subject gets into contact, as a signifier, with another signifier (Lacan, 1970–1971, 10.02.71, p. 52). Besides involving the only possibility of real knowledge for the subject, this contact represents the only opportunity for the same subject to exist. As discussed above, the contact with a signifier subjectifies the individual, who can only be a subject by being subjected *to* the signifying structure, divided *by* it ($) and represented *in* it as a signifier (S1) in relation to another signifier (S2).

Just before stating that an 'individual' is 'subjectified' by his 'introduction to the signifier', Lacan (1958–1959) postulates: 'there is a subject only for another subject' (13.05.59). One year later, he reconsiders this idea and he acknowledges that *there is a subject only as a signifier for another signifier*. The 'subject' becomes a 'signifier' or a 'support of the signifier' in 'direct relation to the signifier' (1959–1960, 11.05.60, pp. 258–264). As for the signifier, it is defined as 'that which represents the subject *to* (*pour*) another signifier' (1960a, p. 299). Furthermore, 'the register of the signifier is instituted on the basis of the fact that a signifier represents a subject for another signifier' (1960b, p. 320). This idea often turns up in Lacan's teachings and writings during the Sixties. In 1970, Lacan still insists on the fact that 'a signifier is articulated by representing a subject for another signifier' (1969–1970, 14.01.70, p. 53). The same year, he puts in plain words that the subject is represented only for another signifier, 'which means: not to another subject' (1970a, pp. 412–413).

Let us take the case of Francisco Javier. The signifier "conviction" can represent him only for another signifier, such as "obligation", and not to another subject, such as María Luisa. However, the signifier "obligation" can, in turn, represent María Luisa to the signifier "conviction". In this social relation between the signifiers, the subjects can be absent in the flesh, but they are symbolically represented by these material words in quotation marks, "obligation" and "conviction", which we have right in front of our eyes. Moreover, even when the subjects meet in person, such as in the face-to-face encounter with hooded Eperrists, they continue to relate through the mediation of their symbolic representatives. These representatives are words, but also other signifying things, such as guns and hoods. In fact, even the bodies and corporeal gestures become signifiers. In this way, the real represented subjects incarnate *literally* their own symbolic representatives. Here is the social situation, well described by Marx, in which 'persons exist for other persons only as representatives' (1867, I, §2, p. 77). The individuals become signifiers, or signifying things, and have 'nothing in their breast' (III, §10, p. 180). Thus, in the signifying social structure, 'the social relations between things' take the place of the 'social relations between persons' (I, §1, p. 73). The signifying relations between structural positions take the place of the social links between subjects.[29] Francisco Javier, for example, should give up his place to the signifier "revolutionary" that may represent him only to other signifiers that may represent us in the signifying social structure.

If 'something is only represented *to*' (Lacan, 1960a, p. 299), the subject can be represented only *to* signifiers in a signifying social structure composed only of signifiers. Similarly, in Parliament, a Member of Parliament can represent a citizen only to other Members of Parliament. Accordingly, in order for a political representative to be considered to be so, there have to be other political representatives. Likewise, for the signifier (S1) to be the symbolic representative of the subject ($), there must be at least another signifier (S2). Besides another signifier, there must be, of course, a represented subject, since a signifier 'represents a subject and nothing else' (Lacan, 1969–1970, 14.01.70, p. 53). This is also the case for the political representative, who must represent someone to be representative. In the same way, the signifier must symbolically represent a subject to be a signifier. Assuming this idea, Lacanian Discourse Analysis must treat all signifiers in full speech, even the most impersonal ones (such as "pillar" or "germ"), as metaphorical symbolic representatives of real subjects (such as a revolutionary or his wife, an architect or a biologist, a German or a Jew for a Nazi).

Since the signifier is that which represents symbolically the real subject to another signifier, its mere existence necessarily requires at least another signifier and a real subject. The existence of the signifier "revolutionary", for example, requires a subject such as Francisco Javier, as well as another signifier, such as the "family". Obviously, as a "revolutionary", Francisco Javier can then be represented to the "family" by other signifiers, such as "the significance of marriage". This "significance" becomes representative of the "revolutionary" that represents the subject. Thus, from our Lacanian viewpoint, the "significance of marriage" does not represent simply a positive attitude towards "marriage", but it also represents the subject as a peculiar "revolutionary" in relation to the "family".[30]

The subject divided between two signifiers

As noted in the last chapter, a thing is a signifier, in Lacan's terminology, when it represents a subject, as a signifier, *to* another signifier. Correlatively, the individual is a subject when he is represented, by a signifier, for another signifier. In this instance, there is 'the emergence of what we call *a subject* because of the signifier that functions by representing the subject for another signifier' (Lacan, 1969–1970, 26.11.69, p. 11).

To be a subject, the individual should be represented, paradoxically, to a 'signifier' and 'not to another subject' (1970a, pp. 412–413). So, as we shall see in the next chapter, the subject is *alone* in his language. In this exteriority of his world, there is nothing but signifiers. This is why the representative of the subject can be only a signifier. This is also why this signifier can only be *oriented to* another signifier.[31]

In the signifying structure of society, there are only signifiers. Therefore, the representative of the subject cannot be oriented to another subject. Nor can it be oriented to the represented subject, who should be absent to be represented.[32] The signifier "revolutionary", for example, cannot represent Francisco Javier to himself, but only to other signifiers, such as "conviction" or "marriage". Similarly, the "revolutionary" cannot represent the subject to us, but rather to the signifiers that represent us, in Francisco Javier's revolutionary language, as perhaps "bourgeois" or "mandarins", or "moral cowards" or "inconsistent revolutionaries", or simply "old men" in contrast with the "new men".

If the signifier represented a subject to us, it would not be a signifier in the Lacanian sense of the word. It would not intransitively and unconsciously signify, but it would transitively signify the subject consciously represented to us. Then it would 'fall' into the status of the 'sign' (Lacan, 1970, p. 413). It would become a sign, in its Peircean definition, as '*representamem*' or 'something which stands for something to someone' (Peirce, 1897, 2.228, p. 135).

The sign represents its signification to someone. Its signification is also its representation. In a sense, by representing its signification, the sign describes it to us. The sign is a sort of *description* of what it signifies and represents to us. On the contrary, the signifier is rather a *definition* of what it represents for another signifier. It is a definition of a position in relation to another position in the signifying structure. In short, the signifier represents symbolically a subject by defining his position in our signifying social structure, while the sign represents imaginarily the same subject by describing his meaning in my individual mind.[33]

Sign	*Signifier*
Represents its signification to someone	Represents a subject for another signifier
Describes a mental meaning	Defines a structural position

By defining the position of the subject in relation to another position, the signifier represents symbolically the subject as a relation between two structural positions. Now, as the literal incarnation of his own symbolic representative, the subject materializes this relation between two signifiers. He materializes their connection, but also their separation, distinction and contradiction. He is thus divided between the two signifiers. Francisco Javier, for example, is divided ($) between the "revolution" (S1) and the Other of "marriage" (S2). Actually, as a subject, our Eperrist is the effect of this division between his identification with a signifier and his alienation in another signifier. At the same time, as an identificatory incarnation of the first signifier, the subject represents this effect of the contradiction between both signifiers. In some way, he is the 'sign' of the 'intermediary effect between what characterizes one signifier and another' (Lacan, 1972–1973, 16.01.73, p. 65). Francisco Javier can be regarded, in that way, as the *intermediary* effect between the "monogamous family" and the "new society", "our time" and the "future", the "obligation" and the "conviction", etc. Between these two sets of signifiers, we appreciate the effect of their partition and separation, that is to say, 'the gap that we call *the subject*' (Lacan, 1969–1970, 18.02.70, p. 101).

In Lacan's terminology, the term *subject* usually refers to a subjective gap or division ($) between the alienation in language (S2), in the predicative multiplicity of signifiers ("family", "marriage", "monogamy", etc.), and the identification with only one signifier ("revolution") that in this way becomes the individual grammatical subject of a statement (S1). As we know, this enunciated symbolic subject (S1) is not the same thing as the enunciating real subject ($). The former, social or individual representative (political state or citizen), does not exhaust the latter, dissociated or divided represented subject (social classes or individual fragments). Although the representative may become the symbolic identity of the real subject who identifies with it, this identification does not eliminate the distinction between the divided subject and the individual identity. So, this identity does not succeed in accurately representing the represented subject. This subject 'is represented' by the identitary signifier, 'of course, but simultaneously he is not represented' (Lacan, 1969–1970, 18.02.70, p. 102). He is not *really* represented. His representative is just symbolic. It has nothing to do with its real represented subject. On the one hand, the representative is a general signifier that may represent several subjects in an individual and univocal way (such as the "revolutionary" that may represent several Eperrists in a "consistent" way). On the other hand, each represented divided subject is not a general signifier, but an enunciating act that is unique, but not univocal (such as Francisco Javier, who is only one of his kind and apparently not too consistent). As evidenced by the object of any discourse (*a*), even the being of the real subject is not univocal, but rather equivocal (such as that which would "contribute to man's development and total fulfilment"). Therefore, it cannot be accurately represented by the univocal identity of the representative (S1). This identity cannot represent the being of the subject (*a*), but only one of his enunciating acts ($). As for his equivocal being, it is an object that can only be represented by the plurivocal alterity of the signifiers (S2). Composing a language, the signifiers actually represent and enchain the 'equivocations' in the 'history' of a subject (Lacan, 1972a, p. 490). This history represents a signifying chain of equivocations (or "inconsistencies"). It displays the discourse of a language, of the Other, as the unconscious.

Enunciated representatives	Univocal identity: a general signifier, an individual symbolic subject (S1)	Plurivocal alterity: a particular language, a predicative multiplicity of signifiers (S2)
Enunciating represented	Unique act: a divided real subject ($)	Equivocal being of the subject: object (a)

Notes

1. Parker (2003) envisages the possibility of 'connecting such an embodied conception of thinking with critiques of cognitive psychology from within philosophy that have taken as their prime target work on *artificial intelligence*' (p. 100). Against this artificial intelligence, we can object that it is nothing as long as it does not materialize, as discourse, in the perceptible form of a rather unintelligible or unconscious body. The corporeal real is necessary to realize literally the symbolic value of the imaginary reality of cognition. With this realization, the body becomes the letter of the thinking language, the real materiality of the symbolic system, the discourse of the Other.

As Parker notes, this discourse passes through 'the body as mediator in the field of the Other as unconscious' (p. 101). The discourse of the Other animates the body and moves its muscles. By moving, the muscles become the device of the system, the articulation of language. They thus belong to the Other and not to the proletarianized subject, who is reduced to the condition of the pure enunciating workforce of language. Now, to do the work of language, this workforce does not need any kind of intelligence. In the work of language, intelligence belongs to language. As for the proletarianized real subject, he is a pure unintelligent workforce applied to the unintelligible corporeal material. His intelligence is atrophied. *It is not.* Among real subjects, intelligence is just imaginary, or artificial.

2. In connection with this, Pêcheux (1975b) observes that the subject should already be the impossible result of his own result in order to 'produce as a result his own cause' (p. 141). This 'contradiction' gives rise to the '*Münchhausen* effect' inherent in every discourse (pp. 141–142).
3. Within the 'limits of discourse', this is how I interpret the situation, described by Hook (2003), in which 'the limitation of culture by nature' would 'determine the conditions of impossibility for the speaking subject and signification' (p. 31).
4. Similar to the subject of Pichonian social psychology, that of Lacanian psychoanalysis is not only a 'relational subject', but an 'agent, producer, protagonist of history, as well as a product formed by linking systems and complex configurations of relations' (Pichon-Rivière, 1975). Now, in Lacan, all those systems and configurations are included in the signifying structure of language.
5. This idea is not really new for discourse analysis in social psychology. Parker (2005a) recently regarded 'the unconscious' as 'what functions as absences in the text' (p. 171). Similarly, Billig (1997) recommended, for the analysis of the unconscious, that we 'examine the absences, rather than presences, in dialogue' (p. 140). Even Potter and Wetherell (1987) already understood that 'the absence is as important as the presence' (p. 31). And before all those authors, d'Unrug (1974) appreciated the necessity of studying the 'omissions' to analyze a 'discourse' as a 'partial actualization of unconscious processes' (pp. 79–80).
6. Together with the analysis proposed by d'Unrug (1974), Lacanian Discourse Analysis must appreciate the 'importance of omissions, errors, failures and everything which may be regarded as atypical in the analyzed discourse' (p. 80).
7. Just as in the Pichonian social psychology, the Lacanian implicit concrete psychology demonstrates here its diametric opposition to the American psychoanalytical or ego-psychological conception of a

'relational subject' who would be 'constituted independently of his external relations', in an 'autonomous mental life' and through the 'internalization of the social world' in the form of a 'super-ego' devoid of 'any kind of material base' (Pichon-Rivière & Quiroga, 1972).

8. In this regard, Hook (2008) speaks eloquently of an 'automatic instantiation of power' in 'an *immediate eventuality* of the subject's engagement with structure' (p. 60). This author discovers here an aspect of power considered by Lacan and ignored by Foucault, who would have concentrated only on its 'preconditions', its 'material causes' and its 'situational variables' (ibid.).
9. When Billig (1987) discusses this relationship in 'the connection between thinking and arguing', he observes rightly that 'there is nothing especially distinct about thinking, as opposed to arguing' (pp. 110–111). Now, unlike the rhetorical approach to social psychology, our Lacanian approach does not lead us to 'expect private thinking to be modelled upon public argument' (p. 111). In our perspective, it is not a question of *modelling*, but of essential indistinction and fundamental determination. Moreover, as will be seen in chapter eight, the *public argument* is neither arguable nor argumentative, but rather tyrannical and unarguable. As for its *public* character, it will be discussed in the next chapter.
10. It follows that only the speech of an individual may get in contact with the speech of another individual. As for their thoughts, they obviously cannot 'get in contact', unless we believe in telepathy (cf. Newcomb, Turner & Converse, 1965, p. 269).
11. According to Parker (2003), this 'Lacanian understanding of thinking in language' would have two important consequences for social psychology (p. 98). On the one hand, it implies that thought is 'an activity that is public and social rather that private and individual' (ibid.). On the other, it 'entails a rejection of notions of *communication* as the transmission of thoughts from one head to another through a transparent medium, with language assumed to be such a medium' (ibid.).
12. This Lacanian idea, which *should be interpreted too literally*, radicalizes a 'paradox' that Billig (1987) does not want 'to be interpreted too literally', namely, that 'humans do not converse because they have inner thoughts to express, but they have thoughts because they are able to converse' (p. 111).
13. Pêcheux (1975b) would observe here that 'thought is determined' by 'the unthinkable' of a 'discursive formation', which 'constitutes' every 'effect of sense', and which decides the 'edges, separations and limits' of what we think (p. 240).
14. When treating thought as a paraphrase of speech, Lacanians are diametrically opposed to cognitive social psychologists who consider

mysteriously that 'speech constitutes a paraphrase of thought' (Bromberg & Trognon, 2000, p. 294).

15. Obviously, I reject the strange Pichonian conception of a 'Lacanian idealism' (Pichon-Rivière, 1975). Even on the subject of desire, Lacan remains faithful to materialism. Just aswith Pichonian need, Lacanian desire is under a material determination (the signifier).
16. On this point, Lacanian materialism is quite the opposite of a cognitive idealism that imagines a 'knowledge basis' on which rests 'the text as superstructure' (Gaonac'h & Passerault, 1998, p. 349). Here is a rather coarse version of the Hegelian 'reversal' already refuted by Marx (1843a, pp. 874–915).
17. In this regard, Parker (2003) notes, with good reason, that 'thinking is understood by Lacan to be something operating within language, and so an activity that is public and social rather than private and individual' (p. 98).
18. According to Sharma (1998), there would be here, in this 'positive aspect' of Lacan, 'a sociolinguistic theory of subjectivity, which is highly compatible with discursive psychology' (p. 56).
19. These two representations of society are incompatible and irreconcilable. Since 'social psychology rests upon an image of individuals existing in social space and interacting with other people in that space, it cannot assimilate a Lacanian view of each individual human subject as always already social' (Parker, 2003, p. 105). By being constituted by the signifying social structure, the Lacanian subject is actually *always already social*. Now, as will be seen, the structure is not exactly the same for each one of its positions. It is not the same for a "psychologist" and for a "revolutionary". Nor is it the same for all "revolutionaries". The signifying social structure treats each subject differently. So, it is particular to each subject. It is its structure, its language, its unconscious. Seen from this angle, the Lacanian subject is *never already social*.
20. This explains 'the ambiguity of the social' that Frosh, Phoenix and Pattman (2003) detect in 'what Lacanians refer to as the accession to the Symbolic, the domain of language and culture' (p. 40). In this 'ambiguity', the 'subject is inserted into an order which lies beyond (pre-dating and post-dating) her or him, and that constrains what can be said and done' (ibid.). Nevertheless, the order resides only in what can be said and done by the force of the subject. This proletarianized workforce is indispensable for the work system of language, the unconscious or culture, which logically needs a workforce to work.
21. Here is the Lacanian version of the classic link that Benveniste (1958a) establishes between 'language' as the 'possibility of subjectivity', since 'it contains the linguistic forms' for 'its expression', and 'discourse' as

the 'emergence of subjectivity', since 'it consists of discrete elements' which fill with 'subjectivity' the 'empty forms' of language (p. 263).

22. In regard to this 'struggle of particular subjects as they locate themselves in relation' to 'social discourses', Frosh, Phoenix and Pattman (2003) assume the Lacanian standpoint to remark that 'there is no such thing as *the individual*, standing outside the social; however, there is an arena of personal subjectivity, even though this does not exist other than as already inscribed in the sociocultural domain' (pp. 39–42).
23. In this respect, D'Unrug (1974) refers to a contradiction and 'separation of the person' in which a separated 'term of the contradiction is assigned to another person' (p. 185). According to the author, this is how a 'speaker' would usually 'cope with the contradictions' of his 'speech' (p. 230).
24. In this view, Parker (1997b) proposes to 'treat the overall text as if it were a *subject*' (p. 488). Thus 'the text is treated as if it were a person, the second analytic move, in the same kind of way that a person is treated as a text in psychoanalysis, the first analytic move, but in such a way as to retain the first analytic move, and to embed the subject as text in text and the text in subject' (p. 489).
25. That is how the 'subject' and the 'subjectivity', in 'Lacanian theory', are 'structured in and by discursive relations which are institutionalized in culture and manifested in linguistic practice' (Frosh, Phoenix & Pattman, 2003, pp. 40–41).
26. Beauvois (1997) acknowledges shamelessly that his 'cognitive paradigm' is there to 'replace the subject of action by the subject of knowledge' (p. 8). In Lacanese: the function of a cognitive psychologist is to replace the real subject with an imaginary subject. So he joyfully throws away the recoverable part of behavioural psychology. Then, to keep himself busy, he kindly recovers the throwaway part of pre-behavioural psychology.
27. In cognitive psychology, this form is the only substance of knowledge. It belongs to the 'psychological event' that 'constitutes the sense, the meaning of the word', which would arise in the 'memory' of Francisco Javier when the 'stimulus-word' of "family" is 'perceived' (Gineste & Le Ny, 2002, p. 11).
28. By the same token, for Berger and Luckmann (1966) 'knowledge objectifies the world through language and the cognitive apparatus based on language' (p. 66). In the final analysis, it is 'language' itself that achieves the 'objectification' and thus becomes the 'basis' and even the 'depository' for the 'collective accumulation of knowledge' (pp. 68–69).
29. In an Althusserian-Lacanian perspective, Pêcheux (1969) would say here that an 'effect of sense' between 'places in the structure of a

social formation' replaces 'a transmission of information' between the 'human individual organisms' (p. 18). This replacement is actually the starting point for the subtle and rigorous *Automatic Discourse Analysis* (AAD) developed by Pêcheux.

30. This does not exclude the psychological idea of the social attitude. The "significance of marriage" can still be regarded, of course, as an attitude that performs its three general functions identified by Alexandre (1996): the 'simple judgment', the 'encoding' of 'information' and the 'token' of 'social membership' of the subject (pp. 30–31). However, in the analyzed discourse, the attitude and its general functions are completely subordinated to the relation between the representatives "revolutionary" and "family". The *attitude* towards "marriage" is nothing but a signifying relation of the revolutionary to "family". The *simplicity of the judgment* is "consistent" with the "consistence" of the "revolutionary". The "significance of marriage" *encodes* the "revolutionary" and its position in the social signifying structure.
31. Contrary to conversational analysis, a Lacanian Discourse Analysis must not treat the representative of a subject as oriented to another subject (e.g., Antaki, 1994), but in 'orientation to later terms in a sequence' (Parker, 2005a, p. 168). It is this 'orientation' which reveals the 'signifying value of a term' as representative of the subject to other terms (ibid.).
32. As Pêcheux (1975b) notes, 'the signifier represents the subject', but 'does not represent anything to the subject' (p. 243). It rather 'acts on him without being seized by him' (ibid.). The signifier is unconscious, in actual fact, precisely because it cannot be seized and it does not represent anything to the subject.
33. This distinction could underpin a reinterpretation of the two-dimensional model of social representations proposed by Moliner (1995, 2001). In the representative core, the 'definitions' and the 'norms' (2001, pp. 27–40) would correspond to the signifying structure and laws of language. In the representational periphery, the 'descriptions' would be signs related to imaginary 'cognitions' that help to 'manage the signification' (2001, pp. 28–33). A 'stereotype' would thus be a sign that 'describes' the signification of somebody to the cognition of somebody else, while the symbolic representative core would 'define' the position of the represented 'at the heart' of his imaginary stereotypical signification or 'representation' (Moliner & Vidal, 2003, pp. 169–171).

CHAPTER SIX

The unconscious as the discourse of the Other

In this chapter we examine the transcendental situation of the subject in the signifying chain. As a temporal unfolding of the spatial environment of language, that signifying chain will appear to us in the form of the unconscious as discourse of the Other. Going deeply into the Lacanian theory of the unconscious, we will find that every analyzable discourse actualizes this *discourse of a language*, a language that is not *the* language of *the* human race, but *a* language of *a* particular subject. We will appreciate how this language forms the outside world of the subject. Unlike some kind of cognitive interior of the consciousness, which is indirectly inferred by content analysis, such a discursive exteriority of the unconscious is directly analyzable by discourse analysis. It *is* discourse. As for its perceptible but unintelligible material structure, it constitutes the field of Lacanian psychoanalysis.

The unconscious locus of speech's deployment

The Lacanian unconscious can be minimally defined as the *discourse of a language*. This language consists of a 'set of signifiers' (Lacan, 1969–1970, 26.11.69, p. 12). The set organizes a place. It is *the place of the Other*. It includes everything that exists for each subject. It materializes through perceptible and unintelligible opaque materials such as ink and blood, textile and skin, steel and living muscles. These materials compose the exteriority inhabited by each subject, his symbolic universe, a signifying social structure for only one position in the structure.

The signifying structure is inherent in the set of signifiers separately used and incarnated by each subject. As the unconscious of only one subject, this structure *for his position* does not constitute a common place. It is an exclusive place for only one subject. Nevertheless, *in itself*, the structure is a public place that contains the social space of culture and civilization.[1] This space is shared by all its positions. It opens around all subjects, but also in each subject, when language 'eats the real' or 'hollows out' the individual nature of the human being (Lacan, 1975–1976, 09.12.75, pp. 31–32).

The social space of culture and civilization is organized by the logic of the signifier. It is thus characterized by its 'articulation according to logical laws' (Lacan, 1956–1957, 05.12.56, p. 51). These laws are the laws of language. They put in order the social space, which is the space of speech, wherein the subject speaks precisely that which he must speak in order to obey the laws of language. Actually, when 'the subject speaks', the place of the 'Other' opens as a 'locus of speech' (Lacan, 1957–1958, 25.06.58, p. 475). As such, as the 'locus of speech's deployment' (1958d, p. 105), the 'Other' is defined by Lacan as 'the locus in which speech is verified as it encounters the exchange of signifiers' (1960b, p. 329). In this exchange, what speech encounters is the structure that gives it form. *When the subject speaks, his own speech is shaped by the unconscious locus of speech's deployment. It is thus articulated by the signifying social structure of language. Now, subjected to this structure, the proletarianized real subject functions as the speaking workforce of language. He gives his breath and his tongue to this Other, as well as his other muscles, his outer and inner senses, his perceptive capacities and mental resources.*

If the subject gives everything to language, it is because the subject himself belongs to language. He is included in language. Just as the Humboldtian man who 'thinks, feels and lives only in language' (Humboldt, 1821, p. 157), the Lacanian human subject, as a speaking being, is a 'living being' who 'stands out from the others because of the fact of living in language' (Lacan, 1973b, p. 554). In actual fact, this language 'is inhabited by everyone who speaks' (1971, p. 15). As a speaking being, the subject is not only subjected to language, but incorporated into it. His life can be regarded as a full speech that is full of the subject. In Lacan, this full speech is the discourse of the Other.

As language, the Other articulates and embraces the lives of all human living beings. *He* surrounds all those beings and comes between them. *He* organizes the environment for each one of their positions. *For each position*, the Other is *himself*, as the unconscious, an organic living environment that lives on the life of an individual subject. At the same time, as a signifying social structure *in itself*, the Other is composed of cumulative laws and wisdom that overdetermine everything in the shared space of culture and civilization inhabited by all subjects.[2] In any case, all individual subjects live within the signifying structure of society. Their place is in this locus of speech's deployment. Actually, '*to be a subject* means *to have a place in the Other*, as the locus of speech' (Lacan, 1960–1961, 26.04.61, p. 299). It is this 'geometrical place' of language where the subject is initially born and is now living 'in the flesh' (Lacan, 1953b, p. 147).

As the 'locus in which is situated the chain of the signifier that governs whatever may be made present of the subject', the Lacanian Other can be described as the 'field of living being in which the subject has to appear' (Lacan, 1964, 27.05.64, p. 228). The Other is actually the only field of emergence and existence of the subject. It is the ecosystem of a subject who is only made of language, who is derived from language and depends on language. In relation to this derived and dependent 'subject', the Other is 'the locus of his signifying cause' (1960b, p. 321).

Arising from the Other, 'the subject cannot be his own cause' (Lacan, 1960b, p. 321). He cannot rise into existence by pulling himself up by his hair. He needs someone else to pull him up. He needs an Other, a language, a creator. The subject alone is not enough to exist. For him, *to be* is not enough *to exist*. Unlike God, the 'essence' of the subject cannot 'imply his existence' (Spinoza, 1674, II, ax., p. 70). This is why the human subject cannot be 'his own cause' (I, VII, pp. 25–26). His cause has to be elsewhere, outside himself, but certainly around him, where his speech resounds, in the exteriority of his unconscious, in his language environment, in the signifying social structure, in this Other who causes the subject by articulating his speech.

As full speech, the discourse of the Other is full of a living subject. To fill the signifying chain, this living subject should occupy, at each moment, one individual position in the signifying social structure. At first sight, the position may be shared between several subjects, such as the position of the "revolutionary", in which Francisco Javier meets with other revolutionaries. However, all things considered, we acknowledge that the position of the "revolutionary" is not exactly the same for all revolutionaries, since the signifying social structure is not exactly the same for all of them. There are as many positions as revolutionaries. In itself, the signifying social structure treats differently each one of these positions of the "revolutionary", as evidenced by the differences between Jacobins and Girondins, Bolsheviks and Mensheviks, Zapatistas and Carrancistas, Che Guevara and Fidel Castro, Trotsky and Stalin, Danton and Robespierre, etc. The disparities between these positions of different "revolutionaries" are as deep as the distinction between the positions of a "revolutionary" and a "counter-revolutionary", or a "proletarian" and a "capitalist". In any case, the same social structure *in itself* is a different structure *for each position in the structure*. The same language 'in general' is in each case *a* 'particular' language (Lenin, 1915, p. 345). The same general structure overdetermines each position in a particular way. For each position, *the* language is *a* language. *The* "revolutionary" is *a* "revolutionary" such as Francisco Javier. The Other is an unconscious, a language, the culture of a subject, the society for a member of society.[3]

The subject in the universal interior of the symbolic exteriority

The Other is the only battlefield where Francisco Javier may act as a "revolutionary". Now, to act as such, the Eperrist shall act in a symbolic way, through symbols, even when these symbols are written in blood. It goes without saying that a non-symbolic action would not be revolutionary, for the very reason that it would not symbolize any kind of revolution, or, what is more, it would not be symbolically signifying as "revolutionary". To put the case clearly, revolutionary actions are nothing but enunciating acts. As for the objective revolution, it constitutes merely an enunciated fact.[4]

The revolution is composed of signifiers. It can only take place within language. This language is the only arena of the revolutionary.

It includes the street for his barricade, the Bastille to be taken, or the palace to be sacked, and not only the rostrum for a verbal discourse. The revolutionary operates inside language. He is language. Why should language be his *Other*? Isn't it rather the Same of the revolutionary? The question may receive two opposite answers:

- *No*, the Other is not the Same of a "revolutionary", but his Other. As language or the locus of speech, the theatre of the revolution is neither subjective nor individual, but rather trans-individual and inter-subjective, or even supra-subjective. This is why language may precede the ontogenesis of the subject. This is also why the social signifying structure, as illustrated by the functioning of the economic system, is beyond the control and the consciousness of each member of society.
- *Yes*, the Other is the Same of the "revolutionary". As a signifier, the "revolutionary" is the same thing as language. *He* is included in language. *He* is thus a part of the Other. Actually, 'a signifier' could 'in no way appear outside that locus', since 'there is no Other of the Other' (Lacan, 1960a, p. 293). In other words, 'there is no metalanguage' (ibid.). Since the "revolutionary" shall remain within *his official* language, *he* cannot belong to an alternative metalanguage. He can only stay in the conventional and conservative language of "our time". To 'speak about' this reactionary language, there is no revolutionary language that could function as a 'metalanguage' (cf. Barthes, 1957, p. 200). There is no such thing, since every language, for one subject, is indistinguishable from *his* one and only language. It follows that the 'linguistic code' does *not* 'differ' from other codes (cf. Anzieu, 1981, pp. 169–170). It does *not* have a 'metacommunicative function' (ibid.). It does *not* 'communicate information' about 'the other codes' that are always the same code (ibid.). At one moment, there is only one code for one subject. For his structural position, there is only one structure. There is only one language. There is *no* 'outside of language' (Derrida, 1967, pp. 227–228). There is no position that would be exterior to the exteriority of the signifying social structure.[5]

Ironically, the Other is everything for a subject. Even the subject is Other to himself. There is thus not a Same in relation to the Other. For the subject, there is only the Other of language. All material things remain in the universal interior of this symbolic exteriority. So, language appears as the 'symbolic universe' of Berger and Luckmann (1966), that is to say, a 'symbolic totality' that 'integrates' and 'embraces everything' (pp. 95–96), that 'puts everything in the right place' (p. 98), that 'legitimates roles, priorities and procedures by situating them *sub specie universi*, in the context of the most general frame of reference that we may conceive' (p. 99). Now, in our perspective, this *universal frame of reference* can only be materialized by *the most particular frame*, the singular one, that of the individual. Together with Marxist-Leninist dialectics, our Freudian-Lacanian dialectics must postulate that 'the general exists only in the particular and by the particular' (Lenin, 1915, p. 345). The generality of *the* universe comes true in the particularity of *an* individual.[6] It is thus particular, but also universal, or 'general' (ibid.). It is only *a* language, but this language is the only one for a certain subject, and there is no metalanguage. There is the Other of only one certain subject, but there is no Other of this Other.

For one subject, there is only one particular Other. Symmetrically, this particular Other is only for one subject. If the social signifying structure exists only as a particular structure, this structure exists only for the position of one individual member of society. Outside this exclusive structure, 'in the place of the Other of the Other, there is no existence' (Lacan, 1975–1976, 13.04.76, p. 134). Even the Same (the "revolutionary") exists inside the Other (in the counter-revolutionary system). Therefore, the Other is not the Other (the Other of the "revolutionary"), since there is no Same, or Other of the Other (an alternative "revolutionary" who would be Other than the official symbolic system of "our time"). Without this 'Other of the Other', the Other cannot 'exist' (Miller, 2002, p. 12). It cannot 'exist as an Other in order to ground an existence' (ibid.).

Since there is no Other of the Other, a "revolutionary" can only exist as a component part of *his* counter-revolutionary Other. Accordingly, this Other is not really the Other of the "revolutionary", who is only a signifier among the other signifiers that compose the Other. In actual fact, there is no real Other of the "revolutionary". Nor is there, consequently, a real revolutionary. The 'always fading' Other puts the revolutionary 'in an always fading position' (Lacan, 1960–1961, 01.03.61, p. 202).

As the fading "revolutionary", the so-called Other is just symbolic. It is just the whole of all signifiers. In relation to the "revolutionary", it is just another signifier of the whole. However, some "revolutionaries" may regard this signifier wrongly as a real counter-revolutionary subject. Just as do these credulous "revolutionaries", we "psychologists" usually take signifiers for subjects. The same is true for the majority of "citizens", "sociologists", "philosophers", "theologians", "priests", "lovers" and all other naïve believers. By treating their symbolic Other as a real Other, all of them confer a certain prestige upon it. In relation to the "human creature", the other signifier can even become the divine Other called "God" or "Creator". The fact remains that this effective Creator is purely symbolic. Therefore, it is totally based on faith. In general, the Other is always based on faith.

As language, the Other is the Creator of everything, including individual subjects and their society. Nevertheless, as a purely symbolic system, the Other is a virtual and uncertain product of convention, confidence, credence, credibility, credulity and even superstition of the same individual subjects and their society.[7] Even though it determines everything, the Other is just symbolic. The real (*a*) fails the Other (S2). The result is loneliness and despair, but also desire, and even love and hatred, faith and frustration, and finally the subject ($) who feels all this and who proves thus to be something more than a signifier (S1). The subject proves this as long as the signifying symbolic relation (S1–S2) is not enough for him, a subject in the flesh, who needs a real relationship (as illustrated by the "sexual love" or the "faithfulness from conviction" of Francisco Javier). Unfortunately, such a thing is impossible, since the Other is purely symbolic.

Apart from the enunciating act, it is impossible for the real subject to establish a real relationship with the symbolic Other. This impossibility justifies all the subject's feelings.[8] Thus, in a sense, it is the symbolic character of the Other that makes possible the real existence of the subject. The symbolic produces the real (*a*) of the same enunciating subject ($) that produces the symbolic (S1–S2). This real corresponds to the object that is always lacking in language. It is the object *a* of Lacan. It is the real being of the subject. As it cannot be included in the symbolic, it has to be excluded from the symbolic. This exclusion *from* language explains its production *by* language. The symbolic universe of language has to produce or *release* a real objective residue that cannot be signifierized or included in language. Somehow or other, this residue lies beneath all subjective feelings.

The personal subjective incarnations of the Other

Once refined or *purified* of any kind of real objective residue, language cannot be purely and entirely symbolic. Its symbolic system requires a real subjective support. There would not be an enunciated fact without an enunciating act. There would not be the symbolic without the real of the symbolic. The letter of the word is essential for its sense. The signifier necessitates the enunciating workforce of a corporeal subject who materializes it through sounds, inscriptions, gestures, behaviours, clothes, buildings, etc. That which is spoken needs a speaker to incarnate it. It also needs a listener, who becomes another speaker during socialization and interaction.

Imaginary other	*Symbolic Other*
Consciousness	Unconscious
Cognitive solipsism	Discursive inter-subjectivity
Individual and solitary knowledge	Social and interacting wisdom

Beyond the individual and solitary knowledge of the imaginary *other*, there is the social and interacting wisdom of the symbolic *Other*, the 'discourse' of language, which 'implies another subject, an interlocutor' (Evans, 1996, p. 44). Beyond the conscious and cognitive solipsism that 'clings' to the objective 'opacity' of the mirror (Lacan, 1967a, p. 354), there is the 'inter-subjective' and 'trans-individual' transparency of 'discourse' and 'language' (Evans, 1996, p. 44). In this transparency of the unconscious, the Other is not personified by only one real enunciating subject, but also by another real enunciating subject, the interlocutor, who can disguise himself and deceive the other subject, manipulate his intentions and conceal his own intentions. In this case, the Other is 'immediately and effectively given as a subject' (Lacan, 1957–1958, 25.06.58, p. 475). *He* is my interlocutor, my adversary, my fellow-creature, but also my Creator, my God. He is the incarnate Other. As such, he can treat me as an object. He can play with me as with a toy, but also mercifully as with another player. He becomes thus my competitor, the 'Other' of my 'strategy', the Other with his stratagems, which can be illustrated by 'chess' (ibid.).

Another subject can become *our* Other as long as he acts upon us, and plays with *us*, whether as toys or players. As toys, we are nothing more than his objects. As players, we are subjects in an inter-subjective relationship with him. But even in this inter-subjective relationship, the Other can always be personified by a subject that misleads us, such as the 'cunning genius' who 'deceives' Descartes (1640, I, p. 75). As the literal incarnation of the Other, Francisco Javier, for example, might tell us all kinds of stories about "marriage" and "faithfulness" with the only purpose being to prompt our bourgeois sympathy. He might also tell us true stories that seem to be false, thus deceiving us by means of the difference between his enunciating act and the enunciated fact. If that is the case, he might take advantage of the incredulity of an avant-garde, mischievous listener, who would congratulate Francisco Javier's false capacity to deceive all the brainless bourgeois, and their conformist ideology, by telling them all kinds of ridiculous stories about "marriage" and "faithfulness". In all these situations, Francisco Javier would be a consummate subject, an Other who enjoys all the privileges of the Other, in particular the right to conceal one's intentions and hide one's cards, which enables him to shy away from those psychologists who would try to know his tactics, his plans, his thoughts.[9]

Besides proceeding secretly, the Other seems to act as a player who deceives by giving credibility to himself. But the player cannot ensure his own credibility. He cannot testify to his own honesty. He cannot be the judge of his own cause. To determine his credibility as a player, the Other should be someone else. He should be language. It is 'language' itself that 'gives credibility to the speaker' (Aristotle, *Rhetoric*, I, 1356).

At the level of an Aristotelian *ethos*, the language is not personified by the speaker, but it materializes a third party that gives credibility to the speaker in relation to the listener. Thus, as language, the Other is something more than a cunning genius. Besides playing and deceiving, the incarnate language acts as the only authority that may supposedly prevent any kind of deception between the players of discourse.

In the arbitration that Lacan proposes instead of the Saussurean arbitrary, the Other is the arbiter of inter-subjective symbolic play. In this way, the Other proves to be *someone*. Language proves to be a third person. *He* is actually the only presence that may guarantee the credibility of the speaker, or the 'sincerity condition' of Searle (1969, p. 60). Obviously, this condition must always exist, even in deception, as the deceived listener would not be deceived if he did not believe to a certain extent in the sincerity and credibility of the deceiving speaker.

To be credible, the speaker is not enough. Besides him, there must be a judge, a witness, a third person, an arbiter, or an Other. Now, leaving aside God, there is nobody who could personify this Other, since there is nobody who could be present at the communication and entirely grasp it, neutrally consider it, and fairly judge it, in a totally impartial way. All subjects have specific positions in the signifying social structure. Accordingly, all subjects are partial. Their partiality corresponds to the bias of a particular signifier. Logically, there is only the totality of the signifiers, or language itself, that can materialize the Other and fairly judge every act of communication in a totally impartial way. It is thus only the channel of communication that may guarantee the reliability of communication. It is language itself, through *its* discourse (the discourse of the Other), which can persuade the listener of the credibility of the speaker. As Aristotle observed, this supposed credibility is an 'effect of discourse', as the 'honesty of the speaker does not contribute to the persuasion' (*Rhetoric*, I, 1356).

When two people interact, their interaction depends on a third person, the Other, who is materialized in the signifying social structure. Thanks to this third party, the inter-subjective relation is not only a mirrored subjective reflection. Thanks to the 'mediation' of this 'third personage', the interaction is not purely imaginary, but instead it acquires its real structure and its 'symbolic value' (Lacan, 1953c, p. 38). It thus becomes 'analyzable' or 'symbolically interpretable' (ibid.).

In a Lacanian perspective, we assume that a discourse is only analyzable when we consider its so-called author as well as the Other. On that assumption, a Lacanian Discourse Analysis must connect three persons, namely, the reader or listener, the writer or speaker, and a third person, the Other, as the personification of language.

To put the case clearly, there must be an explicit connection between the living incarnations of two structural positions and the signifying social structure. In my analysis of Francisco Javier's discourse, for example, I should make explicit the structural interaction between Francisco Javier as the incarnation of his unique "revolutionary" position, myself as the embodiment of my inimitable 'Lacanian' position, and the Other as the personification of the structure *for my position* in the structure, in a signifying structure that is also, *in itself*, a social structure that I share with the Eperrist.

It goes without saying that we cannot analyze a discourse without including the Other in our analysis. In general, two subjects could not even interact through speech without interacting with a third party, a personification of language, *who* speaks through the speaking subjects. On this point, Lacan (1957–1958) observes that, 'since there is a speaking subject, we cannot reduce to an other', to an *imaginary other*, 'his relationship' to his listener, 'but there is always a third party, the Other', the *symbolic Other* (Lacan, 1957–1958, 22.01.58, p. 179). Materialized in language, this Other is obviously none of the subjects who interact through language. To enable inter-subjectivity, the Other has to escape inter-subjectivity. To make possible speech and communication, it must be unspeakable and incommunicable, inexpressible and incomprehensible.[10]

As a necessary condition for interlocution, the Other distinguishes itself from the interlocution itself and not only from the interlocutors.[11] To be sure, the Other does not correspond to the interlocution, but *he* is the one *who* articulates the interlocution through the interlocutors. Logically, *he* is not the same thing as *his* interlocution. Similarly, as part of the interlocution, a discourse is not the same thing as the Other, but it is a *discourse of the Other*, that is to say, a *discourse of language*.

As the personification of the living system that articulates every interlocution, the Other cannot be reduced either to the interlocution or to the interlocutors. Simultaneously, as the personification of the signifying social structure in itself, the Other cannot be reduced to the organization of the structure for the structural position of only one interlocutor. *In itself*, as the impartial guarantee of interlocution, the structure should be the same for the positions of both interlocutors. Generally, and theoretically, the social structure in itself should be the same for all its structural positions. But that is not so.

The same structure in itself is a different structure for each one of its positions. The same economic system of society is not the same for all members of society. Our system does not treat everybody in the same way. The same symbolic universe varies from place to place. It is not the same universe for a capitalist or a proletarian, for an Englishman or an African, for a social psychologist or a hooded revolutionary. The structure for me differs entirely from the structure for an Eperrist. Even if both individual structures belong to the same social structure in itself, both structures are not identical. Accordingly, the unconscious of the Eperrist is not my unconscious. Both intra-subjective languages are not the same, even if they belong to the same inter-subjective language.

In a Lacanian Discourse Analysis, it would be advisable to distinguish between the signifying social structure in itself, as the inter-subjective shared language, and the structure for each structural individual position, as the intra-subjective unconscious language.[12] Besides the subjective roles of the Other in inter-subjectivity, whether as the *interlocutor* or *extra-locutor* that guarantees the reliability of communication, we would thus conceive the subjective role of the Other, as the *intra-locutor*, in intra-subjectivity. In that case, the Other is neither materialized by *the* language nor personified by another subject. Instead, *he* is embodied by *myself* and materialized by *a* language, my language, which expresses itself through my thought and my speech. In Cartesian terms, the Other is neither God nor the cunning genius, but *he* is Descartes (1640) as a speaking and 'thinking thing' (II, pp. 81–85). *He* is the subject of the Cogito, the one who thinks, since 'thought' is just a 'silent interior dialogue of the soul' (Plato, *Sophist*, 263d-e).

As the *interior dialogue* between the identificatory position of the subject (S1) and the alienating structure for this position (S2), the intra-locution reminds us of the Bakhtinian 'hybrid construction', with its 'two perspectives' that 'intersect' in only one 'locutor' (Bakhtin, 1934, p. 125). Beyond this construction, the intra-locution can be also compared, in Bakhtin, to the 'bi-vocal discourse', which is 'concentrated on itself' and 'interiorly dialogized' through a dialogue between 'two locutors' with 'two different intentions' (pp. 144–145). However, unlike this Bakhtinian bi-vocal discourse, the Lacanian intra-locution between *my* position (S1) and *my* structure (S2) not only has 'roots that deeply penetrate into sociolinguistic diversity', but it also 'dips' into 'individual contradictions, misunderstandings and dissonances' (pp. 145–146).

The Lacanian intra-locution is not only social, but also individual. Since the signifying social structure (S2) for an individual position (S1) is not identical to the same structure in itself, the intra-locutory distinctiveness is not a simple internalization of the extra-locutory particularity of a shared objective or inter-subjective system.[13] At the intra-locutory level, the social structure is individualized in a unique way for the individual subject. Correlatively, at the interlocutory level, the individual subject is completely alienated as an element of the social structure. In this structure, he becomes 'another thing different from himself' (Lacan, 1957–1958, 25.06.58, p. 476). He is transformed into 'the Other as himself' (ibid.). The fact remains that this alienation is precisely that which makes it possible for him to dialogue with himself in the intra-locution. Since the individual subject should occupy a structural position (S1) and could never remain *only* 'neutral' as the Other (S2), or the 'third person' of an interlocution (Bakhtin, 1934, p. 135), his interlocutory alienation in the social structure necessarily entails the precondition for his intra-locution, namely, the division ($) of his individuality between his identificatory individual position (S1) and the alienating social structure (S2).

Because of his alienation in the signifying social structure in itself, the subject acquires simultaneously a position in the structure (S1) and an unconscious intra-subjective structure (S2), which is nothing but the signifying social structure for his structural individual position (S1–S2). The enunciating subject is thus divided between his identification with his position (S1) and his alienation in the structure (S2). He is divided between one signifier (the enunciated subject) and all the other signifiers (the predicative language).

As an Aristotelian 'political (*ethos*) animal (*pathos*) with the capacity to speak and think (*logos*)' (Eggs, 1999, p. 47), the subject is not only an alienated (*ethos*) body (*pathos*) with an enunciating power (*logos*), but he is also a body (*pathos*) whose enunciating act (*logos*) entails a division ($) between his individual identity (S1) and his alienation (S2) in the Other (*ethos*). Through the enunciating act, it is this alienation in language that causes a division of the subject. So, in a sense, it is the Other *who* alienates and divides the subject.[14] This alienating and dividing power of the Other is only blatantly observable in his individual function as intra-locutor. However, it is already exerted in his social and cultural function as interlocutor and extra-locutor, as evidenced by Francisco Javier's alienation and division in the answer *of his* language (of the Other as extra-locutor) to María Luisa's question (of the Other as interlocutor).

Let us recapitulate. *We may differentiate between three personal subjective incarnations of the same alienating and dividing symbolic Other, namely, a social interlocutor who may deceive us in his discourse, an individual intra-locutor who shall mislead us in what we take for our own discourse, and a cultural extra-locutor or third person who will ensure the reliability of both discourses. Despite their apparent differences, these inter-subjective, intra-subjective and extra-subjective incarnations personify the same signifying structure of language.* They are living manifestations of the same topological subjective complex of language as the place of 'discourse', or the locus of speech, and not only as the 'subject of discourse' (Althusser, 1966a, pp. 145–146). Thus, in the 'internal region' in which Humboldt (1834) discovered the 'inner form of language' (§21, p. 231), there is not only the intra-subjective exteriority of the individual, but also the extra-subjective and inter-subjective exteriorities of culture and society.[15]

The impersonal incarnate locations of the Other

From our Lacanian perspective, culture and society are facets of the exteriority that deploys in language. They are included in this language that articulates the analyzed discourse. As noted by Benveniste (1968), language 'includes society, but is not included by society' (p. 96). This is why 'one may isolate language' and 'describe it regardless of its use in society', but 'it is impossible to describe culture and society independently of their linguistic expressions' (ibid.). Now, in Lacan, these expressions are individual and not only social and cultural. In this, culture and society are literally included in the language of an individual subject. They are intra-subjective and not only inter-subjective and extra-subjective.

Almost two centuries ago, Humboldt (1821) had already written that 'not only in its exteriority, but also in its interiority, as thought, language is the nation itself' (p. 125). Let us translate: not only in its inter-subjective and extra-subjective exteriority, but also in its intra-subjective exteriority, as the unconscious of an individual subject, language is identical to culture and society.

All things considered, language can basically be described as the cultural, social and individual unconscious structure that determines the position of each subject and organizes the human world in its extra-subjective, inter-subjective and intra-subjective dimensions.[16] This structure forms a matrix that decides everything regarding subjectivity. As a cultural sphere, it can even be compared to a 'natural sphere' of the human subject (Lacan, 1966c, p. 223). Actually, it constitutes the *nature of the subject*, which is also the *culture for the subject*. For the subject, for his structural position, the structure of language thus materializes the 'Other' as 'culture settled in its symbolic order' (Resweber, 1998). Just as society, this culture is only another name for the unconscious exteriority that contains the conscious internal thoughts of the subject.[17]

In a sense, *a* culture *is* language. Francisco Javier's culture, for example, is composed of "marriage" and the "monogamous family", but also of his manners, his clothes and all the other signifiers of *his* language. As illustrated by the hood of the Eperrist, those external opaque signifiers hold the conjectural consciousness of the subject. However, they are not conscious, but unconscious. They are not mentally signified, but physically signifying. They are not intelligible cognitive entities of thinking, but perceptible discursive elements of language.

As *a* culture, *a* language forms the unconscious of *a* subject. It is the social structure unconsciously organized for his individual structural position. It is thus social, granted, but it cannot be assimilated into a 'collective consciousness' (cf. Mukarovsky, 1929, p. 56). As Jakobson (1929) notices, this consciousness represents a 'simple metaphor' of language, of its pure signifying structure, which can be compared to an odd kind of external unconscious 'ideology' (p. 59).

In its unconscious ideological exteriority, language is just the 'locus of speech' (Lacan, 1957–1958, 25.06.58, p. 476). It is just a 'living' structure that is inhabited by the subject, and embodied by his Other, who 'answers' him (ibid.). Whether as interlocutor, extra-locutor, or intra-locutor, this Other is not inside the subject, but outside. He remains outside his consciousness. He personifies the material exteriority of his unconscious. Even as intra-locutor, *he* resides in the exteriority.

As an intra-locutor, the Other may be paradoxically described as an *intra-subjective exteriority*. Berger and Luckmann (1966) would explain this as the 'internalization of language' and the resultant 'formation, in consciousness, of a generalized other' (pp. 133–135). This holds in a phenomenological perspective, but in our psychoanalytical perspective, the intra-subjective exteriority would be explained, rather, by the internal alienation of the subject in the exteriority of language and the ensuing formation, as the unconscious, of a particularized Other.

As an intra-subjective exteriority, the Other is situated in the particular sphere of the individual subject. It embodies the structure *for* the subject, which is the only structure *of* the subject. It is thus in the subject, granted, but that does not mean that it is in his mind. In actual fact, the Other is 'everywhere else' (Lacan, 1953b, p. 148). The unconscious is everywhere outside the mental interiority of the subject. And yet, it is in the subject. It is even what thinks in him. It is his body as the intra-subjective thinking workplace of the unconscious. As the corporeal structure that subjects and subjectifies a subject, the unconscious is the structure *of* its effect of subjectivity. Personified in a divine Other as the 'immanent cause' that exists in its 'effects' (Spinoza, 1674, I, XVIII, p. 43), the unconscious 'exists in its effect of subjectivity' (Althusser, 1966a, pp. 129–131). It exists in all its other effects also. It exists everywhere outside consciousness, which is nevertheless *its* consciousness, 'the consciousness of the unconscious' (Pavón Cuéllar, forthcoming).

Even if the Other, as the unconscious, seems to be 'nowhere', it is in reality 'everywhere', as exteriority (Lacan, 1973a, p. 511). As such, it is deployed everywhere in *our body*, which becomes *his body*, the totality of our material environment, as the corporeal structure in which we exist. As the body of the world, the unconscious is *corporeally written* everywhere in the form of 'the symbolic' as the 'preformed matter' of 'the unconscious' (Lacan, 1972c, p. 548). It consists of a three-dimensional 'archi-writing' that *writes*, engraves or carves the universe for each one of us (cf. Derrida, 1967, pp. 75–88). The characters of this writing spread far and wide, everywhere around us, in the unconscious exteriority of all those things that are written for each one of us. Now, all those things compose an unconscious exteriority precisely because they have been *written*. Just as any other writing, the 'writing' of everything around us 'causes oblivion in our souls', as it proceeds 'on the outside, in foreign characters, and not on the inside, in ourselves' (Plato, *Phaedrus*, 275a).

Instead of consciously thinking, we are always unconsciously reading the foreign characters of the Other. In their spatial geometry, these signifying elements configure our universe, but they cannot become consciously signified. As repeatedly noted before, they are external and not internal, material and not ideal, physical and not mental.

The psychic stuff of the unconscious amounts to the physical stuff of the perceptible world. It is that which is perceived, for instance, in Francisco Javier's "perception of the world". It is the material and external environment of the human being. Thus, in Lacan, the unconscious 'is neither the obscure pulsation of the so-called instinct, nor the core of Being, but a habitat', a 'real medium', a 'bath of language' in which man is 'immersed' (Lacan, 1966c, p. 223). Obviously, this physical bath of language does not reside in the mind of the subject. And yet, it is in his body. As the intra-subjective exteriority, language holds, impregnates and possesses this body, and its real substance, which is thus transformed into the real of the symbolic, the structure of language, the flesh of the word.[18] All corporeal forms, members and movements are signifierized. The resulting literal signifiers are the enunciated gestures of an Other in which the enunciating subject cannot recognize himself. The body of the subject is thus alienated. It becomes the economic system of language, the real structure of the symbolic, the human body of the Other. Henceforth, the Other functions as an unconscious that possesses our body and speaks through it. The body turns into the locus of speech.

As the corporeal individualization of the signifying structure of culture and society, the intra-subjective 'place of the Other' must be situated 'in the body', as 'tegumentary scars, peduncles to be plugged into openings, ancestral artifices and techniques that eat into the body' (Lacan, 1967f, p. 327). Thinking through this 'structure of language' that 'carves his body', the 'subject of the unconscious touches the soul through the body' (1973a, p. 512). He thinks through his body, or, more precisely, he alienates his body in the structure that thinks through it. As an alienated body, the subject becomes the thinking workplace of his unconscious. He turns into a place or a simple structural position. He is absorbed by the structure for his position. In that way, he loses his personality and his subjectivity. He is not a personal subjective incarnation of the Other any more, but he turns out to be an incarnate impersonal place for the Other and *his* personal incarnations. For the subject, this place is basically intra-subjective. It is *his* individual body. However, in itself, the place is also inter-subjective, as the trans-individual body of society.

Impersonal incarnate locations of the Other	Individual Trans-individual
Personal subjective incarnations of the Other	Intra-subjective Inter-subjective Extra-subjective

Besides differentiating between the personal subjective incarnations of the Other, we can make a topical distinction between two impersonal incarnate locations of the same Other as the unconscious locus of speech: one in the individual body of each subject, the other in the trans-individual body of society. The former embodies the signifying social and cultural structure for the individual position of the subject, while the latter embodies the same trans-individual structure in itself. Adding these two locations to the previously examined three incarnations, we have at our disposal five distinct valid dimensions of the same Other that can be separately considered in Lacanian Discourse Analysis.[19] With these five dimensions, we embrace and specify the three conceptions already distinguished by Dreyfuss and his colleagues in Lacan's work, namely, the 'Other as inter-subjective common place', or trans-individual locus of speech; the 'Other in the subjective structure', as the individual locus of speech; and the 'Other in inter-subjectivity', corresponding to the three personal subjective incarnations of the Other (Dreyfuss et al., 1999, pp. 218–225).

Consciousness as an illusion of the unconscious

Whether as an impersonal location or as a personal incarnation, the language of a subject has to exist as an Other for that subject. Actually, for the subject to exist, the Other also has to exist for him, and exist as his Other, since only *something other than he* can be his world and his structure, his matrix and his body, his cause and his condition.

It is true that the signifierized subject becomes the piece of a language that could not then be his Other. However, to exist as a subject, this signifier has to be something different than its language. It has to be something more than a signifier. In a sense, the subject as a signifier should be signified as a subject in order to be a subject and not only a signifier. Now, as a signifier, the subject 'cannot signify himself', but he needs an Other to 'signify him' (Lacan, 1966–1967, 07.12.66). The Other is necessary for the signifier to exist as a subject, since the signifier can 'signify everything, except itself', or *himself*, as a subject (Lacan, 1969–1970, 18.02.70, p. 103). The "revolutionary", for example, cannot simply signify himself as Francisco Javier. For the "revolutionary" to *be* a subject and not only a signifier, it must be signified as a revolutionary subject by an Other, a language, a predicate. This predicate enables the "consistent revolutionary", as an enunciated grammatical subject, to represent the signified enunciating subject. This real subject "would not be a consistent revolutionary if his conceptions of marriage and the couple were not based on love, respect and faithfulness". Correspondingly, the signifier "consistent revolutionary" would not be embodied by a subject (Francisco Javier) if the Other ("conceptions of marriage and the couple…") did not signify the signifier as a subject whose "conceptions of marriage and the couple are based on love, respect and faithfulness". The Other is thus necessary for the signifier to exist as a subject.

To exist as a signified subject, the subjective signifier shall represent the subject in a predicative 'repressed' language (Lacan, 1967e, p. 277). This language is repressed, or unconscious, because its signifiers can only signify a subject who is nothing more than a signifier, a signifier that is also a subject, of course, but a subject who is nothing more than a signifier, and so on. Besides signifying this subject *on the horizon*, each signifier of a language, such as an entry in a dictionary, does not signify a conscious signified entity, but it refers to another signifier of the same language, which in turn refers to another signifier, which refers to another one, and so on. This is why language, by definition, is an unconscious language.

In order to approach the psychoanalytical certainty of unconscious language, we may proceed like good psychologists and start from the psychological reality of conscious thought. We may thus take the path already cleared by Sapir (1921, pp. 16–17):

- We begin by 'suspecting that the symbolic expression of thought may in some cases run along outside the fringe of the conscious mind'.
- To justify our suspicion, we might concede that 'the auditory or equivalent visual or motor centres in the brain, together with the appropriate paths of association, which are the cerebral equivalent of speech, are touched off so lightly during the process of thought as not to rise into consciousness at all'.
- If we consider that all strong and complex analogical processes of thought can be decomposed into their light and simple discrete components, we will understand that 'the most rarefied thought may be but the conscious counterpart of an unconscious linguistic symbolism'.
- Regarding thought as the derived conscious counterpart of a basic unconscious language, we can acknowledge that 'thought processes set in, as a kind of psychic overflow, almost at the beginning of linguistic expression'.
- As the psychic overflow of thought depends necessarily on the physical flow of language, we should not reject the definition of the unconscious linguistic symbol as that which 'makes possible' the conscious mental 'product'.

At the end of this path, we arrive at the unconscious language that produces consciousness. However, to our surprise, this productive language turns out to be essentially the same thing as the produced consciousness. As the overflow of the flow of language, the conscious mental product does not depend only on the unconscious language, but it consists only of this language. As the unconscious language, consciousness is composed of signifiers. Its signified character is just imaginary. In truth, the signifiers make up consciousness as well as the unconscious. So, strictly speaking, the 'bar' between the 'signifier' and the 'signified' does not correspond exactly to the 'barrier' between the 'unconscious' and 'consciousness' (Lacan, 1970c, p. 400). And yet, the former may help us to discern the latter. Although consciousness really consists of signifiers, it distinguishes itself from the unconscious because the signifying elements are erroneously regarded as signified realities. These *realities* are just imaginary realities. *Conscious reality is just a reified imaginarized part of the unconscious language. Apart from this illusion of the unconscious, supposed consciousness consists of nothing more than unconscious language. Its imaginary reality is thus, in truth, nothing but its symbolic value.*

Tongue and language, the symbolic linguistic system and the real structure of the symbolic

Defined as the discourse of the Other, *the unconscious* is nothing but the discourse of the unconscious language. It is only here, in this analyzable discourse, where 'we can find the unconscious' (Lacan, 1969, p. 389). The 'structure' of the 'unconscious' is 'isomorphic to discourse' (1967c, p. 341). As discourse, the unconscious is articulated by the signifying structure. Besides presupposing a sort of *primary repression*, this structure of language accomplishes *the repression* according to the strictest definition of the term, that is to say, a sort of *secondary repression* from which arises *the unconscious*.[20]

From the Lacanian point of view, the unconscious is shaped by language. It is 'fundamentally structured, woven, chained, meshed, by language' (Lacan, 1955–1956, 01.02.56, p. 135). It 'plays only with effects of language' (1967g, p. 334). It consists of an 'alluvial deposit of language' (1970a, p. 417). Essentially, and by definition, the unconscious *is* a language. It is 'a structure, that is, a language' (1973a, p. 513), since 'a structure means a language' (1966c, p. 225). The Lacanian principle of the 'unconscious structured as a language' thus amounts to a 'pleonasm' (p. 223). The 'structure' of the 'unconscious' can only be a 'structure' of 'language' (1966b, p. 208). Structured as a language, the unconscious 'can only be translated into knots of language' (1965a, p. 199). These knots are woven in the real and material structure of language, the only structure of the unconscious, that cannot be reduced to the symbolic, and purely formal, linguistic system.

Formal system of a tongue	*Material structure of a language*
Symbolic system	Real structure of the symbolic
Linguistic variety	Infra-linguistic and supra-linguistic unconscious

In Lacan, the unconscious is structured as a language, but not as a tongue or a linguistic variety of language. Strictly speaking, the structure of the unconscious is not a symbolic linguistic system as the formal system of a tongue, but a material structure of a language as the real structure of the symbolic. On the subject of this structure in which 'unconscious symbolism is revealed', Benveniste (1956) points out that it is not linguistic, but rather 'infra-linguistic and supra-linguistic' (p. 86). *Beyond* a tongue, the unconscious language is 'supra-linguistic' as it 'uses' overdetermined or 'extremely condensed' signifiers (ibid.). *Beneath* a tongue, the same language is 'infra-linguistic', since it 'uses signs that cannot be decomposed and imply several individual variations' (ibid.).

The supra-linguistic and infra-linguistic structure of the unconscious can be simply defined as a *non-linguistic structure*.[21] Logically, this structure cannot be studied by linguistics. Even if the unconscious is the condition of linguistics, 'there is no way for linguistics to grasp the unconscious' (Lacan, 1970a, p. 410). Nevertheless, the non-linguistic structure of the unconscious may be studied, outside linguistics, by other disciplines and techniques, such as our Lacanian Discourse Analysis.

To analyze the unconscious in a Lacanian perspective, we must begin by understanding that its structure is the structure of language (*structure langagière*), which *is not* the same thing as the linguistic system (*système linguistique*) of the tongue (*la langue*).[22] Structured as a language (*langage*), the unconscious is not structured as a tongue (*langue*). It is not a purely formal system of homogeneous signs. It is not organized in a stable and uniform way for only one linguistic community. It is not independent of variations between speeches of diverse individuals in different circumstances. Nor is it independent of subjective particularities and vital or mortal contingencies. Contrary to the linguistic symbolic system, the real structure of the unconscious language is not beyond life and death, but it 'brings death' and 'plugs into' a 'life' (Lacan, 1975, p. 313). As the structure of the symbolic, this structure is not just a symbolic system, but it 'knots' the real and imaginary 'places of life' (ibid.). Thus tied to life, the unconscious language is not purely formal, but it depends on a living materiality. It consists of specific materials found in all symbolic, real, and imaginary domains of life, namely, the textiles for a hood, metal for a gun, stones for a barricade, muscles for rebellious behaviour, air for a dissident voice, ink for seditious writing, but also already existing revolutionary slogans, insubordinate feelings and egalitarian ideas, fancies of revenge and memories of humiliations. In the unconscious, all these materials are symbolized or re-symbolized. They are iteratively signifierized. They are tied and tied again to heterogeneous systems, to multiform and unstable overdetermining structures that present different aspects at each moment, according to the position of the speaking subject at each link in the signifying chain.

As Althusser (1966a, 1966b) notices, the signifiers of unconscious language 'can be words, but also many other things' (1966b, p. 102). They can be 'fragments of the imaginary' (p. 106), that is, 'forms, elements and relations' of an 'ideological imaginary' (p. 109). They can be 'ideological formations' as 'feelings, impressions, ideas, objects, images, open or closed directions' (1966a, p. 143). The Lacanian unconscious includes all this and much more. Actually, as a symbolic universe, it is supposed to be an exteriority that includes everything. So, unlike the Althusserian unconscious, the Lacanian one can be regarded as a language that embraces every ideological discourse, as well as any other discourse, speech, or tongue.[23] As the 'field of language', the unconscious of Lacan (1953b) embraces any tongue, but also 'spreads' beyond all tongues (p. 139). Beyond the spoken and written words of a tongue, the 'signifying materials' of the unconscious language can be 'functions of an apparatus, illusions of consciousness, segments of the body or its image, and social phenomenon' (ibid.).

Containing and surpassing all tongues, the unconscious may be regarded as 'a tongue heard in all other tongues' (Lacan, 1953a, p. 292). Now, as a Humboldtian 'language', our Lacanian unconscious 'combines individual specialization and universal convergence in such a way that it can be rightly defined both as a language of mankind and a language of only one individual' (Humboldt, 1834, §12, p. 188). Likewise, even if the Lacanian unconscious language can be 'heard in all tongues', it is nevertheless 'absolutely particular to the subject' (Lacan, 1953a, p. 292). And yet, it embraces everything for the subject. It materializes the totality of the structure for his structural position. It contains a symbolic universe that can only exist concretely for a real individual point in the universe.[24]

The unconscious holds everything that language holds. However, it is not structured as *the* language in general, but as *a* language, *a* particular and limited language that particularizes *my* thoughts and limits *my* world:

- A *particular language*, my language, which constitutes my thoughts in a 'particular' way (Lacan, 1953a, p. 292). This is logical, given that 'thought does not depend only on a general language', but 'also' on the 'particular feature' of each language (Humboldt, 1820, §17, p. 85).
- A *limited language*, 'my language', whose 'limits mean the limits of my own world' (Wittgenstein, 1921, 5.6, p. 141). This is also logical, seeing that *my own world* is a 'discursive world' entirely 'constructed by a determinate language' (Melo, 2000, p. 618).

If 'the language' is 'the structure that causes an effect of languages', the unconscious is only 'one' of these 'languages' (Lacan, 1972a, p. 489). As *one* language, the unconscious is not *the* language, but *a* language. The singular indefinite article *a* indicates that the unconscious is neither 'the language' nor 'all languages', but only 'one language among others' (ibid.). As *a* particular and limited language, it is language, of course, but it is not identical to *the* unlimited language in general.

The 'particular is general', but it 'is incompletely included in the general' (Lenin, 1915, p. 345). In this way, as the unconscious, the signifying social structure *for a structural position* is incompletely included in the same structure *in itself*. *A* language of an individual is not identical to *the* shared language of our time or culture. Nor is it identical to *the* language as a human transcultural and ahistorical faculty. Although the observable fact of the unconscious may be as universal as the human faculty of language, *the* unconscious is always *a* concrete individual unconscious, that is to say, a particular language that speaks, in a cultural and historical precise context, through only one individual subject.[25]

The tangible particularity and intangible universality of language

Everywhere, and not only in works of art, the unconscious functions as a 'tongue spoken by only one person' (cf. Anzieu, 1981, p. 175).

It can be described as a tongue 'made to measure' (ibid.). It is an 'idiolect' (ibid.). It is the idiolect of a subject that 'speaks just for himself, as everybody does, if the unconscious really exists' (Lacan, 1975–1976, 13.04.76, p. 129). Logically, this idiolect is not speech. Nor is it an 'intermediate entity between speech and tongue' (cf. Barthes, 1964, p. 26). Beyond speech and tongue, the unconscious is a language. It is a full language. And yet, it is used by only one subject. It is his particular unconscious language. In its particularity, it belongs to *the* language in general. But this unlimited language in general is only a speculative abstraction. As the structure in itself that exists only for each one of its positions, the language in general exists only through each particular language. *The language* is a theoretical essence that remains beyond all its particularizations. It cannot be known. Therefore, it has nothing to do with the already known 'universal language' of a generalized individual subject, *the normal human being*, who is artificially forged by the 'psychology of the masters' denounced by Barthes (1957, p. 52) and evidenced by the psychological models that tend to universalize a particular white heterosexual male of modern capitalist societies.[26]

To make a proper use of Lacanian Discourse Analysis, our psychology must not proceed as an abstract *psychology of the masters* that would look for an already known universal language behind the analyzed discourse of a particular language. Our *concrete psychology* must rather acknowledge, in the enunciated 'psychological fact' of the analyzed discourse, a 'segment' of a particular language inherent in 'the life of a particular individual' (Politzer, 1947, I, XII, pp. 59–60). This particular language is the only knowable language for Lacanian Discourse Analysis. Now, for the purpose of reaching a 'psychological knowledge' of this language, we must 'attain' the enunciated 'dramatic facts in their individual singularity' (1947, I, XII, p. 60). We must attain them at the level of an 'unconscious' that 'already heralds a concrete psychology', *a* psychology of *a* singular individual subject (1928, V, II, p. 222), which has nothing to do with '*the* psychology' (Barthes, 1957, p. 89), *the* 'abstract psychology' of *the* normal generalized subject, of his consciousness and the universal language of this consciousness (Politzer, 1928, V, II, p. 226).

The unconscious that heralds the still expected Politzerian concrete psychology is the unconscious of Freudian and Lacanian psychoanalysis. It is the material discourse of a corporeal Other, a real structure, a tangible particular language that makes it possible for us to get out of the intangible universal language of consciousness imagined by classical or cognitive abstract psychologies. The psychoanalytical evolution from the *universal language of consciousness*, that underpins communication, to the *particular language of the unconscious*, which is intrinsically incommunicable, involves a 'progression from abstract psychology to concrete psychology' (Politzer, 1928, V, II, p. 226). After this progression, we attain the particular concretion of an unconscious articulated by only one language among a plurality of languages. At the same time, unfortunately, we attain a situation of irremediable non-communication.

If there are as many languages as individuals, then communication between individuals is not viable. And if this is the case, the linguistic system proves to be useless and even non-existent. The 'plurality' of individual 'languages' therefore raises a 'problem for the linguist' (Arrivé, 1994, pp. 126–127). It is the problem of the uselessness and non-existence of a tongue, or a linguistic system, which cannot exist without a linguistic community that shares it and uses it to communicate.[27] This problem cannot be solved, but it must be reconsidered in the light of two circumstances. On the one hand, there is theoretically an unknowable signifying social structure *in itself* that establishes all kinds of connections or *communications* between its individual positions by embracing all of its particular materializations or languages for these positions. On the other hand, besides the totally shared structure in itself, its particular materializations or languages are partly shared by individuals who occupy close positions in the structure, namely, real subjects represented by the same signifier or symbolic subject (such as "revolutionary", "Lacanian" or "English-speaking"), who may partially *communicate* in their *collective particular languages* (such as English, Lacanese or the revolutionary jargon).

Whether faced with individual or collective particular languages, we must recognize the modern 'partition' of *the* language, that which 'exists only' in a 'dispersed way' (Foucault, 1966, p. 315). Independently from the specific feature of modern times, we must resign ourselves to the old heritage of Babel (*Genesis*, 11: 1–7), that is to say, the 'split' and 'externalization' of 'the only language' (Boehme, 1623, II, §35, p. 124), the 'multiplication' of 'external languages' that are 'perceptible' but 'unintelligible' (Saint-Martin, 1775, pp. 455–497), the 'transition from unity to multiplicity, from understanding to misunderstanding', from the only universal 'interiority' of 'consciousness' to the multiple 'exteriorities' of the 'unconscious' (Pavón Cuéllar, 2007a, pp. 30–32). After this transition, we must assume the plurality of languages and the partial noncommunication between subjects.[28] We must be prepared to deal with a plurality of 'idiolects' and 'languages' of 'linguistic communities' (Barthes, 1964, p. 26). That is the case of the languages of different classes, with their own 'phrases' submitted to 'grammars of class' (cf. Stalin, 1950a, pp. 157, 162). Even if those languages can be regarded as simple 'branches' of the signifying social structure in itself, they *do not* only consist of a 'selection of specific words that reflect specific tastes' (p. 157). Far from it, they constitute the symbolic universe of the members of each class. Their signifiers correspond to all the signifierized things related to the members of each class, which include those that enter through the eyes and ears, those that come out of the mouth or the pocket, those that garnish living rooms and clothes and personalities, those that open or close paths and destinies, those saved or spent, those who work in the factory or the office, those that kill or die or make a revolution, etc.

The plurality of languages creates a contradictory *coexistence of symbolic universes*. As universes, each one excludes the others. The universes cannot coexist. Nor can they communicate. Without a 'single common symbolic universe', there is a failure of the 'aptitude to communicate' (Anzieu & Martin, 1968, p. 194). There is not only the 'disparity of languages', but also 'their impenetrable closure' (Barthes, 1957, p. 51). There is an abyss of incommunication. Communication inevitably fails between a Georgian and a Russian, a moujik and an intellectual, a bureaucrat and a proletarian, Stalin and Trotsky, etc. When language is not 'a common instrument of all people', it 'cannot be used any longer to communicate' (Stalin, 1950a, p. 151). The result is incommunication, the dissociation of society, civil war, exile, loneliness, misunderstanding, disagreement, and discord. However, to compensate, there are false accords, artificial agreements, imaginary understandings, content analyses, cognitive psychologies, effective psychotherapies, successful manipulations, addictive companionships, strong unities, United States or Kingdoms, European or Soviet Unions, globalization, Nazism, the necessity for dictatorship and totalitarianism, the power of fashion, the flock of sheep, shared errors, collective silliness and stupidity.[29]

In spite of the plurality of languages, we may have the impression that we are able to communicate with each other. This agreeable illusion arises from the fact that each language is not only individual, but also partly general and specific, that is, characteristic of a circle of family and friends, and also of a neighbourhood, and furthermore of a job, a social class, a nation, and humankind.[30] Simultaneously, communication fails all the time, since each language is not only human, but national too, and also regional, local, professional, familiar, etc. The worst is that each language is ultimately individual. Each language is an unconscious of only one individual subject. Therefore, 'there is no collective unconscious', but only 'particular unconsciouses, as each individual, at each moment, gives the finishing touches to the tongue he speaks' (Lacan, 1975–1976, 13.04.76, p. 133).

To 'understand' a language, it is not enough to know its 'social presuppositions', but we must also discern its 'individual presuppositions' (cf. Goffman, 1981, pp. 205–206). Now, to this end, it would be necessary to share the same structural position of the real speaking subject who enunciates the analyzed discourse. This is the only way, however impracticable, to know the signifying structure for the subject, that is, the 'language' that 'constructs' his 'discursive world' (Melo, 2000, p. 618), which is precisely the 'world' that is 'presupposed' by the analyzed discourse (cf. Goffman, 1981, p. 207).

As I cannot put myself in the position of Francisco Javier, I cannot know his "perception of the world". I cannot know the perceptible structure for his position. I can understand neither his language nor his world or the individual and social presuppositions of his enunciated discourse. Therefore, he cannot really communicate with me. Between his position and mine, there is always an incommunication, a rupture, an impassable gap of information.[31] The structure for his position is not exactly the structure for my position. His language is not identical to my language. Both languages are not identical to *the* language. Arising from an 'incidence of the real', they are not identical to the 'structure' *in itself* 'from which this incidence of the real is motivated' (Lacan, 1972a, p. 490).

A language is not the same thing as *the* real unknowable language. Nor is it the same as *the* already known imaginary language of the generalized normal subject, as the only foundation of '*the* psychology' (Barthes, 1957, p. 89). This is why *a* language 'diverges' from 'common sense' (Lacan, 1972a, p. 489). This is also why *a* language cannot be used to communicate, but it involves a retreat to 'solipsism', an impossibility of going beyond its 'limits', which are 'the limits' of the 'world' of the enunciating subject (Wittgenstein, 1921, 5.62, p. 142). When *a* language exhibits a 'semblance of communication', it appears only as 'dream, lapsus or joke' (Lacan, 1972a, pp. 490–491). Behind this semblance, *a* language cannot be communicated. It is only for one subject. It constitutes, for him, a closed universe.

Enunciation: Expression by the subject and articulation by the structure

If there were only *a* language for a subject, then this language constitutes a universe. It includes everything for the subject. Therefore, the language cannot get out of itself. It cannot become another language, a metalanguage, in order to refer to itself. So, in a sense, it escapes itself.

By indicating that there is just one language for one subject, the Lacanian postulate 'there is no metalanguage' also implies that 'something escapes language, that is, language itself' (Milner, 1978, pp. 78–79). As language escapes itself, it cannot become a metalanguage in order to signify itself. Its signifying elements cannot be signified by it. Therefore, they cannot be signified in any way for the subject, since there is only one language for him.

The signifying elements of a language cannot become consciously signified by a metalanguage. There is thus nothing outside the signifying exteriority of the unconscious. This exteriority constitutes a symbolic universe. It symbolically includes everything for the subject. There is no place for the metalanguage of consciousness. Therefore, in spite of Barthes, there are neither myths nor semiologies:

- There is no 'myth' defined as 'metalanguage' (Barthes, 1957, p. 200). There is only one language for the mythologist. The result is that this language cannot be a metalanguage.
- There is no 'semiology' defined as 'metalanguage' (Barthes, 1964, p. 79). There is no 'second system' that would 'undertake a first language' (ibid.). There is only one system for the semiologist. The so-called *first system* is not signified, but is signifierized and thus incorporated into the *second system*, which then becomes the only system, that is, a language without a metalanguage.

For a subject, there is only one language. For his position, there is only one signifying structure that signifierizes or incorporates all other structures into itself. Instead of a conscious signification, there is only an unconscious signifierization. Even the powerful 'language' of Barthes (1964) does not have the power to become a 'metalanguage' and thus 'signify' the elements of other languages, 'isological systems', whose signifiers would inevitably need a 'metalanguage' to be 'signified' (pp. 44–47).

In the perspective of Lacanian Discourse Analysis, a language is an isological system. That means that all its signifiers obey the same (*iso-*) logic of the signifier (*-logos*). In contrast to a 'non-isological' cognitive-linguistic system composed of signifiers and signified elements 'undertaken' by the signifiers, a language is an isological system that consists only of signifiers that 'have no other materialization' than themselves (cf. Barthes, 1964, p. 44). When a signifier signifierizes a thing, this thing is incorporated into the *same logic* (*iso-logic*) of the first signifier. It thus becomes a material signifier in the same logic of the signifier, and not an ideal signified of the signifier in another logic. In Francisco Javier's discourse, for example, the "pillar" is *not* a different materialization of the "family" that would be related to the signification and idealization of the "family" in a cognitive logic. Instead, the "pillar" is materialized and signifierized by the "family" and thus incorporated into the same discursive logic of the signifier. For the Eperrist, at each moment, this logic is the only existing logic. It is *the* logic of the signifying structure for his structural position. This structure of the unconscious is then isological. As *a* language, all the unconscious obeys the same discursive logic of the signifier.

Everywhere in the exteriority of the unconscious, the same logic of the signifier 'plays the fundamental role' (Lacan, 1955–1956, 01.02.56, p. 135). The isological signifying structure of a language is the only structure of the unconscious. Therefore, the unconscious is not merely structured *as* a language, but it is totally structured *by* a language. This language structures the unconscious by particularizing the structure for the position of a subject. By deploying thus a symbolic universe all around the subject, the language opens for him the exteriority of the unconscious.[32]

Leclaire reasonably stated against Laplanche that the 'origin of the unconscious' must be situated in the 'process that introduces the subject into the symbolic universe' (Leclaire & Laplanche, 1961, p. 117). This process can be described as a '*languagization*' that 'establishes the unconscious' (Resweber, 1998). The process can be also described as a *signifierization* that generates unconscious perceptible signifiers without a conscious intelligible meaning. In any case, as the process is accomplished by the signifiers of language, Lacan (1970a) concludes rightly that 'language is the condition of the unconscious' (p. 406).

The Lacanian unconscious is defined as the *discourse of the Other*, that is, the *discourse of a language*, of *a language* that represents correspondingly the condition of *its discourse*. As the *discourse of a language*, the unconscious is articulated by this language. In actual fact, the unconscious results from this articulation. It results from the fact that *a language speaks* through the subject. Lacan compares this *speaking language* to the Freudian *id* (in French *ça*, or *that*). Since '*that* speaks' (*ça parle*) through a subject who functions just as the speaking workforce of *that*, then there is an 'unconscious' for the subject (Lacan, 1973a, p. 511). This unconscious resides in the speech uttered *through* the individual subject, but articulated *by* a language whose perceptible complex social structure could never be intelligible for the subject. Thus, in speech, the subject experiences the unconscious. But the 'right of speech' of this 'unconscious' is conferred by 'its structure of language' (1966b, p. 204). The unconscious 'depends' therefore 'on language' (1973a, p. 511). It depends on it as an effect depends on its cause and its condition. As an 'effect' of language, the unconscious 'supposes the structure of language as a *sine qua non*' (1971, p. 14).

Since '*the* language' is 'the structure that causes the effect of languages', and since an unconscious is only one of those languages, then '*the* language' explains 'the unconscious' as '*a* language' (Lacan, 1972a, pp. 488–489). The signifying social structure *in itself*, as the trans-individual system of *the* language, explains its particular structuration, as *a* language or *an* unconscious, *for* an individual position in the structure. Accordingly, 'the language is the condition of the unconscious, and not the contrary' (Lacan, 1970c, p. 400). To be sure, it is *not* 'the unconscious' that is 'the condition of language', as claimed by Laplanche, who failed to notice that repression, intrinsic to language, is the condition of the unconscious (cf. Leclaire & Laplanche, 1961, p. 109).

As the condition of the unconscious, language cannot operate without repressing.[33] Its symbolization amounts to a derealization. Its enunciation already implies a primary repression. It involves the hollowing out of the real, or the real differentiation of the symbolic in relation to the real. To exist, language necessitates this differentiation between the 'sounds' and the 'sound properties of things' (Deleuze, 1969, pp. 212–217). This pure 'distinction' of language is that which 'makes language possible' (ibid.). This explains the pureness of language, as pure structure, purely determined by itself. This 'pure structure of language' is *that* (*ça*) which 'speaks' through the mouth of the speaking subject (Lacan, 1966–1967, 12.04.67). *That* is the language that articulates *its* discourse, the unconscious discourse of the Other, which outwardly seems to be the enunciated discourse of the enunciating subject.

In Lacanian Discourse Analysis, we may immediately *know* the real 'subject' who utters or pronounces a 'sentence', but 'the question' is 'who' conceives and creates this 'sentence' (Lacan, 1966–1967, 12.04.67). As noted above, the real subject is only the enunciating workforce of his unconscious. He is the proletarianized force that does the work of the signifying structure for his structural position. Correlatively, this real structure is the Other *who articulates* the discourse that is only *expressed* by the real subject.

The enunciation of a discourse can be divided between its articulation by the real structure of a language, as the enunciating work system of the unconscious, and its expression by the real subject, as the enunciating workforce of the structure. Logically, this enunciating workforce cannot be the subject matter of the resulting enunciated discourse. This workforce is nothing besides its force. There is nothing to say about this nothingness. A discourse cannot refer to the nothingness of the proletarianized subject who simply voices it. Francisco Javier's discourse about "marriage", for example, cannot refer to the real subject who identifies himself as a "revolutionary". The discourse, in actual fact, does not refer to this subject who *expresses* it, but it refers to the Other who *articulates* it. Francisco Javier's discourse thus refers to the structuration, for his structural position, of the signifying social structure inherent in a precise Mexican traditional and conventional culture.

As the discourse of the Other, the unconscious does not speak of the individual speaking subject, but of the Other that personifies a language, a locus of speech, a signifying social structure that configures a cultural environment and decides the structural position of the subject in this environment.[34] When the subject seems to speak of himself, this structure is that which speaks of itself through the structural position of the subject. The so-called *discourse of the subject* is thus a *discourse of the Other*. It is the predicative discourse of the structure for the structural position of the subject. It is the alienating discourse of a culture (S2) for the cultural symbolic identity (S1) of the real subject ($). This can be illustrated by Francisco Javier, by *his* discourse, as the discourse of the traditional Mexican culture of "marriage" *for* the cultural identity of the "revolutionary". Now, between the culture and the cultural identity, there is a flagrant contradiction, but also an attempt at a compromise and reconciliation. The revolutionary tries to come to an arrangement and acts in concert with his counter-revolutionary culture. To this end, he undertakes a sort of dialogue that is, in reality, a monologue of the culture with itself, or, more precisely, a monologue of the structure with one of the structural positions that compose it.[35]

The 'autistic monologue' of the structure demonstrates the impossibility of 'dialogue' for a language without a metalanguage (Miller, 1996b, pp. 13, 16). Without an Other of the Other, the Other can only soliloquize to himself. Thus, in Lacan, the unconscious is confined to a monologue. However, as the discourse of the Other, it is not confined to silence. It can be heard everywhere and all the time. It is always *here*. It is not in oblivion. Unlike the unconscious in the banal sense of the word, the Lacanian unconscious 'is not a loss of memory' (Lacan, 1967g, p. 334). It is not a silence caused by a memory lapse. It is rather an appreciable 'misrecognition' that resounds with a 'deafening voice' (Althusser, 1964, p. 36). It is the resounding materialization of an Other in *his* discourse, in *his* monologue, in which the speaking subject cannot 'find himself', but only the Other that soliloquizes (Lacan, 1967g, p. 334).

Individual speaking positions as mouths of the signifying social structure

When a subject speaks, he cannot find himself in his speech. This speech does not speak about him, but it is objectively a discourse about 'the Other' (Lacan, 1960a, p. 295). It is a discourse in which the subject cannot recognize himself. However, the 'subject' is 'a party to' the 'Other's discourse' (Lacan, 1958e, p. 27). Even if the discourse referred to an Other and were articulated by this Other, the subject is, nevertheless, the speaking workforce that enunciates the discourse. The proletarianized subject does the work of the unconscious. He is the support of the letter, the incarnation of the language, the fullness of the full speech articulated by the Other. The subject thus fills the 'empty locus' of speech (Lacan, 1967a, p. 356). This locus, as the 'mark' and 'lack' of the real, takes hold of the real subject as the 'effect of the mark and support of the lack' (1965a, p. 200).

The speaking subject alienates his body in the locus of speech. At each moment, he embodies a signifier in the signifying chain. He actually exists because of this embodiment of language. His embodiment amounts to his subjectivation through his subjection to the signifying structure. This subjectivation begins with an identification with a 'signifier' that 'makes manifest the subject' (Lacan, 1964, 27.05.64, pp. 227–233). But this signifier 'produces itself in the field of the Other' (ibid.). The voluntary identification of the subject to a signifier (S1) would not be accomplished without his necessary alienation in all the other signifiers, in a language, as the field of the Other (S2). This can be exemplified by Francisco Javier, who "would not be" *consistently identified* with a "revolutionary" if he was not *inconsistently alienated* in a language, in a locus of speech, in which we find his "conceptions of marriage and the couple". In this void in the structure, unfortunately, there is the reactionary 'Minus-One' that reacts against the 'One' of the "consistent revolutionary" (Lacan, 1970a, p. 409). As the individual identity of the subject ($), this revolutionary One (S1) encounters a violent and tenacious resistance in the reactionary Other, in the signifying social structure, in the *status quo* of the Mexican traditional and conventional culture (S2).[36] This is only natural. The necessities of the unconscious shall naturally resist the willpower of consciousness. In actual fact, this willpower is nothing more than a privileged necessity of the unconscious. The structural position of the subject belongs to the signifying structure of a language. The "revolutionary" takes part in the traditional cultural system of "our time". Francisco Javier embodies a signifier of language.

The structure of language 'reduces the subject to a signifier' (Lacan, 1964, 27.05.64, p. 232). In so doing, the structure 'petrifies' the same subject that it 'drives to function, to speak, as a subject' (ibid.).

The structural petrifaction of the enunciated subject (S1) coincides with the structural animation of the enunciating subject ($). Thus, in Francisco Javier's discourse, the petrifying identification with the "consistent revolutionary" coincides with the animating impulse to enunciate a revolutionary discourse. Paradoxically, by enunciating this discourse, the real subject proves to be a "consistent revolutionary". Thus, he proves to be a signifier, a word, an enunciated symbolic subject (S1). And yet, this subject is still conscious. With *his* consciousness, *he* even 'imagines that he is master of his being' (Lacan, 1967f, p. 324). He imagines that 'he is not language' (ibid.). Now, to imagine such a thing, he should not think. In general, *he should not think in order to be.*

As discussed before, the Cartesian Cogito can be translated in Lacanese as: *The language thinks in my place, therefore the language is*. When I think, the Other *thinks* and *is* instead of me. So, when I think, I am not. In a Lacanian perspective, the Cartesian Cogito can be inverted: *I think, therefore I am not*. Actually, to be, I should not think. I should be reduced to the identificatory conscious position of the 'I am' (S1), in which 'I do not think', in contrast with the alienating 'unconscious' position in which 'I think' (S2), so that 'I am not' (Lacan, 1967f, p. 324). To be a "consistent revolutionary", for example, Francisco Javier should be reduced to the identificatory position in which he would not think about his "conceptions of marriage and the couple". When he thinks about these conservative conceptions, he cannot be a "consistent revolutionary" any more. His alienation in the conservative language keeps him from being the revolutionary signifier. The fact remains that he cannot consciously be identified with a signifier (S1) without being unconsciously alienated in a language (S2). He cannot be a "consistent revolutionary" without his "conceptions of marriage and the couple". He cannot be without thinking, but his thinking prevents him from being, and his being prevents him from thinking. Between those two poles, there is a 'temporal pulsation' that is inherent to 'the unconscious' (Lacan, 1964, 27.05.64, p. 232). It is the pulsation between the subject and his Other, the signifier and the language, consciousness and the unconscious.

In the pulsation of the unconscious, I express a discourse and I cyclically misinterpret it, as it is not my discourse, but the discourse of the Other. And yet, I express the discourse. I express it because it is my unconscious, that is, the particular discourse of the structure for my individual position in the structure. *Unsurprisingly, the structure for my structural position can only be expressed through my position, that is to say, through my mouth, that functions as one of the multiple mouths of the signifying social structure. Each individual position of a subject constitutes, so to speak, a mouth of the Other. In my position, I am nothing more than this mouth, a speaking power of the system, a proletarianized enunciating workforce that expresses the discourse articulated by the structure.* This discourse belongs to the structure. It is a work of genius that belongs to the cunning genius of language. But it is done by me. I thus do work that does not belong to me. To be sure, this work of my unconscious is not my work, but the work of the Other, that I do not know how to interpret.

When I interpret the work of *my* unconscious, I misinterpret it, or, more correctly, I interpret it accurately, and even with astonishing exactness, but in the wrong way. For example, I regard a conservative reaction as a revolutionary action. I take the discourse of the Other for my own discourse. Then, predictably, I fail to 'recognize' myself in what I take for my own discourse (Lacan, 1957–1958, 25.06.58, p. 476). In this discourse, at the same time, I catch a glimpse of someone or something that I 'do not know' (ibid.). By going deeply into what I glimpse, it should be possible for me to positively recognize the presence of the Other and not only negatively recognize the absence of myself. However, instead of this hard recognition, I obviously prefer a comfortable misrecognition in which I misinterpret the Other and I treat its discourse as my own discourse. That is how the symbolic Other becomes the 'structure of misrecognition' of the imaginary (Althusser, 1964, p. 46). That is also how the conscious subject ends up being unconscious of the unconscious.

Despite our widespread misrecognition, we are always, in part, conscious of the unconscious. We are constantly somewhat aware of our alienation in the discourse of the Other. Behind the imaginary certitude of being in discourse [i(*a*)], each real enunciating subject ($) experiences, at least to a certain extent, the absence of his real being (*a*) in the symbolic universe of the enunciated discourse (S1–S2). Furthermore, as the absent being should be logically present, each one *desires* its presence. This desire maintains the attachment of the subject to discourse. It may also eventually drive the subject to transgress the structure of misrecognition, to contravene its laws, to break the rules of discourse.[37]

The political personification and animation of the signifying social structure

The enunciated discourse may be disrupted by the desire of the enunciating subject. The fact remains that the enunciation of discourse depends directly on this desire. If the subject were not stimulated by the desire of his being, he would not be motivated to do the enunciating work of language. By doing this work of the unconscious, the subject tries to obtain a real being from discourse. However, in the symbolic universe of discourse, every ostensible real being is a purely symbolic being that rests solely on the recognition of the Other. This applies to words, titles, qualifications, rights, money, etc. In any case, the being is purely symbolic. But the subject is deceived. He gives an imaginary reality to the symbolic being. He takes the symbolic being for a real being. And since he desires this real being, he desires the recognition from the Other, on which rests the existence of the symbolic being that he takes for the real being. The desire for the real being is transformed into a desire for the symbolic recognition from the Other. Driven by this desire, the subject expresses the discourse of the Other. Thus, in Lacan's early work, the 'desire for recognition' can function as the 'ultimate motive of the unconscious' (Lacan, 1957–1958, 05.03.58, p. 256).

The subject can only be something in the symbolic universe. But here, in order to be, he needs to be recognized by the Other, and to this end, he has to be alienated in the Other.[38] This can be illustrated by Francisco Javier, who can only be something, such as a "revolutionary", through the symbolic recognition of a signifying social structure in which "marriage" plays a crucial role. In a sense, Francisco Javier cannot be a revolutionary without negotiating his recognition as a revolutionary with the counter-revolutionary language. Even if he refuses any kind of negotiation with the system, he cannot be a revolutionary without negotiating with the system. That is a language. That is also what we call politics. Actually, as 'the unconscious', the Lacanian Other 'is politics' (Lacan, 1966–1967, 10.05.67). In the structure, it is what 'links men' and 'opposes them' as signifiers (ibid.). *As the living unconscious Other, the political thing results from the personification and animation of the signifying social structure through those who desire and negotiate their symbolic recognition in the structure. That involves a personal action that is unconsciously executed, by the structure, through its structural positions, or political positioning, such as that of the revolutionary.*

When Lacan states that 'the unconscious is politics', he thereby 'situates the unconscious in a trans-individual dimension' (Miller, 2003, p. 112). In this dimension, the unconscious can be regarded, at first sight, as a 'relation' (ibid.). It can be regarded as a social interaction or a dialogue between internalized individual subjects.[39] However, on second thoughts, we have already understood that this dialogue represents, rather, a monologue of the structure, since the internalized individual subjects are nothing more than positions that belong to the same signifying social structure. Even if the positions are occupied by different external or internalized subjects, these subjects are nothing more than mouths of the same structure that articulates that which is expressed by its mouths. And yet, when we deal with external subjects, each mouth expresses only a unique structure for a particular position. Therefore, different mouths express different structures. However, these partial structures compose the same total structure in itself. Their dialogue amounts to its monologue.

The monological structure in itself is a theoretical abstraction that cannot be known. But we can always know the monological structure for our structural position. We can always perceive its unconscious monologue, which stages a dialogue between different signifiers that may represent different subjects. Even if those symbolic representatives were confined to a language for only one individual position, they can nevertheless be personified by the political representatives in the public arena. Besides being the constituent elements of the languages of the represented people, these representatives are actually nothing but their individual positions in their respective languages. This is why the so-called *political dialogue* constitutes whether a monologue of one language or a simultaneousness of monologues of different languages expressed by different political representatives. It is always the same monologue articulated by the structure. It is always the same 'spectacle' that Debord (1967) describes as 'the order's uninterrupted discourse about itself, its laudatory monologue' (§24, p. 26). This monologue obviously has nothing to do with the represented people. It is not for nothing that so many brave citizens, such as Francisco Javier, resort to violence as a last resort to attain the symbolic recognition of the Other in the political stage of the unconscious. This must give us food for thought. Somehow or other, politics enables us to visualize the unconscious. If the unconscious *is* politics, then 'politics', of which 'we have an idea', may help us to get some idea of 'the unconscious', of which 'we don't have any idea' (Miller, 2003, p. 112).

The structure of articulating absences and the chain of articulated presences

As the discourse of the Other, the unconscious can be materialized by a political discourse, but also by any other discourses, such as an ideological one. So, in a sense, ideology is included in the unconscious. The "proletarian ideology" of Francisco Javier, for example, is included in the discourse of the signifying social structure for his individual position. As discussed before, this inclusion of ideology in the unconscious is opposed to the Althusserian theory in which the 'structure of the unconscious' is 'produced' and 'articulated' within an 'ideological discourse' (Althusser, 1966a, pp. 136–139). This theory could only be acceptable, in the Lacanian perspective, if the ideological wisdom were identical to the symbolic or *the language*, in general, as the condition of the unconscious as *a language*. In Althusser (1966b), unfortunately, 'the ideology' is regarded as 'the imaginary' (p. 109). It is 'the imaginary' in which 'the unconscious' can 'select forms, elements or relations that *suit* it' (ibid.).

In the Althusserian theory of 1966, 'the unconscious runs on the imaginary' (Althusser, 1966b, p. 109). Since 'the imaginary' is the same thing as 'ideology' (ibid.), then the 'unconscious' is 'a mechanism' that 'runs on ideology', or '*functions* massively with ideology', such as 'an engine that functions with fuel' (1966a, p. 141). In a Lacanian reinterpretation of Althusser, we might say that the imaginary fuel acquires a function, a symbolic value, a signifying structural position. The ideology is thus symbolized, signifierized or incorporated into the structure. However, before being iteratively symbolized, the ideology, as ideology, already had a symbolic value. It was the wisdom of language. It was overdetermined by the signifying social structure for an individual position. It was a component of this structure of the unconscious. If the unconscious runs on ideology, this means that it runs on signifiers, on a language, on the symbolic wisdom of the same language. As one might say, *the unconscious runs on the unconscious*. Since there is no metalanguage, ideology belongs to the same unconscious language. In spite of Althusser, ideology does not come from the exterior of the exteriority of the unconscious, but it is already a part of this unique individual exteriority of the symbolic universe.

In the Lacanian perspective, the ideological and the unconscious are not two discourses that can refer to one another. They are only one discourse of only one language that cannot be simply enunciated, but that has to be constantly enunciating itself, since there is no other discourse of another language to enunciate it. *Without a metalanguage, the discourse of a language has to be simultaneously enunciated and enunciating. This is why it is unconscious. It is unconscious because the explicit enunciated discourse always involves an implicit enunciating articulation by the structure. This unconscious structure of the unconscious involves a surreptitious negative language of merely signifying wisdom that may be ideological, but also moral, economic, historical, etc. In any case, it is a structure of articulating absences that shape the analyzed discursive chain of articulated presences, a chain that may be, in turn, ideological, but also moral, economic, and historical.*[40]

Our Lacanian representation of ideology, whether as an unconscious discourse or as an unconscious language, differs radically from that of Althusser. In Althusser (1966a), there would be an 'overlap' or an 'encroachment' between the ideological and unconscious levels, so that 'some elements' and 'some relations' would 'belong at once to both the discourse of ideology and the discourse of the unconscious' (Althusser, 1966a, p. 146). Instead, in Lacan, there would be a sort of inclusion of ideology in the unconscious, so that all elements and relations of ideology, whether as discourse or language, would belong to the unconscious, as prominent features of every discourse or language. From this point of view, ideology constitutes just one dimension of the unconscious. As for the unconscious, it results from the necessary enunciating articulation of all discourses by the structure. In actual fact, it *is* also this articulation. It *is* thus the 'first articulation' of every explicit enunciated and articulated discourse (cf. Althusser, 1966a, p. 161). Before 1966, Althusser (1964) understood all this, as evidenced by his definition of the 'unconscious', in relation to 'language', as the 'absolute condition of every discourse' (pp. 37–40).

Notes

1. This social space corresponds approximately to the 'social place' that Bronckart (1985) proposes, as a substitute for the 'social institution', to describe the 'zone of cooperation wherein takes place the activity of language' (p. 31).
2. Thus, in social psychology, we can regard 'the Other as a social substance, as the amassed roles, traditions, understandings, and unwritten obligations that define a given societal situation' (Hook, 2008, p. 55). As in Durkheim, all this transcends each individual. Now, in Lacan, all this is particularized for only one individual. The signifying social structure, as the unconscious, constitutes the trans-individual universe of only one individual subject. In this, the Lacanian Other is Weberian rather than Durkheimian. The fact remains that the Other 'amounts to more than the sum total of a society's individuals' (ibid.). He is not only *more* than their society, but also *more* than their individualities. As Marxian surplus-value or Lacanian 'surplus-enjoyment' (Lacan, 1968–1969, 13.11.68, p. (11–25), this *surplus* divides Weberian individuals and dissociates Durkheimian society. It is a social object (surplus-value) that divides from the individual subject. It is also an individual object (surplus-enjoyment) that breaks away from the social subject, which is thus dissociated. By considering this object (*a*), we acknowledge that the Lacanian Other is Marxian and Freudian rather than Weberian or Durkheimian. We see also how this Other, which dissociates society by dividing the individual, functions 'as the mediator between the societal and the individual' (Hook, 2008, p. 58).
3. This explains what Frosh, Phoenix and Pattman (2003) regard as 'the ambiguity' of the Lacanian 'account of the social or cultural' (p. 40). From our viewpoint, this ambiguity lies in the fact that the 'regulatory' existence of 'the social or cultural' may be only individual, while the individual is produced and constituted by the social or cultural, as 'productive or constitutive of subjectivity' (ibid.). This is why Lacanian 'subjectivity', though 'founded in the social link', cannot be 'dissolved into social praxis' (Malone, 2000, p. 81).
4. In this manner, the Lacanian perspective radicalizes the ethogenic approach, in which 'the first step is to think of a social episode, a sequence of acts-actions, as analogous to a sentence composed of words, phrases, clauses, and so on' (Harré, Clarke & De Carlo, 1985,

p. 100). In the Lacanian perspective, the sequence of acts-actions *is* a sentence. When it seems to be *analogous*, it is rather *identical* to a sentence.

5. This implies, in Lacanian Discourse Analysis, that 'there is no external point from which it is possible to speak that is not necessarily implicated in a certain kind of position' (Parker, 2005a, p. 174). Accordingly, 'there is, simply, no external point from which the true story of the subject can be told' (Frosh, 2007, p. 638). Each *point* can only give a partial version of the *story of the subject*. This is so because all points are included in language. Thus, when we analyze discourse, our viewpoint is a position in the signifying social structure. If we perceive a reactionary aspect in a revolutionary discourse, this aspect is not unrelated to our viewpoint. The perception concerns our structural position. We must assume explicitly this position to turn it into an 'ethical position' in which we are 'reflexively positioned in relation to the text' (Parker, 2005a, p. 175). We can thus acknowledge our position within a signifying social structure that also expresses itself through the analyzed discourse. But this structure is not the same for our position and for the position of the author of the analyzed discourse. *The* same language *in itself* is *a* language *for* me and *a* different language *for* Francisco Javier. It is an unconscious for the former and another unconscious for the latter. Unfortunately, for each one of us, there is only one unconscious. There is only one language. There is no metalanguage.
6. By demonstrating the absence of 'contradiction between the general validity of a law and the concrete validity of an individual case', that idea shows that our Lacanian orientation would be situated, according to Lewin (1931), in the 'Galilean way of thinking' in contrast with the 'Aristotelian' one (p. 63). In the form of a concrete psychology, this Galilean way of thinking must be adopted by a Lacanian Discourse Analysis that examines 'the integrality of the total concrete situation', as the discursive occurrence of the symbolic universe of a particular language, instead of a 'collection' of 'frequent historic cases' (ibid.).
7. In Lacanian Discourse Analysis, we must never forget this 'paradox' well formulated by Hook (2008): 'The Other rises at the same time, lacking a domain of presumption and fiction, and yet, it nonetheless remains the anchoring point that a given society relies on to maintain its coherence' (p. 61). We may even radicalize this paradox by regarding the alleged Other as that which maintains, not only the *coherence*, but the *existence* and *subsistence* of society and its members.
8. As Malone (2000) observes, it is precisely this 'impossibility of our relationship with the Other' that 'creates relations of hatred, of love,

of power, that both intersect and partially define the political terrain that psychology so deftly navigates' (p. 83). In all those relations, the 'problematic nature of one's address to the Other creates a particular set of effects Lacanians call the subject' (p. 84). Actually, this subject results from a sort of insubordination against the necessity of the signifying relation and the impossibility of the sexual relation with the Other. The subject appears thus as a *subversion* of the truth against wisdom, the enunciating act against the enunciated fact, "conviction" against "obligation".

9. This futile attempt at intrusion can be observed even in the most serious and reasonable cognitive psychologists, such as Ghiglione (1997), whose 'cognitive social psychology of communication' aims at interpreting *only* the 'indexes' of the 'intentions', the 'strategies' and the 'representations of the stake' (pp. 238–239). If we consider the Peircean distinction between the real of 'indexes', the imaginary of 'icons', and the symbolic of 'symbols' (Peirce, 1903, 1.552, p. 292, 1.558, p. 295), we can criticize Ghiglione for treating discursive symbols as real indexes of inaccessible imaginary icons.
10. To be 'the very stuff—the social substance—of my attempts at comprehension', the Other should be 'always somehow enigmatic', as 'an absolute Other' with 'a fundamental alterity' (Hook, 2008, p. 54). If 'the big Other exists' thus 'at a step removed from the dialectics of inter-subjectivity despite that it grounds the coherence of any such interchange', it is precisely because it constitutes that which 'grounds the coherence of any such interchange' (ibid.). Now, this structural coherence is the justification for the *domestication* of the Other in social psychology. However, as the grounds for this 'psychological domestication' (ibid.), the Other should escape it and resist it. The Other should remain 'beyond the horizon of any conceivable inter-subjectivity' (ibid.). This is how the Other can be the 'point that provides the coordinates for inter-subjectivity' (ibid.).
11. Thus, in Aristotle, the '*ethos*' is different from both the '*logos*', which 'demonstrates or seems to demonstrate', and the '*pathos*', which 'puts' the interlocutors in a certain 'disposition' (*Rhetoric*, I, 1356).
12. This distinction recovers and simplifies the differentiation, proposed by Pêcheux (1975b), between the 'pre-constructed inter-discourse', and the 'intra-discourse' of 'each subject', as the 'effect of inter-discourse on itself', or the 'interiority determined by the exterior' (p. 152). Now, unlike Pêcheux, Lacan does not reduce this intra-discourse to its conscious imaginary content, but he regards it as an unconscious symbolic form or container, situated in the exteriority of the structure for each subject. By contrast, the 'oblivion

number 1' of Pêcheux refers to a shared social unconscious situated in the 'exterior' objective inter-discourse (p. 159).

13. Although socialization gives to a subject the 'rhetorical devices that can be applied to his own internal thoughts' (Billig, 1998, p. 41), there is a particular socialization for each subject and therefore the rhetorical devices are also particular to each subject.
14. Paradoxically, such an alienating and dividing Other personifies, in Aristotle, the 'entirely evolved nature' of the 'human being' (Hermosa Andújar, 2006, pp. 35–37). This 'perfect' nature constitutes the ethical and political nature of each divided and alienated subject, that is, his *cultural nature*, as the 'moral biology of the individual in the *polis*' (ibid.). Now, externally materialized by this *polis*, the alienating and dividing Other becomes 'Civil Society' (S2) whose ulterior 'dissociation' from the 'Political State' (S1) is logically correlative to a 'division of the individuality' ($) between his civil alienating 'situation' and his political identificatory 'position' (Pavón Cuéllar & Sabucedo Cameselle, 2009). This can be illustrated by considering the division of Francisco Javier between his alienated 'material life' in the structure of *our time* (with "marriage" and other "familiar obligations") and his 'affirmation' or positioning ("from conviction") as a *revolutionary* 'communitarian being' (Marx, 1844, III, p. 356).
15. All this is not unrelated to the concept of 'diatext' that Minnini (1994) proposes, in social psychology, to describe the relocation of 'the two exteriorities of the subject and the situation' into the 'internal context of a text' (p. 130). As the signifierization of Lacan, this 'internalization' of Minnini transforms the 'extralinguistic context' into an 'intradiscursive context' (p. 132). In this context, we may even come across the incarnate Other in the form of an 'intralocutor' who becomes an 'interlocutor through his text' (p. 131).
16. Exactly as the 'linking structure' in the social psychology of Pichon-Rivière, the signifying structure of Lacan includes the 'inter-subjective and intra-subjective dimensions' and 'explains the relation of the subject to the world' (Pichon-Rivière & Quiroga, 1972). However, unlike the Pichonian structure, the Lacanian one is not essentially a structure of social links, but it is an individual, social and cultural structure of signifying relations that may be interpreted as social links. Furthermore, the Lacanian structure includes a cultural-extra-subjective dimension and may thus explain the human world and not only the relation of the subject to *the world*.
17. The 'notion that the unconscious is exterior to the subject, as an Other to the subject, as the discourse of the Other', makes it possible for us to 'conceive *mental* processes as culturally-embedded'

(Parker, 2000). In this way, it enables the opening of a field in which 'Lacan connects with some of the discursive and feminist work in psychology' (ibid.).

18. This symbolized form represents the only analyzable form in which Lacanian Discourse Analysis can approach 'the indeterminate fleshiness of our own bodily matter', that is, the '*corporeal suit* that we need to psychically take on' (Hook, 2003, p. 28).
19. These distinct dimensions of the Other correspond to distinct levels in the analysis of the discourse of the Other. They can be conceived, consequently, as a reinterpretation of the levels of socio-psychological analysis distinguished by Doise (1982). In addition to the 'intraindividual' and 'interindividual levels', equivalent to the intra-subjective and inter-subjective-extra-subjective personal dimensions, a Lacanian must also differentiate between the individual and trans-individual 'positional' dimensions (pp. 28–33). As for the 'ideological level' of Doise (ibid.), it concerns the ideological *wisdom of the Other* in Lacan, as we shall see later.
20. Likewise, in the Psychoanalytic Discursive Psychology of Billig (2006), 'unconscious factors' are 'understood' in relation to 'the activity of repression that itself operates through language' (p. 18). At least on this general point, Billig's position coincides with that of Lacan.
21. This definition is diametrically opposed to the linguistic unconscious of Billig (1998), who even claimed to show that 'conversations which Freud presented as evidence for an essentially non-linguistic unconscious should also provide evidence for the operations of repression being constituted in conversation' (p. 14). In a Lacanian perspective, we must raise at least two objections to this claim. On the one hand, the linguistic sphere *is not* the sphere of conversation, as demonstrated precisely by the fact that Freud presented conversations *as evidence for a non-linguistic unconscious*. On the other hand, even if we conceded that some *operations of repression* may have a linguistic character, this character is not inherent in repression, as demonstrated by the insufficiency of the purely symbolic linguistic system to explain repression, which can only be explained by the *real* conversational enunciating act of a *real* subject determined by the *real* structure of language. If the unconscious were just linguistic, there would be only as many samples of the unconscious as there are varieties of tongues. There would be a French unconscious, an English one, etc. And if the conversation were furthermore reduced to its linguistic ingredient, there would be only conversational monologues *of* soliloquizing tongues, without any intervention of a real

speaking subject. Our interview with Francisco Javier, for example, would have been just a soliloquy *of* our Mexican tongue.

22. We might hope that Billig would be more receptive to Lacanian psychoanalysis if he did not wrongly imagine that 'Lacan, in discussing the structure of language, was referring to *la langue*, which, following Saussure's distinction, is presumed to lie behind utterances (or *la parole*)' (Billig, 1998, p. 13). In contrast with Saussurean *langue*, one of the main features of the Lacanian *langage* is precisely that it *does not lie behind utterances*. If the 'combinatory operation' of 'linguistics' gives 'its status to the unconscious', this does not mean that such an operation 'includes' the unconscious (Lacan, 1964, 22.01.64, pp. 20–21). In Lacan, 'the unconscious' is 'something different' than everything studied by 'linguistics' (ibid.). But one thing remains certain: the Lacanian unconscious *is not* 'the total linguistic structure' (cf. Billig, 1997, p. 141).
23. On this point, our Lacanian orientation diverges from the Althusserian orientation of Pêcheux and Fuchs (1975), who presuppose that 'discursive species belong to the ideological genus' (p. 11). Instead, we assume that the ideological species belong to a discursive genus that belongs in turn to the symbolic universe of an unconscious language. And yet, this universe is always individualized for each subject. It is the structure for his unique individual structural position. In Pêcheux (1975b), it corresponds to a 'discursive formation' (p. 146). As for the signifying structure in itself, it refers to the Pêcheuxian 'material contradictory objectivity of inter-discourse' that 'determines' each 'discursive form' (p. 147).
24. Thanks to this 'Galilean way of thinking' inherited by Lacan, Freud 'contributed to the abolition of the frontiers between the normal and the pathological, the usual and the exceptional' (Lewin, 1931, p. 45), the universal and the individual, *the* language and *a* language, culture and the unconscious, the social structure in itself and the same structure for a structural position.
25. In this manner, the idea of the unconscious structured as a language 'suggests that the unconscious, though universal, is a sociocultural construction and not innately determined, just as repression may be universally occurring but not uniform across cultures' (Sharma, 1998, p. 55). In this, as Sharma observes, the Lacanian theory of the unconscious seems to be close to that of Billig (1998), in which 'dialogic repression is universal, but what is to be repressed, and how it is to be repressed, will vary culturally' (p. 42). Billig (1997) justifies this variation by reasoning: 'if repression is dialogically and socially constructed, then topics of repression will vary culturally and

historically' (p. 155). But dialogue and society are never constructed in the same way for all participants in dialogue and members of society. Therefore, we may add to Billig's assumption that *topics of repression will also vary individually.* In our Lacanian perspective, this variation explains the variety of individual unconscious languages that represent configurations, determinations, and manifestations of the same structure for different individual positions in the structure.

26. As Hayes (2003) notices, 'we glimpse only a partial subject of modernity, and more specifically capitalist modernity, if our (research) gaze is mostly directed at the universalising form of what a person is, instead of what constitutes the myriad subjects of humanity'. Now, in the mirror, the *universalizing form* becomes 'the autonomous and coherent ego of the bourgeois individual, so decried by Lacan' (ibid.). Unfortunately, 'lacking a social theory of subject formation, psychology has been prone to the construction of this abstract and idealised subject divorced from the materiality of everyday life' (ibid.).
27. Instead of a functional communicational system that would be 'common to speakers and listeners', there is only a plurality of idiolects that prevent us from being able to 'communicate by means of language' (cf. Bromberg, 2004, p. 104).
28. On this point, our Lacanian Discourse Analysis differs from the Althusserian-Lacanian Discourse Analysis of Pêcheux and Fuchs (1975), who reject the 'plurality of languages' and the idea that 'bosses and workers don't speak the same language' (p. 22). Of course, they speak French, but they speak neither the same collective language of class nor the same individual languages. It is not only a matter of different 'discursive processes' in the same 'linguistic base' (pp. 22–23). What is at stake here is the literal and corporeal 'materiality' of different basic structures of language (ibid.). In each base, for example, the 'strike' occupies a different place. Its place is not the same for the boss and for the worker. Nor is it the same for all the workers or bosses. Pêcheux (1975b) himself recognizes that 'the sense of a signifier changes according to the positions of those who use it' (p. 144). Therefore, despite Pêcheux, bosses and workers do not speak the same language. This is more than enough to justify the refusal of Francisco Javier and other "consistent revolutionaries" to dialogue with the bosses.
29. One head thinks better than a million heads because the million heads do not share *enough language* to constitute even one little head. Since every thought is based in language, the insufficiency of

shared language entails a deficiency of collective thought, that is to say, a group mental deficiency. This is not unrelated to the 'groupthink' of Janis (1973), as 'a deterioration of mental efficiency, reality testing and moral judgment' (p. 329). If this deterioration 'results from in-group pressures' (ibid.), it would seem that these pressures result, in the final analysis, from an attempt to compensate for the insufficiency of a shared language.

30. Here is the reason why the 'content of the unconscious', which is nothing more than language, can be described by Freud (1939) as 'collective' and 'belonging generally to all human beings' (p. 237). Accordingly, the unconscious can involve communication, but also consciousness, since consciousness cannot be separated from communication. This is so because the *conscious imaginary thing* always refers to the meaning of discourse, to the signification of the signifiers, to the supposed communicable consciousness of the unconscious. As noted by Nietzsche (1887), 'consciousness is nothing but a net of communication' (§354, pp. 218–219). It is thus nothing but an imaginary representation of the signifying social structure of a language. That amounts to saying that consciousness is '*a* consciousness of the unconscious' (Pavón Cuéllar, forthcoming).
31. This 'gap' excludes the possibility of an 'equalization of information' between the 'transmitter' and a 'receiver' who is always only 'potential' (cf. Newcomb, Turner & Converse, 1965, p. 244).
32. Chauchat (1999) acknowledges this when she asserts, in her social psychological theory of subjective identity, that 'language enables', not only 'the emergence of consciousness', but also 'access to the symbolic order' and 'the formation of the unconscious' (p. 19). Synthetically, we may say that language generates the symbolic exteriority of the unconscious and not only the imaginary consciousness of this exteriority.
33. In social psychology, this has been recognized by Billig (1998), who notices that 'language is not only expressive, but also repressive', since it 'provides the crucial rhetorical devices for the operation of repression' (p. 12). According to Billig, his disagreement with Lacan, on this point, resides in their respective approaches to language. Billig 'roots the study of language in the details of dialogic utterances', while Lacan 'pays scant attention to the detail of actual conversations' (p. 13). From our point of view, we would rather say that Lacan has doubts about his own capacity to understand the meaning of details in a language that is not his own. Furthermore, Lacan is suspicious of the *actual presence* of what is enunciated in the *actual conversations*. He prefers to consider their

enunciation, as well as the implicit *virtual presences* and *actual absences*. Billig (1997) is also interested in these absences (p. 140), granted, but only at an enunciated level on which they function as negative and secondary effects of a 'repression formed in dialogue' (p. 151). Instead, in a Lacanian perspective, we must regard the absences, at the level of enunciation, as causes of repression, positions in the structure of the unconscious, positive entities that shape the dialogue. If Billig analyzed the symbolic effects of repression, a Lacanian must also analyze the real causes of these effects. If the condition of the Billigian unconscious resided in the articulated details of dialogic utterances, the condition of the Lacanian unconscious resides in the articulating features of a language, of its 'structure', that must not be reduced to 'the micro-details of what people actually say' (cf. Billig, 2006a, p. 22). Besides the *micro-details* of the signifying chain, there is the signifying structure that determines the enunciation and articulates the enunciated signifying chain. From the Lacanian viewpoint, this structure is the only real 'dialogical and pragmatic context' of 'details of language' (cf. Billig, 1998, pp. 42–43).

34. In Parker (1997b), the Lacanian unconscious, as the 'discourse of the Other', is similarly related to 'the symbolic system that holds culture in place and determines the location of each individual speaking subject' (p. 486).
35. In the *rhetorical approach* of Billig (1987), 'what seems to be a monologue' would be, rather, a dialogue, since 'the monologue possesses the content of a dialogue' (pp. 116–117). On the contrary, in the Lacanian perspective, *what seems to be a dialogue* is, rather, a monologue, a monologue of a language with itself, of the unconscious with the unconscious, of the system with the system. To be sure, there is no dialogue between the identification of the subject with an element of the system (S1) and his alienation in the other elements of the same system (S2). There is only a monologue of the same system incarnated by the same subject. When this subject 'divides in order to become his own critic and admirer' (Billig, 1987, p. 117), he does not become two subjects in dialogue, but two signifiers (S1–S2) of the same language whose monologue is the unconscious of the same divided subject ($). In a Lacanian Discourse Analysis, we shall deal with this *monologic unconscious* instead of Billig's 'dialogic unconscious' (1997, pp. 152–156).
36. As evidenced by Francisco Javier and his comrades, this resistance entails a downright 'guerrilla battle' between 'the individual and the social order', a battle that we must analyze with the

'great sensitiveness' that certain social psychologists recognized in psychoanalysis on that score (Deutsch & Krauss, 1972, p. 189).

37. In so doing, the subject justly disobeys 'prohibitions' that bear no relation to him (cf. Billig, 1998, p. 19). In my opinion, this lack of relation is enough to explain that the prohibitions 'create their own desires' (ibid.). The prohibitions create a desire for transgression in the subject, because they concern the Other and not the subject. Nevertheless, what is prohibited also concerns the Other, so that the transgression can only satisfy the desire of the Other. Since everything comes from the Other, everything returns to the Other. The desires as well as the laws and rules are decided and used by the structure. The transgressions as well as the prohibitions take place in language. They concern the Other, the personification of culture, and not a subject who may only be driven by the desire of the Other. The so-called *desire of the subject* may revolt against this alienation, but it is ultimately alienated, even in its revolt. Thus, in Francisco Javier's discourse, the "consistent revolutionary" is, in the end, reabsorbed by the system of "our time".
38. Taking a legitimate short cut, Frosh (2007) observes that 'we are called into being through the process of being recognized, and this in itself means we have some of that otherness laid upon us' (p. 642). In a Lacanian perspective, that *otherness* resides fundamentally in the symbolic universe of the Other. In this signifying social structure, 'the subject' is constantly 'produced as something else by what the other does' (ibid.).
39. Thus, in the *psychoanalytical discursive psychology* of Billig (1997), the unconscious is regarded as a 'dialogic unconscious' that is 'dialogically constituted' (p. 151), 'constituted in dialogue', 'constituted in interaction' (p. 140) or 'within social activity' (p. 152).
40. It follows that Lacanian Discourse Analysis cannot examine ideology without considering the level of *articulating absences*. As Billig (2006) notices, an 'ideological analysis' must go 'beyond what is said in interaction in order to examine significant absences' (p. 21). We must then go beyond the articulated facts in order to reach the absent articulating acts. Now, rather than 'discovering how shared patterns of action might be preventing other patterns from occurring' (ibid.), we must *discover how patterns that are not occurring may really be occurring by generating patterns of action*.

CHAPTER SEVEN

The representative of the subject

This chapter compares, with respect to discourse, the fundamental components of material structure and ideal content. On the one hand there is the symbolic representative of the subject, as a physical signifier in the signifying real structure of the unconscious. On the other hand there is the social representation of an object, as psychic information in the signified imaginary content of consciousness. I discuss why this conscious representation of an object can only be gathered, in the analyzed discourse, from its unconscious representatives, which are always the representatives of a particular subject. Following Lacan, I examine how these representatives link up and make up the real structure of the outside world, the literal exteriority of the unconscious, the discourse of the Other where the subject exists.

The real presence, the imaginary representation and the symbolic representative

If *the* language is the condition of an unconscious defined either as *a* language, or a discourse of this language (discourse of the Other), then this unconscious is, in turn, the condition of every discourse, as every discourse is an unconscious discourse of an unconscious language. To be sure, every discourse consists of unconscious words without an intrinsic conscious meaning. These words come from a language that involves wisdom (*savoir*), but the subject has no knowledge (*connaissance*) of this wisdom, which belongs to the language, to its structure, to its personification as *the Other*.

In each word, 'it is not' the subject who knows, but a 'certain state' of his (Kleist, 1806, p. 17). This state can be characterized as a *state of alienation*. It is an alienated state of the subject. It is not he, but his Other. However, it may be his representative. Besides alienating the subject, a signifier may symbolically represent him. It may be a symbolic enunciated representative (S1) of the real enunciating presence of the subject ($). The fact remains that the signifier belongs to a language that appears as Other than the subject (S2), that is to say, as an unconscious language in which the subject cannot recognize his real being (*a*).

Accordingly, the conscious representation of the subject ($) by his representative (S1) cannot be real, but rather it has to be just an imaginary representation, an image in the mirror, an idea of the ego (*moi*). Similarly, any conscious representation of the real being (*a*) symbolically represented by all the other signifiers of language (S2) also has to be a purely imaginary representation [i(*a*)]. Besides the imaginary conscious representations of the subject and the being on the surface of the mirror [*moi* | i(*a*)], there are only the symbolic unconscious representatives that compose the enunciated discourse (S1–S2), as well as the real presence of an enunciating subject in relation to the absent being ($◊*a*).

Imaginary representations	*moi*	*i*(*a*)
Symbolic representatives	S1	S2
Real presences	$	*a*

Within the context of a concrete discourse, everything begins with the symbolic identification of the enunciating subject ($) with a selected signifier (S1). Due to this identification, the selected signifier becomes the *master-signifier*, the enunciated grammatical subject, and the symbolic representative of the subject (the "revolutionary" in Francisco Javier's discourse). By imagining the signification of this signifier, the subject becomes conscious of himself. His symbolic unconscious representative (S1) is invested with an imaginary conscious representation of his ego (*moi*). This is how the master-signifier turns out to be the signifier of the 'consciousness that masters' (Lacan, 1969–1970, 11.02.70, p. 79). Through an imaginary mental signification, it becomes the signifier of consciousness in the unconscious of language. In this discourse of the Other, the master-signifier signifies consciousness. It signifies the awakened consciousness of the "revolutionary" in the sleep of the conformist system. It opens the conscious interiority in the exteriority of the unconscious. It hollows out the individual position of the subject in the signifying social structure.

In the alienation of language, the master-signifier indicates the symbolic identification of the enunciating corporeal subject ($) with an enunciated grammatical subject (S1). This identification enables the subject to hold on to language. Thus, from the symbolic angle, the master-signifier attaches the subject to the system. But at the same time, from the real angle, it attaches the system to the subject. From this same angle, the master-signifier is a real point of attachment for the imaginary and the symbolic. It is a point of fact, a point of truth in the symbolic stuff of wisdom, a point of real signifierization in the imaginary field of signification. In this field, the master-signifier functions as 'an anchorage point (*point de capiton*), by which the signifier stops the otherwise indefinite sliding of signification' (Lacan, 1960a, p. 285). As the point that anchors signification to signifierization, the master-signifier corresponds to the symbolic that fixes the imaginary in the real. It corresponds thus to the subject of the enunciated fact, as the link between the subject of the imagined knowledge and the subject of the enunciating act. By representing this real subject in discourse, the master-signifier constitutes an 'organic point of reference' for the signifiers, a sort of umbilical cord through which the 'drive' (*pulsion*) intervenes as the 'enunciation' in that which is 'enunciated' (pp. 297–299).

Against all expectations, the master-signifier is neither unique nor alone. Actually, it functions as an anchorage point among other anchorage points. All the points are required for the system to hold up. They function as the multiple necessary hooks of the structure. They appear as the reference marks for the exteriority of language. They are the points of contact between wisdom and truth, the symbolic and the real, sense and nonsense, the discursive sliding and that which always returns to the same place.[1]

As the point of contact with a recurring nonsensical real, an anchoring point could be represented by Francisco Javier's "monogamous family". We are familiar with single-parent families. From time to time, we even meet monogamous individuals. But what exactly is a "monogamous family"? What may a family be with only one (*mono-*) partner (*-gamous*)? Such a thing can be compared, in its nonsensical side, to the well-meaning man who would not be a "consistent revolutionary" if he did not deliver his discourse on "marriage". In both cases, there is a sort of real impossibility. But in the case of the revolutionary, we at least see what is at stake. It is the nonsense of the enunciating real subject who means to produce himself, as his own cause, through his identification with the master-signifier of the "revolutionary".[2] By the way, this signifier is not enough to represent the subject. Hence the necessity of alienation in the discourse on "marriage". To be sure, Francisco Javier has to be alienated by language because of the insufficiency of only one signifier to represent him. And yet, if the Eperrist is insufficiently represented by the "revolutionary", he is not better represented by "marriage" or the other signifiers of his discourse. All these signifiers cannot represent anything real of the subject. Their value is purely symbolic. Therefore, this value cannot be attached to the real presence of the subject, but only to the imaginary reality of his representation.

A signifier is a symbolic representative that represents only the imaginary representation of a real presence. In a sense, the representative represents the presence through the representation, but only in a symbolic way. This means that nothing real supports its representativeness. Apart from a purely symbolic value, the presence and its representative have nothing real in common. The presence is completely absent in its representative. Therefore, the representative cannot present what it represents. It cannot be evidence of it. It cannot even give an idea of it. *The value of the representative is purely symbolic. It is the value of being for the presence, of being instead of it, and in its place. Besides this symbolic value or representativeness, there is nothing more in common between the real presence and its symbolic representative. Between the thing and the word, the supposed mental representation is just imaginary.* It is just a mental image. It is nowhere outside the mind. The symbolic representative does not show it. Nor does it show a real presence. Actually, besides itself, the representative does not show anything. Even when it is personified by the subject, it does not let us see him. It is rather his mask, or, to be more precise, his face turned into a mask.

Following Marx, who would have been the first 'structuralist' in the eyes of Lacan (13.11.68, pp. 16–17), a Lacanian must not take words for persons, but he must treat the signifiers as 'masks' that subjects 'wear' in 'society' (Marx, 1867, I, §1, p. 73). In the signifying social structure, the signifiers must thus be treated, not as real presences, but as 'representatives' of subjects (II, §2, p. 77). Of course, the representatives are 'personified' by the represented subjects themselves (ibid.), but this does not change anything. In Lacanian Discourse Analysis, the real represented presence must not be confused with the real literal presence of the symbolic representative. Behind the hood, the real Francisco Javier is not the same thing as a hooded "consistent revolutionary". The divided subject in the flesh is not identical to his individual position in the structure. The subject is not what he incarnates. He is not the role he plays in discourse. Of course, *he is represented by what he represents*, but *he is not what he represents*.[3] Despite the symbolic identification of the enunciating subject with the enunciated subject, the former is not identical to the latter. The real subject is not exhausted by his symbolic identity. Nor is he exhausted by the predicate in which he is symbolically alienated. He is divided ($) between the grammatical subject (S1) and the predicative language (S2), but he is neither the *One* nor the *Other*, but rather the difference between them (*a*).

Since 'the subject is divided between the S1 and the S2', he cannot be entirely 'represented' by 'only one of those two signifiers' (Lacan, 1977–1978, 15.11.77). He has to be represented by both of them. The fact remains that both signifiers are completely different, and even contradictory. This is why only their difference may represent the being of the subject (*a*). This is also why the subject has to be divided ($). He has to be divided because he has to be represented simultaneously by two contradictory signifiers (S1–S2). Besides being a "revolutionary", Francisco Javier must conform to "our time". Besides conforming to "our time", he must construct "the new society and the new man". He must thereby distinguish himself from the same language that he embodies. Paradoxically, he must *also* be one signifier and not *only* all the other signifiers.

Besides 'disappearing into' the multiplicity of the 'binary signifier' (S2), the 'subject' needs to 'appear' as the singularity of the 'unary signifier' (S1), which functions as his representative in the strictest sense of the word (Lacan, 1964, 03.06.64, p. 243). But this representative cannot be the only one. Nevertheless, it can be different from all the others. It can be the grammatical subject, the most insistent and recurrent signifier, the prevailing and commanding master-signifier, the emblem of evidence and fixity for the consciousness, the only point in which the imaginary ego representation is anchored to the represented real subject.[4]

If the master-signifier is the only anchorage point of the ego representation, the other signifiers can be anchorages of other imaginary representations. In any case, the anchorage ensures the real foundation and symbolic determination of the imaginary representations. Thus, if the representative cannot really represent anything, in compensation it can determine the imaginary representation. Actually, as discussed in chapter two, this determining power of the signifier is precisely that which prevents a real signification, a clear presentation, or effective communication, as the neutral flow of information.[5]

Determined by the symbolic representative, the representation can only be imaginary. Between the real undetermined presence and the symbolic determinant representative, there is nothing real, but only this imaginary determined representation. Unlike the representative, this representation is not something perceptible. It is not something that we can locate somewhere. Like those who situate their God in the Kingdom of Heaven, cognitive psychologists locate their representation in the Kingdom of Mind, as if everybody knew its location. As for us, until there is a precise location of such a place, we must assume that the representation is nowhere, which is only natural, since it is imaginary. On the contrary, everybody knows the location of the representatives. They are everywhere. Actually, they are everything, since all things represent, even if we do not know exactly what they represent.

In spite of Derrida (1967), the symbolic representative has nothing to do with the imaginary representation. The former is everything and everywhere, while the latter is nowhere, since it is nothing but imaginary. In the outer world, even the 'reflecting picture' or image in the mirror supposes a 'metaphor' (p. 412). However, if that is the case, then the picture is *not* a 'pure representation without metaphorical displacement' (ibid.), but it is rather a *symbolic representative resulting from metaphorical substitutions and metonymical displacements.* In a *reflecting picture,* of course, the representative is similar to the represented. It thereby seems to also be a representation. But that makes absolutely no difference. The representative seems to be a representation just as it also seems to be the represented presence. Independently from what it seems to be, the representative is only what it is. It is nothing but a representative.

To 'represent what it represents', the Lacanian representative does not need to be a Cratylean 'representation of the object' (Plato, *Cratylus,* 433b). Thanks to the metaphorical substitution and the metonymical displacement, the signifier can be representative without any kind of representation. Its representativeness does not reside in its representation. Its symbolic value is not the same thing as the imaginary reality of its representation. Its structural position is not a question of resemblance, likeness, reflection, suggestion, etc. Its function as a signifier is *not* its supposed signification. As a symbolic representative, the signifier cannot be either reduced or subordinated to the imaginary representation.[6]

The subject may claim to *have* a representation, an idea or a reading of something, but before this he needs to *be* represented by a signifier that functions as his representative, his agent or his figurehead, as well as the active support of any hypothetical passive representation. Now, in the symbolic universe, the subject personifies his representative. Francisco Javier, for example, incarnates the "consistent revolutionary". He identifies himself with the role he plays. And to play this role, he must pretend to have something in his mind. As a signifier *who* pretends to have a signification, the actor must pretend to have mental representations (such as the "conceptions of marriage") that explain his literal behaviour (his discourse about "marriage") by connecting his real presence to the symbolic representativeness of his role (the "consistent revolutionary" who "would not" exist without his "conceptions"). Actually, since the actor is identified with his role, he *must have* the mental representations. The fact remains that these representations are nothing but words. Besides these words, the representations are just imaginary. Their value is purely symbolic. They simply form part of the role. Their 'life' depends exclusively on the 'actual human behaviour' inherent in the 'role' of the subject (Berger & Luckmann, 1966, pp. 75–76).

The representation depends on the representative just as the signification depends on the signifier. If the signification is nothing but its imaginary representation, this mental representation is always a signification dependent on a discursive signifier. Now, to have this signification, the signifier has to be wrongly regarded as a 'sign' whose 'nature consists of arousing' the 'represented thing' through the 'representing thing' (Arnauld & Nicole, 1683, p. 80). Through this representative or representing thing, the *subject of knowledge* supposedly knows what is represented. The representation actually refers to this knowledge (signification) of the represented (signified) through its representative (signifier). In all this, however, the only evident thing is the representative, whose perceptible symbolic representativeness permeates everything present, everything real, the real *subject of the signifier* as well as the real signifying structure of his environment.

Contrary to the pretentious imaginary *subject of knowledge,* the real and realist *subject of the signifier* does not know anything. His 'role' does *not* give to him any kind of real 'knowledge' (cf. Berger & Luckmann, 1966, p. 78). Even the *know-how* of the role does not become genuine knowledge of the subject, but it constitutes a discourse without meaning, an unintelligible script to be followed without thinking, a set of incomprehensible instructions that belong entirely to the wisdom of the Other. In its involvedness, this wisdom is exterior to the involved subject. It is *the wisdom of the system.* It is inherent in the social signifying structure for the individual position of the subject. As for this subject, he plays his role in the dark. He functions mechanically as a piece of the system. He works for the system without any knowledge of it. He is thereby a proletarianized workforce that unconsciously does the work of the unconscious. In this work, the subject deals with all kinds of symbolic representatives, but he does not know what they really represent. This real representation can only be embraced by the wisdom of the Other. *It can only be conscious for the unconscious.* It is the unreachable operating information of the system. In a sense, this information is too rich, too subtle and too complex for the weak cognitive capacities of the individual subject. When this subject pretends that he knows the real representation of a symbolic representative, we can be sure of the imaginary reality of this real representation.

Unapproachable determined representation and approachable determining representative

Taking the subject for the Other, devout psychologists take the human imaginary representation for a divine real representation. In that way, the 'representation' becomes the matter of a 'psychology' in which 'the objects of the world are taken in charge', not by the Other, but 'under the parenthesis of a subject' (Lacan, 1964, 03.06.64, p. 246). Filling this parenthesis, the objective representation has always benefited from the 'religiosity' of psychologists (Politzer, 1928, 1947). In the form of the *social representation*, it is the substance of social psychology for a number of researchers.[7] Funnily enough, even among psychologists who specialize in the symbolic representatives of discourse and language, the imaginary representation occupies an unmerited privileged place.[8]

To prevent an 'annexation' to the psychology of consciousness, a Lacanian must resist the psychological 'dictatorship of representations' (Resweber, 1998). In a Lacanian Discourse Analysis that must be focused on the unconscious, the prioritized element must be the symbolic representative, and not the imaginary representation, which involves necessarily a consciousness that imagines what is unconsciously represented by the symbolic representative.[9] From our point of view, this consciousness is nothing but a device of the unconscious. It is *the consciousness of the unconscious*. In actual fact, it forms part of a particular symbolic representative. It is included in the role of the subject identified with the master-signifier. To play his mastering role, the subject has to be conscious. His identification with the master-signifier entails a 'consciousness that masters' (Lacan, 1969–1970, 11.02.70, p. 79).

The master-signifier is 'the first signifier, the unary signifier' (S1), which 'emerges in the field of the Other' (S2) and 'represents the subject for another signifier' (Lacan, 1964, 03.06.64, p. 242). In the signifying social structure, this advantaged representative acts in the name of the subject. It also acts through him, since the subject himself personifies his own representative. Therefore, his consciousness, with its representations, may be *possessed* by his representative.

With this consciousness, the master-signifier (S1) makes its way into the unconscious, which consists of all the other signifiers (S2). In this manner, the "revolutionary" struggles his way, his *conscious way*, through the unconscious exteriority that comprises "marriage" and "monogamy". Resisting the consciousness of the "revolutionary", those opaque and impenetrable signifiers constitute his culture and his outer world. They materialize through all things and persons. They are everything perceptible and unintelligible in Francisco Javier's "perception of the world". They function thereby as the 'support of the unconscious' (Lacan, 1969–1970, 11.03.70, p. 131). At the same time, they represent the conscious representations or "conceptions" of the "revolutionary". In the exteriority of the unconscious, they are the uncommunicative, reticent, reserved, *repressed* symbolic representatives of the imaginary contents of consciousness.

According to Lacan (1964), 'what is repressed', as the 'discourse of the Other', is not 'the represented, but the representative of the representation' (03.06.64, p. 242). Located in the Other as the 'special site' of repression (1959–1960, 16.12.59, p. 78), the representative is 'that which is repressed' (1958–1959, 26.11.58). Now, even if the representative is 'repressed' or 'hidden', it is nevertheless 'located in spoken, enunciated discourse' (1959–1960, 16.12.59, p. 78). It is here, in the open air, all around us. It can be perceived everywhere. Unlike the imperceptible conscious representation, the unconscious representative is completely perceptible. However, contrary to the same understandable or intelligible representation, the perceptible representative is completely unintelligible. Of course, it is discursively interpretable, but that does not mean that it is mentally understandable or intelligible.[10]

Understandable conscious representation:
intelligible but imperceptible

Interpretable unconscious representative:
perceptible but unintelligible

Defined as a mentally intelligible object, the representation is either conscious or preconscious. When it is not yet an object of consciousness, it can become one. Nothing opposes its consciousness. By definition, the representation is *not* repressed.[11] On the contrary, and also by definition, the representatives are 'repressed' (Lacan, 1959–1960, 16.12.59, pp. 77–78). Therefore, they are 'unconscious' (ibid.). They are unconscious because they cannot really represent anything for consciousness, because their conscious representation is just imaginary, because the representatives themselves are purely symbolic.

As a succession of perceptible signifiers without an intelligible real signification, the signifying chain of symbolic representatives cannot really represent any kind of real presence apart from its own literal unintelligible presence. For instance, Francisco Javier's discourse can only really represent itself, and not the being of the "consistent revolutionary". Now, by representing itself, the conformist discourse about "marriage" presents the non-revolutionary Other of the "revolutionary". And yet, the "revolutionary" tries to represent his own being through this discourse. Despite his conscious identification with the "revolutionary", the subject makes this conformist discourse of the Other precisely because the perceptible presence of this discourse is unintelligible, unconscious, repressed for him, as evidenced by his funny conviction that he "would not be" a "consistent revolutionary" without such a discourse.[12] In other words, the subject does the work of the unconscious precisely because he is unconscious of the unconscious. This is why he can involuntarily become, even against his interests, the proletarianized enunciating workforce of a system, of a language or a culture, by making a discourse that enables the reproduction of the signifying social structure for his individual position.

In his individual position, the presence of the real subject cannot be directly analyzed by our Lacanian Discourse Analysis. This analysis can only reach the representative of the subject, as well as his discourse, which is not actually *his* discourse, but the discourse of the Other. If this *symbolic unconscious of the subject* is directly analyzable, the *real subject of the unconscious* can only be indirectly analyzed, through the analysis of the unconscious. As for the *imaginary ego of consciousness*, it cannot even be approached by a discourse analysis.[13] This analysis can only approach the 'representative of the representation', as 'that which takes the place of representation' (Lacan, 1964, 12.02.64, p. 70). If the imaginary representation stays in the inaccessible mental interiority of our neighbour, the representative escapes this interiority and comes out here, to the partly shared exteriority of our signifying social structure. In this symbolic universe, the representative links up with other representatives to compose the analyzed discourse.

Unfortunately, just like the structure, this discourse of the structure is not the same for my neighbour as it is for me. And in itself, of course, it cannot be known. However, it can be simply analyzed from our position. From this point of view, we can break the discourse down into its elements and the relations between these elements. In that way, we can make our *analysis,* in the strictest sense of the word (from the Greek *analusis*, separation into parts). This analysis is better than nothing. As far as I know, it is actually the only direct way to explore our only universe, which is the symbolic one.

In our universe, we can only have symbols *at our disposal.* The imaginary representations of our neighbours are simply unreachable, but we can reach, in compensation, the symbolic representatives of these representations. The symbolic representatives are actually the only things that we can directly analyze in our Lacanian Discourse Analysis.[14] But this is not at all regrettable. *Besides being the only approachable data in discourse, the symbolic representative determines the unapproachable imaginary representations of consciousness. Moreover, it composes the unconscious of our neighbour, as well as the partly shared exteriority of our signifying social structure.*

Paradoxically, the unconscious of our neighbour is *less inaccessible* than his consciousness. To explore Francisco Javier's consciousness, for instance, we must necessarily be him and share his interiority, which is naturally impossible for us. On the other hand, to explore the signifying social structure of his unconscious, we must only take his discourse literally. We must analyze this discourse, which is already the unconscious, as the discourse of *a* language. As the structure for the individual position of our neighbour, this language cannot be known by us, of course, but it can be partly explored, since it is also our language to a certain extent. Now, through the exploration of this language, we can go deep down into the heart of hearts of our neighbour, which is strangely outside him, in language. On this point, Humboldt (1834) noticed, a long time ago, that 'nothing in the heart of man' should remain outside 'language' (§21, p. 231). Everything 'in the heart' should 'enter language' (ibid.). But language is outside. Therefore, everything in the heart should be outside, in the exteriority of the unconscious. Paradoxically, the heart or core of the individual interiority, the Augustinian *intimum cordis,* resides in the transindividual exteriority of language. The exteriority thus contains the deepest motivation of consciousness, the innermost interior determination, which resides in the symbolic external representative that determines all imaginary internal representations.

Individual conscious representation and social unconscious representative

The main responsibility of the representatives of a country, such as ambassadors and other diplomats, lies in their power to determine the representations of their countries. Similarly, any other symbolic representative has the power to determine its imaginary representation.[15] Actually, representations 'gravitate, operate exchanges and are modulated' under the power of their representatives and 'according to' the 'laws of the signifying chain' of these 'representatives' (Lacan, 1959–1960, 16.12.59, p. 77). As is the custom of Lacan, the symbolic determines the imaginary.

Representation of the ego (*moi*)	Representations of all things [*i*(*a*)]
Representative of the subject (S1)	Representatives of the object (S2)

If we examine the two categories of symbolic representatives distinguished by Lacan (the S1 and the S2), we may see that each one involves a determination of specific imaginary representations. On the one hand, as master-signifier (S1), the *representative of the subject* (the "revolutionary") determines the representation of his objective ego (*moi*), whose figure displays the made-up signification of the master-signifier (the image of a revolutionary). On the other hand, as language as a whole (S2), the *representatives of the object* (such as "family") are all the other signifiers that determine their own significations, or what they seem to represent, the representations of all things of the world [i(*a*)], their mental or internal realities (the image of a family).[16] In any case, the representations are retrospectively determined by their representative. Although they are projected by it onto an imaginary depth behind it, they arise from it. As remarked by Deleuze and Guattari (1972), the imaginary representations for our consciousness 'result' from 'the symbolic', from 'the unconscious', from the 'pure representative' (p. 364).

Besides determining the representations, the representative constitutes their symbolic value, which is actually their only value, their sense or the reason why they make sense. Now, unlike the intrinsic imaginary reality of the representations, their symbolic value is an extrinsic thing that can be separated from them and break out of the individual consciousness to which they are confined. As noted in chapter two, the symbolic value can be transmitted, exchanged and put into circulation. It can be attached to different representations imagined by diverse individuals. That way it can become the social value of those representations. The symbolic value materialized in the word "family", for example, can become the unconscious transmissible representative of different conscious intransmissible representations of the family. But these representations stay in your individual mind, in mine or in that of Francisco Javier. In these individual minds, there is evidently no *social representation* of the family. Until there is proof of the contrary, we must grant that all mental representations, including the so-called *social representations*, are individual representations. They are individual because they cannot get out of the individual mind. They cannot be *socialized*. What can be comparatively socialized is not their intrinsic imaginary reality, but their extrinsic symbolic value, their name, the word.[17]

Individual conscious representation:
imaginary reality in the cognitive interiority

Social unconscious representative:
symbolic value in the discursive exteriority

What is relatively social is not the determined representation, but its determining representative. Society resides in the unconscious word and not in its conscious meaning. Unlike the imaginary reality of this meaning, the word is not isolated in the cognitive interiority of the individual, but it constitutes a symbolic value that can be shared and communicated in the discursive exteriority of society. At any rate, in this exteriority of the signifying structure, the structural interaction between symbolic values is that which determines the passive imaginary realities represented by their own symbolic values. As usual, the active determining pole is the symbolic one. The symbolic elements actively determine the appearance of imaginary entities. Now, for this determination to be possible, the symbolic elements have to be independent from the imaginary entities. The words of discourse cannot depend on their cognitive meaning.[18]

Paradoxically, the representatives cannot depend on what they represent. The symbolic value of an imaginary reality cannot depend on this reality, but on other symbolic values of other realities. To illustrate this, Lacan (1964) refers to 'diplomats', who 'simply exercise, in relation to one another, that function of being pure representatives and, above all, their own signification must not intervene' (03.06.64, p. 246). Therefore, in an 'exchange of views' between two diplomats, 'each must record only what the other transmits in his pure function as signifier' (ibid.). On this point, Lacan emphasizes that 'the term *representative* is to be taken in this sense', as 'a signifier', and on the 'opposite pole from signification', which 'comes into play in the representation' (ibid.).

The same social representative for two distinct individual positions in the structure

Signification comes into play in representation, but this does not mean that representation involves communication. Even though the signifiers are communicated, they do not carry their own signification with them. This signification is just its imaginary representation, which is inseparable from the mind that imagines it. This mind has to detain *its* signification. Therefore, signification cannot take part in communication. Its imaginary representation cannot be communicated. In spite of cognitive psychologists, this representation is confined to the mental interiority of an individual subject. It cannot get out of this interiority. Without telepathy, it cannot be conveyed to another interiority. It cannot even be compared to the representation of another subject.[19]

When we analyze a discourse, the representation of the speaking subject is beyond our scope. It is the private business of the subject. It stays in his inaccessible interiority. It cannot be present in language. In this locus of speech, the only matter for our analysis consists of symbolic representatives that communicate nothing but themselves, their own real presence and not their imaginary representation. It is nevertheless the case that the analyzed representative arouses a representation in our individual interiority. As discussed in the first chapter, this representation of the listener could bear a resemblance to the one of the speaker. Both representations could be similar, granted, but not identical, since they are determined in two different ways by the two divergent particularizations of the signifying social structure for the two distinct positions of the speaker and the listener. Put differently, even if a signifier such as "family" is the same in itself, it cannot be the same for two different structural positions, so it cannot arouse the same representation of the family in both of them.

In two distinct structural positions, there have to be at least two different representations of the family. The representation of the speaker must not be regarded as a cognition that would pass through the structure, inside a communicative capsule, to be received in an unchanged state in the position of the listener.[20] Even if we believed in a sort of telepathic transmission, we should grant that the received representation would be at least influenced and modified by what it would encounter in its transmission channels within the structure. In these channels, the representation would be decomposed and recomposed in a different way. It would not be only transmitted, but also transformed by the interactions that would transmit it. In the signifying social structure, these interactions would shape the representation.[21] Now, if we reasonably reject a telepathic transmission of the representation, we must recognize, nevertheless, that the representation is an effect of the structure for its position. It is an effect of that which converges in this position. It is then an effect of this position, which is materialized by the representative. The representation is thereby totally determined by that which is intertwined *in* its determining representative.

In the representation, the representative determines everything, including the hypothetical resemblance to other representations. As we know, two determined representations of the family could be similar because of the identity of their same determining representative ("family"). Now, if the two determined representations are not identical, it is also because of their determining representative, which cannot be exactly the same representative for two different structural positions. The signifier is the same in itself or in the structure in itself, of course, but it is not the same in the two manifestations of the structure for the two positions. For these two positions, the same value of the "family" has two different signifying exchange values (symbolic values) and not only two different signified use values (imaginary realities). Similarly, the same amount of money *in itself* has two different social values for two distinct individual positions. Thus, even money, as a 'universal equivalent', is still a 'relative value' that differs qualitatively and quantitatively in relation to different individual positions (cf. Marx, 1867, I, §1, pp. 51–68). This difference opens a gulf between the individual subjects, their symbolic universes, their enunciating workforces and their enunciated discourses. Although this gulf cannot be systematically analyzed, it must be acknowledged by a Lacanian Discourse Analysis that proves to be, on this particular point, Freudian rather than Marxian.

In a Freudian-Lacanian perspective, the same social representative in itself cannot be exactly the same for two distinct individual positions in the structure. It cannot present the same symbolic value for both positions. Nor can it represent the same imaginary reality for both of them. This conception involves a structuralist reinterpretation of the classical distinction between the Thing in itself and the thing for the subject.[22] In this reinterpretation, the thing for the subject is either the representation, which is just imaginary, or its symbolic representative for the subject. As for the real Thing, it is the real structure in itself, with the real presence of its structural elements, or symbolic representatives in itself. In the literality of its real presence, each one of these symbolic representatives *is* in itself the real presence. It cannot be differentiated from it. However, the real presence must be differentiated from the imaginary representation. Unlike the representative, this representation does not have a real presence. This is why it is just imaginary. It is just imaginary precisely because its *reality* cannot constitute a real presence. Unlike the letter of the symbol, the reality of the image *cannot be real*. Thus, paradoxically, the represented imaginary reality cannot be as real as its literal symbolic representative. As Bakhtin (1938) intuitively remarked, 'however realist the represented world can be, it could never be identical to the real representative world, in which we find the author that has created this image' (p. 396).

Together with Bakhtin, and contrary to common sense, Lacan situates the real presence, not in what is represented, but in what represents it. From a Lacanian viewpoint, the represented thing is just imaginary, while our attention is turned to the real presence of its symbolic representative. This representative presents everything, even the subject, who presents himself by embodying the signifier. Therefore, in a sense, everything is present. The so-called representation becomes just imaginary. The real presence is in the representative. The real Thing 'is the signifier' (Pavón Cuéllar, 2005, p. 13). This signifier is the Thing 'to which all signifiers refer' (ibid.). This Thing must remain the 'beyond-of-the-signifier' precisely because 'it is itself the signifier' (ibid.). To signify, the signifier goes round in circles. It circles round itself. Here is the reason why we are condemned to the monologue of the Other without an Other of the Other. In this language without a metalanguage, the only real is the real of the symbolic. The signifier is always referring to another signifier. The discourse consists always of words about words. Consequently, the Thing escapes the signifier. But it must be stressed that it escapes the signifier because it is itself a signifier. Logically, this signifier cannot completely turn towards itself. Therefore, the Thing cannot be entirely signifierized by itself. There is always a non-signifierizable residual product (*a*).[23]

Notes

1. When Parker (2005a) turns his attention to these points of contact, he perspicaciously describes them as 'points of blockage where nonsensical signifiers may be at work', as 'quilting points that keep the fabric of the signifying system in place', or as 'fixed points' represented by 'signifiers or metaphorical substitutes' that 'recur in a text' (p. 169). On the assumption that 'specifying these points may be the furthest we can go in any particular analysis', Parker believes that such a specification 'is useful for locating fixed points around which one text may revolve, locating a text in broader patterns of discourse, and examining how the temporal logic of a text is constructed' (ibid.). To this end, a Lacanian Discourse Analysis must detect those signifiers that recur in a text, but also certain *hapax* and other signifiers that present a rather suspect frequency in the analyzed discourse. With that in mind, we may even take the liberty of making an enlightened use of lexical statistics and all those prodigious pieces of software that delight the well-behaved social psychologists.
2. In the Althusserian-Lacanian Discourse Analysis of Pêcheux (1975b), this nonsense corresponds to the 'Münchhaussen effect' of the 'subject-form of discourse, in which there is a coexistence of interpellation, identification and creation of sense', that involves

the 'nonsense of the production of the subject as his own cause' (p. 245).

3. In this, our Lacanian Discourse Analysis differs from the Lacan-oriented analysis of Georgaca (2003), in which 'positions in speech do not represent', but 'articulate subjectivity' (p. 544). We would rather say that *positions in speech simultaneously represent and articulate subjectivity*. Accordingly, we assume the existence of an 'underlying' subject who 'plays the roles' and 'represents' himself through his representatives (ibid.). However, since the subject is divided by his representatives, our viewpoint does not 'presuppose' a 'unified underlying self' (ibid.). The representatives of the subject may be *unified* (S1), but the subject has to be divided ($) between his representatives (S1–S2). If the signifier cannot really *unify* the subject, it is precisely because the subject is not really presented by the signifier, but only symbolically represented by it. If the subject could be identical to the signifier, then there would be a *unified self*. But this is not possible. The player cannot be the same thing as his played role. He cannot be only his structural position. This is precisely why he can always 'maintain a reflexive stance' in relation to his 'position' (cf. Georgaca, 2003, p. 556).
4. As Parker (2005a) notices, 'the master-signifier functions as an anchor of representation in a text through such rhetorical tropes as the insistence that *this is the way things are*, that is not subject to challenge or dissent' (p. 170). The master-signifier (S1) functions in this way, as the anchor of the imaginary representation, because of its steady foundation in the ground of the represented real subject ($\S1). Here is what ensures the indisputable evidence and dogmatic fixity of the master-signifier, in contrast with all of the other signifiers (S2), which cannot have a steady foundation in a being that is constantly slipping (S2/*a*).
5. With good reason, Potter and Wetherell (1987) remark that our signifier is not a 'transparent information channel', but a 'potent, action oriented medium', that must be approached 'in its own right and not as a secondary route to things *beyond* the text' (p. 160).
6. The 'differentiation between the presentation and the representation' has nothing to do with the 'difference between the signified and the signifier' (cf. Derrida, 1967, p. 418). Actually, the representation appears only as a signifier when it is signifierized or symbolized, when it becomes a symbolic representative, when it is no longer a representation in the strictest sense of the word. And yet, as the representation, the representative 'represents something other than itself' (Lacan, 1953c, p. 25). Therefore, as the representation,

the representative is 'analyzable' (ibid.). However, the representative can only be analyzed with a discourse analysis, while the representation requires a content analysis.

7. It must be granted that the concept of *social representation* implies in itself, from the outset, the intervention of the symbolic representativeness of the signifier. This representativeness has been implicitly recognized by Moscovici (1961) when he considers that the representation represents 'someone' and makes 'signifying' that which is represented (pp. 62–63). This leads Moscovici to distinguish, in 'the representation', the 'passive pole of the impression of the object' and the 'active pole of the choice of the subject' (p. 63). Even if those poles of 'representing' and 'representing itself' (ibid.) correspond approximately to the representation and the representative, the distinction between imaginary and symbolic is not yet involved. To find this distinction, we must look for it elsewhere, as in Jodelet (1984), in her differentiation between the 'imaginary (*imageant*) feature' and the 'symbolic' or 'signifying feature' of the representation (pp. 362–363).
8. For instance, 'language' is treated as 'that which accomplishes the union of communication and representation' (Champagnol, 1993, p. 45). Both functions can also converge in the analysis of 'discourse' as that which 'conveys' the 'representations' (Ghiglione et al., 1980, p. 100).
9. Being imaginary, the representation can only be conscious, since it cannot be anything outside the imagination of consciousness. Hence the absurdity of the concept of 'unconscious representation', which means an unconscious that has been imaginarized, psychologized, disciplined, tamed, so that 'it doesn't produce any more, but it is satisfied with believing' (Deleuze & Guattari, 1972, p. 352).
10. In social psychology, we may say that the interpretable representative is not mentally intelligible because it does not correspond to a 'mental entity' such as the 'social representation', but to the discursive elements, 'terms and metaphors', that are either *interpreted* or *used to interpret* in the 'interpretative repertoire' of Potter and Wetherell (1987, pp. 138–139).
11. As noticed by Kaës (1985), the 'representation' is 'more or less available for the consciousness of the subject', that is to say, 'free from any effect of drive (*pulsion*) and repression' (p. 120). And yet, the representation is used to repress and cover the impulsive and pulling void of drive. From this angle, it functions as a 'plug' for the 'unthinkable' (p. 124).
12. This conviction constitutes manifestly an effect of repression that can be recognized by other analysts of discourse. However, they

would not call a spade a spade. They would recognize the effect, but not the cause of the effect. Thus, in general, 'discursive psychologists, not to mention conversation analysts, might exclude the concept of repression from their theoretical vocabulary, but, occasionally, the repressed repression can be detected, lurking on the edges of analysis' (Billig, 1997, p. 143).

13. If we trust Kaës (1985), we may grant that this 'ego' is approached 'by the psychological research of the representation' (p. 120). Discourse analysis must be focused on the 'discourse of wisdom (*savoir*)' that represents symbolically the imaginary 'ego' (ibid.). But this representativeness does *not* mean, as Kaës believes, that the discourse 'is produced by' the ego (ibid.). From our Lacanian viewpoint, it is rather the ego that would be produced by discourse.
14. In the terms of Potter and Wetherell (1987), our analysis can only come into contact with the 'interpretative repertoires' that represent the 'social representations' (pp. 138–157). We can thus attain the 'way accounts are constructed', but not the 'mental entities' represented by 'language use' (p. 157).
15. In Potter and Wetherell (1987), this power corresponds to the 'performative and indexical nature of language' in relation to social representations, as 'cognitive or mental states' (p. 145).
16. Both categories of representatives might also explain two angles that Flament and Rouquette (2003) distinguish in every representation. While the S1 would bear the 'implication' of the representation, which involves the 'personal identification', the S2 would articulate the 'context' of the same representation, as the 'conditions' for its 'actualization' (pp. 117–134).
17. Calling into question the social character of social representations, Harré (1985) observes that their 'implementation' is a 'symbolic activity' (p. 149). In this activity of the representatives as 'supports of social representations', we find the 'linguistic practice, which is social in the strictest sense of the word' (ibid.).
18. In this, our Lacanian Discourse Analysis just follows the classical orientation of a discourse analysis that has providentially 'eschewed any form of cognitive reductionism, any explanation that treats linguistic behaviour as a product of mental entities or processes, whether it is based around social representations or some other cognitive furniture such as attitudes, beliefs, goals or wants' (Potter & Wetherell, 1987, p. 157).
19. We must reject the idea of a conscious 'communication' by which 'representations' would be 'compared' (cf. Almudever & Le Blanc, 2000, p. 290). All the same, we can take for granted an unconscious

'co-construction', in different structural positions, of *incomparable* conscious 'representations of the interlocutors, the object and the situation' (ibid.).

20. By rejecting this idea, Lacanian Discourse Analysis stands apart from a Propositional Content Analysis in which 'representations' are moved, transferred, 'carried' or 'transported' (*véhiculées*) by 'discourse' (cf. Ghiglione et al., 1985, p. 100).
21. Kaës (1985) is aware of this, as evidenced in his description of the 'group shoring' (*étayage*) as a 'codification' that 'gives a support, a shape and a credit to the intrapsychic representation in a retaking by speech that makes it signify in the interpersonal or social link' (p. 113).
22. In social psychology, this reinterpretation can be compared to the classical one of Wagner (2001), who regards our *social structure in itself* as 'something' that is 'beyond the social' (p. 117) and about which 'people cannot speak' (p. 94). As for the same real structure for each structural position, it is described as an 'imaginary or symbolic object' about which 'people can discuss' (p. 93). On the basis of this distinction, Wagner concludes that 'the representation is the same object that it represents' (p. 97). To escape this vicious circle, we must recognize the real social presence of the symbolic representative, as well as the difference between the imaginary representation and its symbolic representative.
23. In a Lacanian Discourse Analysis, this is how we may interpret 'the experience' that 'somehow language never quite encompasses reality, that the way we talk about things might indeed have all the performative, effective and constructive functions described in the literature—that we might indeed be positioned by language—and yet the feeling remains that whenever we try to say something completely, the saying of it misses the point' (Frosh, 2007, pp. 640–641).

CHAPTER EIGHT

The discourse of the master

In this chapter I display the matrix in which Lacan formalizes the relations between four positions he distinguishes in the discourse of the Other as *discourse of the master*. I indicate simultaneously the occupants of these positions in a discourse which is considered by Lacan not only as the framework for politics and society but as the fundamental discursive unconscious configuration that precedes and underlies any other kind of discourse. In this configuration, we will observe how truth is embodied by the real subject of the enunciation. We will then see how the subject is divided between their representative and all the other signifiers, between the agent and the Other of discourse, between the symbolic subject of the statement and the statement itself. We will finally grasp why the product coming away from this division corresponds, in Lacanian theory, to a remainder of the real subject, a surplus that cannot be assimilated by the signifiers and that coagulates as an object of desire overflowing all being in discourse.

Enunciation, identification, alienation and deprivation

Since the signifier cannot completely turn towards itself, there must be a difference (*a*) between the signifier *itself* (S1) and its turn, flexion or inflexion, towards itself or *for itself* (S2). In other words, there must be a displacement between the enunciated subject and its predicative explanation, between a signifier and a language, between the structural position and the structure for the structural position. This can be illustrated by Francisco Javier's displacement between his identification with "the revolutionary" and his alienating self-justification in terms of "marriage" and "faithfulness". We can indicate this *metonymical movement* by an arrow (S1→S2). This arrow leads from the enunciated individual subject (S1), as the subjective representative of the enunciating divided subject ($\$\backslash S1$), to the predicative representative (S2) of a remaining object (S2/*a*), *the* object of Lacan (*a*), which results precisely from the difference between both representatives (the S1 and the S2). All this can be described by a formula ($\$\backslash S1 \rightarrow S2/a$) that reproduces, in a linear form, the Lacanian matrix of the *discourse of the master*, whose four elements can be illustrated by Francisco Javier's discourse:

$$\frac{S1}{\$} \longrightarrow \frac{S2}{a}$$

Subjective representative	→	Predicative representative
Enunciating subject		Remaining object

"Revolutionary"	→	Discourse about "marriage", "faithfulness", etc.
Francisco Javier divided between the "revolutionary" and the discourse about "marriage", "faithfulness", etc.		Difference between the "revolutionary" and its discourse about "marriage", "faithfulness", etc.

The four elements indicate four features of the same individual subject: his enunciation of discourse ($), his identification with the master-signifier (S1), his alienation in language (S2) and his deprivation by discourse (*a*). The four *elements* can also be described in relation to the four discursive *positions* (truth, agency, necessity, product) that are occupied by the four features of the subject: the truth of his division ($), the agency of his individualizing sameness (S1), the necessity of his dividing otherness (S2) and the product of his division (*a*). In Lacan, these four features ultimately refer to the desire of the subject, his conscious intention, his unconscious structure, and the cause of his desire. In the intricate relations and tensions between the four subjective elements, we can appreciate the complexity of the Lacanian theory of subjectivity[1]:

Identification with a signifier	→	Alienation in a language
Enunciation of discourse		Deprivation by discourse

Agency	→	Necessity	Conscious interior	→	Unconscious structure
Truth		Production	Subjective desire		Cause of desire

To orientate ourselves in the matrix of the discourse of the master, we must begin by distinguishing the two levels of the enunciating act and the enunciated fact, which were already introduced in the fourth chapter:

- At the level of the enunciated fact ($S1 \rightarrow S2$), in the symbolic, there is a permanent movement from the master-signifier (S1) to all other signifiers (S2), from the individual identity of a signifier to the dividing plurality of a language, from the structural position to the structure for this position, from an intentional agency to a structural necessity, from an identificatory sameness to an alienating otherness, from the One of consciousness to the Other of the unconscious, from the "revolutionary" to the system of "our time", etc.
- At the level of the enunciating act ($\$ \lozenge a$), in the real of the symbolic, there is a division of the subject between his enunciation *of* discourse ($) and his deprivation *by* discourse (*a*), his speaking workforce and the lost product of this workforce, his desire and the cause of his desire, the reason for his identification with a signifier and the consequence of his alienation in language, the supporting body of the signifier and the remaining difference between signifiers, the truth of the "revolutionary" and the object of his revolution, etc.

The *discourse of the master* is thus an enunciated fact that implies an enunciating act. It is an articulation between two symbolic representatives (the S1 and the S2) that represent successively a real presence ($\$$) and a real absence (*a*). *As a specific discursive form, the discourse of the master functions as the predicative unconscious discourse of a subjective conscious master-signifier that represents the speaking subject, makes him work and dispossesses him of the product of his work. As a general discursive matrix, this predicative discourse* ($\$\backslash S1 \rightarrow S2/a$) *carries out the passage from the symbolic identification with a signifier* (S1), *which presupposes a real enunciation of discourse* ($\$\backslash$), *to the resulting symbolic alienation in language* ($\rightarrow S2$), *which entails a real deprivation by discourse* ($/a$). In the next four sections, we will separately examine these four elements in their logical succession: first the presupposed enunciation ($\$\backslash$), the identification ($\backslash S1$), then the resulting alienation ($\rightarrow S2$) and finally the entailed deprivation ($/a$).

The truth: Enunciation of discourse ($\$$)

In the discourse of the master, the position of truth is occupied by the real subject, the proletarianized subject, who is reduced by language to his enunciating workforce. With this workforce, the real subject does the work of the unconscious, of a language, of the signifying social structure for his structural position. Logically, this work is also the work of the structure in itself, that is to say, the work of culture or civilization. Hard at this work of culture, the subject becomes a 'cultural animal' whose working 'life' is totally 'dominated by the verbal substitutes for the physical world' (Sapir, 1931a, p. 42). This domination is usually implicit, but it becomes explicit in the master-signifier (S1). When encountering this signifier, the labouring subject comes to terms with being dominated by it, in exchange for his symbolic identification with it ($\$\backslash S1$), which makes him feel that he is dominating through it ($\$\backslash S1 \rightarrow$). In this way, the signifier becomes a sort of underlying permanent grammatical subject (S1) of the predicative discourse ($S1 \rightarrow S2$), as evidenced by the "revolutionary" in Francisco Javier's discourse. Under the power of this enunciated subject ($\$\backslash S1$), the enunciating subject is just 'supposed' (Lacan, 1969–1970, 26.11.69, p. 12). Nevertheless, this supposition of the 'master-signifier' involves a structural position that determines the subject's point of view, his consciousness and his 'illusions' (18.02.70, p. 106).

From the "revolutionary point of view" of the master-signifier, Francisco Javier is just a revolutionary whose "conceptions of marriage and the couple", whatever they may be, must automatically be revolutionary. Following this axiom, the enunciated 'discourse of the master' aims at 'masking the division' of the enunciating subject, the intrinsically divided subject (Lacan, 1969–1970, 11.03.70, p. 118), who cannot only be a "revolutionary", but must also be someone else, an Other that may even be regarded as conformist or simply non-revolutionary. Divided between this Other (S2) and the "revolutionary" (S1), the enunciating subject ($) constitutes *the truth*, the 'truth' of the discourse of the master ($\S1→S2), the 'truth' that is 'concealed' by the individual master-signifier ($\S1) of the enunciated subject (18.02.70, p. 102).

The truth can be compared to the face covered by the hood of the revolutionary. Like this hood, the enunciated subject covers the enunciating subject. The individuality of the "revolutionary" covers the division of Francisco Javier. By covering this deep wound, the signifier protects the raw nerve of the subject. It protects the sore point of the *inconsistent* truth of the "revolutionary". It protects it from our prying eyes. The cover is thus protective, while the covered subject is protected.[2] Now, besides being covered and protected by the "revolutionary", Francisco Javier expresses it and is in return symbolized by it. He enunciates a "revolutionary" that tentatively represents him. In return for this enunciation, the enunciated signifier represents the enunciating subject. In exchange for this representativeness, the represented subject enunciates his representative. The representativeness of the enunciated "revolutionary" involves an enunciation for the represented Francisco Javier. The position and identity of the former simultaneously reveals and conceals the positioning and identification of the latter.[3]

If the *identity of the signifier* (S1) conceals the *identification with the signifier* ($\S1), it is because this identification allows us to see the distinction between the signifier (S1) and the subject ($), as well as the alienation of the subject in language and his division between his identification and his alienation ($\S1→S2). To succeed in concealing all this, the master-signifier (S1) may be repeated at the expense of all other signifiers (S2). For instance, in Francisco Javier's discourse, the occurrence of the "conceptions" of the "revolutionaries" functions as a recurrence of the "revolutionary point of view". In some cases, the discourse of the master (S1–S2) may even be transformed into a simple reiteration of the master-signifier (S1–S1). This reiteration of the same signifier avoids the necessary 'contradiction' between 'different' signifiers (Mao Zedong, 1937, II, p. 60). Actually, for all I know, repetition is the only effective intra-discursive remedy for the contradiction that divides the subject.[4]

In the enunciated discourse, the contradiction has to be remedied, since it is responsible for the problematic division of the enunciating subject. Identified with the signifier, the subject inevitably divides ($) when the signifier (S) contradicts itself by differentiating from itself (S1→S2). Thus, when the "revolutionary" has some "conceptions", Francisco Javier splits between the "revolutionary" and its "conceptions". The symbolic contradiction implies a real division between the contradictory terms. Actually, besides this real division, the symbolic 'contradiction' implies a real 'impossibility' (Wittgenstein, 1921, 5.525, p. 130). Now, paradoxically, this impossibility is required for the real subject to exist. It corresponds to his 'impossible truth' (4.464, p. 101). It amounts to the fullness and truthfulness of his full speech.

In the essentially contradictory discourse of the master, the 'impossibility' of the real subject 'fills the entire logic space' (Wittgenstein, 1921, 4.463, p. 101). To be empty, a discourse should not be contradictory, but repetitive. To a certain extent, the discursive emptiness can be assured by the recurrence of a signifier in a 'tautological' discourse that 'leaves' the 'entire logic space' to the imaginary 'reality' (4.463, p. 101). Strictly speaking, this *recurrence of the master-signifier* (S1–S1) is not the same thing as a *discourse of the master* (S1–S2). However, it can be described as a degenerative radicalization and simplification of this discourse, as evidenced by a 'revolutionary' theory without a 'theory of contradiction' (Lacan, 1975–1976, 13.04.76, p. 136). Besides its theoretical deficiency, this 'revolutionary theory' also suffers from 'emptiness' in the position of the 'truth' (1966b, p. 208). The 'revolution' lacks 'support' (1975–1976, 13.04.76, p. 136). It is not only a signifier without a language, a power without wisdom, an agency (S1) without necessity (S2), but also, as a consequence, an agency (S1) without truth ($), or a power without 'the basic supposition of its efficacy' (1966b, p. 208). Without this supposition, the only remaining efficacy of this power is obviously its power. Its only argument is the reiteration of its claim to authority.[5]

Tautological discourse (S1→S1)	*Geometrical discourse (S2→S2)*
Recurrence of the master-signifier	Discourse without a master-signifier
Partial and committed subjective slogan	Impartial and neutral predicative language
Power, authority	Science, reason

In the tautological discourse of the master-signifier, there is repetition of an argument of authority that takes on the character of a cyclic and rhythmic demonstration of power (S1→S1). Poles apart from this recurrent 'performative command', there is the geometrical discourse of Spinoza, the strictly logical discourse of a pure science, which has been described by Žižek as a *'perfect rational knowledge'* that 'is not obliged to have recourse to a master-signifier, to a point of order' (Ayerza, 1992). In this *geometrical discourse*, we restrict ourselves to 'interpret the world' without the aim of 'transforming' it (Marx, 1845, XI, p. 1033). Instead of making the "revolution" by making the "theory of the revolution" (S1→S2), it is only a question of making this theory by making it and nothing more than it (S2→S2). As an impartial and neutral predicative language, this theory is quite the opposite of the partial and committed subjective slogan, as the inveterate choice of a signifier (S1→S1). Against this choice, the geometrical discourse is a choice of all signifiers, a choice of reason, a choice of non-choice. Now, this rationalist and bureaucratic ideal choice of modern scientific absolutism can only be practically realized (e.g. through a serious journal of psychology) in the form of the university discourse (S2→*a*). But this discourse fails in its attempt to symbolize the real (*a*), which unavoidably escapes all signifiers, their language and their reason, the perfect wisdom of the pure symbolic totality (S2). After the failure of this discourse, we appreciate the necessity of a master-signifier whose tautological functioning manages to exclude the real and thereby ensure the cohesion and conformity of the symbolic logic.

Besides being one of the terms of the subjective division, the master-signifier *wants* a tautology, or at least a compromise between the divided terms. It thus *wants* a symbolic identity, or at least an imaginary equivalence. This *will* can be illustrated, in Francisco Javier's discourse, by the "revolutionary" that aims for the synthesis between the revolutionary thesis and the anti-revolutionary antithesis. In such an ideal *new deal*, there would be a "new society" and a "new man", a non-dissociated society and a non-divided individual, who would save us from the *dissociated society* and the *divided individuality* that have been respectively explained by Marx and Freud.

With the aim of healing the individual division and social dissociation, the master-signifier aroused the discursive movement that led to the nightmares of Western Individualism and Eastern Socialism. In this movement, which takes place on a small scale in every discourse, the master-signifier hides the division and the dissociation behind the 'illusion of being One' (Lacan, 1967e, p. 277). Actually, to create the illusion, the master-signifier makes two moves. First, it imposes a *joining* 'consciousness' in which appears a 'unity' that *sews up* the 'conflicting tear' of society and individuality (Althusser, 1976, p. 239). Then, through this consciousness, the master-signifier tries to get rid of the *imaginary conscious dissonance* that expresses the *real conflicting tear*. Ironically, this aggravates the tear by deepening the contradiction between the *joining consciousness* of the master-signifier and the *tearing unconscious* of all of the other signifiers, as the discourse of language, whose symbolic alterity and multiplicity involve the real tear.[6]

The agency: Identification with a signifier (S1)

When we pass from the real subject ($) to the master-signifier (S1), we are moving from the *tear* to the *joining*, from dissociation to society, from division to individuality, from the enunciating subject to the enunciated one. In that way, in the discourse of the master, we rise from the position of truth to the 'dominant position' of agency, which is logically occupied by the 'master-signifier' (Evans, 1996, p. 45). In this *position of power*, the master-signifier gets its power from the subject's identification with it.

S1	*Agency:* enunciated subject Individuality, society
$	*Truth*: enunciating subject Division, dissociation

By virtue of the identification of the subject with the master-signifier ($\S1), this signifier (S1) distinguishes itself from the other signifiers (S2). It becomes *the* signifier, *the* choice of the subject, *the* support of his consciousness, *the* representative of his presence. It becomes itself a subject, *the* underlying enunciated subject, which moves apart from the predicative discourse. With all these dignities, the master-signifier stands out in the crowd of all other signifiers. It is *the* signifier that refers to the set of signifiers. It defines this set. It signifierizes its elements, 'which become signifiers under the action of this despotic symbol that totalizes them in the name of its absence or withdrawal' (Deleuze & Guattari, 1972, p. 369).

At first sight, the master-signifier seems to embrace all signifiers that are referred to it, or signifierized by it. For instance, the "revolutionary point of view" seems to embrace everything exposed to its view, including the "family", "marriage", and "our time". On second thoughts, we understand that the 'solitary' master-signifier is nothing more than a *hood* or an 'empty bag' (Lacan, 1975–1976, 18.11.75, p. 18). It is an 'empty set' (S1) whose only element cannot be its element, since it is its 'couple' (S2), that is, its Other materialized in all other signifiers (Miller, 2005, p. 214). Without an Other of this Other, the Other is the real set that contains the master-signifier, which is only an element, a signifier among others. Just as for the others, the master-signifier 'has no corresponding signifier' (Ragland-Sullivan, 1992, p. 73). In Lacan, to be sure, the enunciated symbolic subject does not signify the enunciating real subject. *The hood does not signify the face*. The "revolutionary" does not signify Francisco Javier. Nevertheless, it can represent him in relation to the "family", "marriage" and the rest of the signifiers. Among those elements of the unconscious, the "revolutionary" can act in the name of the consciousness of the subject.

The master-signifier acts in the name of consciousness. It actually possesses the consciousness of the subject who identifies with it. The fact remains that it forms part of the unconscious. Thus consciousness belongs to an element of the unconscious. To be sure, this element is just a signifier among other signifiers. Despite its position of agency, the master is just a slave among other slaves. As for its consciousness, it stages the realization of an ideal of mastery over the unconscious enslaved embodiment of the material signifying structure. Since this realization is just imaginary, the consciousness of the master-signifier can be described as 'a dream, the dream of the slave, the dream of mastery over the body' (Miller, 2005–2006, 07.06.06, p. 6). With such a dream, the master-signifier drags the body through the symbolic universe of language. Objectively, or *in itself*, this concrete universe precedes and comprises the rather abstract master-signifier (Condillac, 1746; Marx, 1843b). However, from the viewpoint of the subject, there is first his subjective identification with the master-signifier, and then the resulting predicative alienation of his body dragged through language by the master-signifier (Rousseau, 1781; Hegel, 1820). From this viewpoint, the master-signifier is present before undertaking its discursive route through the symbolic universe. The *revolutionary avant-garde* heads the *social movement*. The position precedes the structure for the position. The signifier already exists before its own internal differentiation from itself and its ensuing transformation in discourse. On that assumption, paradoxically, the ideological materiality of the signifying metonymical chain follows from an ideal metaphor. Even if this first metaphor is the 'most abstract term', it is not the most 'derived' (cf. Condillac, 1746, X, §102, p. 283). On the contrary, it is the less derived, the most original, *the first*. From this angle, 'figurative language was the first to appear' (Rousseau, 1781, p. 45).

The first signifier can only be figurative because it must already be symbolic. Therefore, it cannot really present the subject, but it has to be a figurative substitute for his presence. It has to be just a symbol of the enunciating act. As a pure symbolic representative, it has to represent nothing more than an imaginary representation, a conception, a *semblance* of that which is symbolized. Its 'semblance resides in the fact that it pretends to nominate and thus directly translate into the symbolic fidelity the dimension of the act' (Žižek, 1999a). Its 'gesture' is a symbol that 'changes the act into a master-signifier' (ibid.). In relation to the enunciating act, this master-signifier is an enunciated metaphor, a purely symbolic representative, necessarily exterior to the enunciating subject. And yet, the subject identifies with this exterior signifier. He is then automatically alienated by it. The first identification already implies alienation. In other words, the master-signifier (S1) can only represent the subject ($) in the exteriority of the unconscious ($\S1→S2). Francisco Javier's revolutionary hood is an enlightening example of this exterior representativeness of the master-signifier. By covering the 'supposed' speaking subject, the hood externally 'represents' him 'through an intervention' in the spoken 'field of wisdom' (Lacan, 1969–1970, 26.11.69, p. 12). This exterior field comprises the hood, which is after all an article of clothing, a garment among other garments, a signifier among other signifiers. Similarly, the "revolutionary" forms part of the wisdom of "our time". The One is a piece of the Other. Everything in the One belongs to the Other. The consciousness of the One is a consciousness of the unconscious Other. Even the One's desire is a desire of the Other. No matter how revolutionary the 'master's desire' may be, it has to conform to the conformist system of the 'Other' (17.12.69, p. 41). In general, 'the desire of man' always amounts to the 'desire of the Other' (18.02.70, p. 106).

In a Lacanian perspective, man's desire is embraced and determined by the signifying social structure of language. It is a desire felt through the signifiers, for them, by them and because of them. Man's desire belongs to the signifier. This also applies to man's power, authority, agency, or mastery. According to Lacan (1969), 'the signifier' is the only 'master' (p. 387). The signifier masters man. To be a master, a man has to be a signifier. The 'master-signifier' indicates precisely this 'function of the signifier that underpins the essence of the master' (1969–1970, 26.11.69, pp. 20–21).

Even the most elementary essential feature of the master depends entirely on the signifier. For instance, the signifier is necessary for the 'master' to be One, to have an identity, as well as a conviction of being One, 'identical to himself' (Lacan, 11.03.70, p. 118). The identity and the identitary conviction are both determined by the signifier, by discourse, specifically by the supposed 'univocal' attribute of the 'discourse of the master' (ibid.). To be sure, this attribute determines the social or individual character of the master, the coherence and unity or unanimity of what it materializes, the personal or interpersonal "consistency" of the "revolutionaries".[7] Now, to succeed in the determination of all this, a discourse may reinforce its univocal attribute by having recourse to stratagems such as the 'perfect definition' (*definitude*) that Damourette and Pichon (1911) call 'notoriety' (I, §366–367, pp. 470–471). With this notoriety, *a* signifier becomes *the* signifier. With the [definite] 'article *the*', the master-signifier obtains a 'substance' that cannot be 'equivocal' (ibid.), but only *univocal*, as evidenced by "*the* revolutionaries" (*los revolucionarios*) for whom "marriage" has "importance and significance" in Francisco Javier's discourse. The definite article, in this instance, confirms the univocal attribute of the master-signifier that may then ensure the consistency of the "consistent revolutionaries".

The divided or dissociated enunciating subject ($) can only be represented by the univocal master-signifier, in a purely symbolic way, as an individual or social enunciated subject (S1). As noted many times before, this unbroken representative is not *really representative* of the broken presence. Its purely symbolic representativeness refers rather to a merely imaginary representation. Actually, as a signifier of 'the consciousness that masters' (Lacan, 1969–1970, 11.02.70, p. 79), the master-signifier *is* an unconscious symbolic representative of the conscious imaginary representation of the *psychological ego*. With the power of this alleged *individual representative* of the subject, the *psychological ego* functions in the same way that the *political state* does with the power of the alleged *social representatives* of its subjects. As a matter of fact, there is a fundamental fusion and confusion between the *psychological ego* and the *political state.*[8] This state may be understood here in the strictest sense of the word, but also in a broader sense, as any group that takes the form of a powerful and authoritative substance, such as the European Union, the United Kingdom, the global market, the international community, the scientific community, the psychoanalytical organization or school or association, as well as the party, the university, modernity, democracy, globalization, civilization, humankind, etc. When those *signifiers* become *signs of* a substance comparable with that of the *psychological ego*, then they can be examined in the light of the *political state* that Hegel 'substitutes for the master' (Lacan, J. 1969–1970, 11.02.70, pp. 89–90).

As the 'objective spirit', the ideal political 'state' of Hegel (1820, §258, pp. 313–314) is substantiated in such a way that it represents a sort of psychological ego, it occupies the position of the enunciated subject (S1), and it thereby precedes the predicative material actualization of the signifying social structure (S2). This is how the Hegelian 'speculation', according to Marx (1843b), 'inverts the relationship' between the political ideality of the master-signifier and the social materiality of language (p. 875). On the one hand, the 'idea' of 'the state' becomes 'the subject' (ibid.), so that its predicative 'exterior necessity', the necessity of the structure, is regarded as a subjective 'superior power' (Hegel, 1820, §261, p. 325). On the other hand, the 'real subjects, in civil society', are 'transformed into the objective elements of the idea', or 'the predicate' (Marx, 1843b, pp. 876–878). In that way, in Hegel, the discourse of the Other (or *discourse of a language*) becomes the discourse of the master (or *discourse of a signifier*). From this subjective viewpoint of the structural position, as discussed above, the position precedes and determines *its* structure. The signifier (S1) heads language (→S2), in the same way that the "revolutionary" *heads* "the constitution of society", or the "scientist" *heads* the "fabrication of wisdom". As for the real subject ($) represented by the "scientist" or the "revolutionary" ($\S1), he must be submitted to the signifier that represents him and dominates him through the signifying structure of wisdom or society.[9]

In Hegel, *the* signifier dominates through all other signifiers. The One asserts itself through the Other. The State exercises its power through civil society. However, as objected by Marx (1843b), 'the State is an abstract thing, only the people are a concrete thing' (p. 899). In our terms, only the signifying social structure is a concrete material thing. As for the State, it is just an ideal signifier abstracted from the structure. It is just one idea in the mind of the corporeal Other. Unfortunately, Hegel does not regard this Other 'as the real person', but 'as a real person that only has the element of its personality in an abstract manner' (p. 912). In itself, the Other would lack this element, as if it were the case that the signifying social structure needed the abstract master-signifier in order to realize its material concreteness. And yet, that is the case. The structure in itself can only materialize *for* one structural position, *in* this position, *as* it. Put differently, *one* concrete language can only become *one* as *one* abstract signifier. As a universe, the symbolic universe must form part of itself. The set of all existing things can only exist if it is an element of itself. The social plurality can only acquire a personality through one of its constituent elements, such as the Church, the Nation, the Revolution, the State and other master-signifiers. The 'multitude' can only be 'united in one Person', namely, the 'Leviathan', the 'Mortal God' of Hobbes (1651, I, §17, p. 120). This political master-signifier gives a unity to the plurality of individuals who identify with it. On the basis of this collective symbolic identification, the master-signifier ensures the subjection of its represented subjects to a *partly shared* signifying social structure.[10] This *partly shared* structure is not the structure in itself, of course, but the structure for the *partly shared* position of the political master-signifier. Leaving aside the individual differences between the positions of different revolutionaries, we can theoretically assume that all identify with the same political master-signifier of the "revolutionary". As Francisco Javier notes, this identification with the same signifier involves "an identification in the perception of the world". The revolutionaries share the viewpoint of the revolutionary structural position (the "revolutionary point of view" in Francisco Javier's discourse), as well as the signifying social structure for this position. That being so, they share the same space, the same world, the same structural emptiness. Actually, they are here to fill this emptiness.

To fill the structural emptiness, we need a real subject. Conversely, to give a consistency to this emptiness, we need a symbolic subject, a master-signifier, as evidenced by the "consistent revolutionary" of Francisco Javier. The consistency of the master-signifier coagulates the structural emptiness and transforms it into a structure. Therefore, in a sense, this structure *consists* of nothing but the *consistency* of the master-signifier.[11] The fact remains that this signifier is nothing but a constituent element of the structure. Its consistency comes from the structure. This objective side of the question is still forgotten by Hegelians and Lacanians. Accordingly, the Marxian critique of Hegel is still relevant. It demonstrates 'the biased, partial and incomplete character' of the Hegelian discourse of the master that still justifies our 'bourgeois State' (Lacan, 1959–1960, 04.05.60, p. 247).

Marx 'definitely refuted' the Hegelian discourse of the master (Lacan, 1969–1970, 11.02.70, p. 90). However, after this Marxian refutation, there has been a reactionary anti-Marxist restoration of the same discourse. There has also been a revolutionary Marxist restoration of it. In this case, ironically, Marx himself functioned as the 'restorer of order' (Lacan, 1979–1980, 18.03.80). His theory 'consolidated a discourse of the master' (1971–1972, 08.03.72). In this discourse, the subjective position of agency, authority, and power can be still occupied by *the* signifier, a master-signifier, such as the "revolutionary" in Francisco Javier's Marxist-Leninist discourse. As for the predicative position of structural necessity, it still corresponds to signifiers such as the "society" and the "family", as evidenced again by Francisco Javier, whose discourse, on this point, mysteriously reminds us of the Hegelian dialectical synthesis of the 'family' and 'civil society', as predicates of the subjective master-signifier of the 'state' (Hegel, 1820, §156–157, pp. 305–306).

The necessity: Alienation in language (S2)

In the discourse of the master, the two positions at the enunciated level are always occupied by the successive linked elements of an ostensibly conscious subjective signifier (S1) and a truly unconscious predicative language (S2). Composing a signifying chain, these linked elements can be found everywhere in modern and contemporary political thought (Pavón Cuéllar, 2005; Pavón Cuéllar & Sabucedo Cameselle, 2009). Their metamorphoses include, for instance, 'political movement' and 'civil movement' (Tocqueville, 1840, I, pp. 253–254), 'exercise of power' and 'class struggle' (Marx, 1847, p. 136), 'spiritual life' and 'economic regime' (Lenin, 1913, p. 15; Stalin, 1938, p. 212), as well as 'direct domination' and 'cultural hegemony' (Gramsci, 1930, p. 28; 1932, p. 314). In any case, regardless of the important discrepancies between these conceptual pairs, we always find the same subject and the same predicate, which can also be described in terms of mastery and slavery, oppression and exploitation, position and relation, consistency and structure, 'topography' and 'logic' (Laclau, 2000b, p. 58). In Lacan, as we know, both places concern 'a single subject' in two distinct 'relations to himself', or, more correctly, in two distinct relations to the Other, namely, the identification with one of its signifiers and the alienation in all of the other signifiers (Miller, 2005–2006, 07.06.06, p. 6). Logically, without the accurate detection of these two enunciated relations in the analyzed discourse of the master, a Lacanian Discourse Analysis cannot even approach the enunciating subject, or *the truth* of discourse, whose existence resides in the real division between the two distinct symbolic relations.

Subjective signifier (S1)	*Predicative language (S2)*
Political state	Civil society
Exercise of power	Class struggle
Domination	Hegemony
Oppression	Exploitation
Identification	Alienation
Position, consistency, topography	Relation, structure, logic

Let us take the case of Francisco Javier. As noted many times before, he is divided ($) between two distinct relations to the signifying social structure, namely, the political relation to his identity as a "revolutionary" (*domination* of the S1), and the civil, economic, or cultural relation to "family" and "society" in terms of "marriage" and "monogamy" (*hegemony* of the S2). These relations divide the subject because they are mutually exclusive, and they are so because they impose contradictory conditions on the subject. In the final analysis, the real division of the subject results from the symbolic 'contradiction' between the conditions of the 'citizen' and the 'bourgeois', the 'political man' and the 'religious man', the 'generic life and the material life' (Marx, 1844, pp. 356–357), the 'ethereal' or 'aerial life' (1843b, p. 959) and the 'commercial' or 'industrial life' (1846, p. 1068). Divided between 'a celestial and a terrestrial life', the individual subject has a 'double life' (1844, p. 356). He is in the service of 'two rival armies' (1843b, p. 926). On the one hand, he is consciously integrated into the celestial Popular Revolutionary Army. On the other, he is unconsciously included in the terrestrial counter-revolutionary *army* of his cultural environment, his economic system, and his civil society in the strictest sense of the word.

To be politically represented in the signifying social structure, the subject must individualize himself through a symbolic identification with *One* signifier, such as the "revolutionary". Since other subjects identify with the same signifier, the individualization implies socialization. The transformation into a "revolutionary" involves the incorporation into the social group of "revolutionaries". All things considered, the symbolic identification with the master-signifier can be regarded as *socialization through individualization.*[12] At the same time, on the basis of this symbolic identification, there is also the imaginary identification between the psychological ego and the political state. In any case, the symbolic or imaginary socialization results from an individualization of the enunciating subject as an enunciated subject. Now, this individualization *as* a symbolic subject (S1) necessarily involves a division *in* the real subject ($). Since this subject cannot be entirely reduced to one univocal signifier, he must 'accomplish an essential separation from himself' (Marx, 1843b, pp. 957–962). He must 'deprive himself' of his 'substantial being' (*a*), 'leave' it in the 'empirical reality' of the signifying social structure (S2/*a*), and 'disappear from this organization to take refuge in his individuality' ($\S1), that is to say, in the individuality of his symbolic political identity (ibid.). This is how the signifying social structure becomes the exteriority of the unconscious for the subject.

The individualization (S1) involves a division ($\S1) because the identification with *a* signifier (S1) involves an alienation in *a* language ($\S1→S2). This dividing alienation is inseparable from the individualizing identification. The real subject cannot have a symbolic identity without functioning as a piece of the symbolic system. Francisco Javier himself acknowledges that he cannot be a "consistent revolutionary" (S1) without his "conceptions of marriage and the couple" (S2). In general, one cannot take up a structural position without bearing the structure for this position. To be symbolically represented, the real subject must take the 'symbolic universe' upon himself (Berger & Luckmann, 1966, pp. 97–100). The articulated fact implies a 'legitimization' of the articulating structure (p. 94). The signifying chain actually appears as a *demonstration* of the signifying social structure. The 'message materializes the organization' of the 'code' (Martinet, 1960, p. 25). The discourse is material evidence of a language. It is an occurrence of the cultural environment. It is a performance of the symbolic system. Now, as it happens, our system is willingly or unwillingly Christian and monogamous, essentially patriarchal and homophobic, arrogantly western and European, traditionally racist and ethnocentric, instinctively liberal and free-market, providentially capitalist and bourgeois, etc. This is why Francisco Javier's revolutionary message, like 'everything that is not bourgeois, has to borrow from the bourgeoisie' (Barthes, 1957, p. 226). It has to borrow from the bourgeoisie because the bourgeois code precedes the revolutionary message. This precedence can be described in different ways:

- Pre-existence of the bourgeois 'civil society' in relation to the idea of a revolutionary 'state' that would 'make itself society' (Marx, 1843b, pp. 875–907).
- Pre-existence of the bourgeois 'hegemony', as 'educator', in relation to the revolutionary 'wish' to 'dominate' or 'educate the educator' (Gramsci, 1931, §18, p. 185).
- Pre-existence of the counter-revolutionary bourgeois 'society' in relation to the 'counter-society' proposed by the revolutionary (Berger & Luckmann, 1966, pp. 127, 144–145).

All these descriptions refer to the same pre-existent signifying social structure as the precondition of any particular signifying chain. They thus refer to the same preceding Other as the prerequisite for the discourse of the master. Now, since this Other is also the 'receiver' of discourse, Lacan assumes here an 'antecedence' of the 'receiver', of language or the locus of speech, in relation to the 'transmission', as discourse or speech (Lacan, 1958b, p. 167). Paradoxically, to 'communicate the message', the transmitter 'has to receive it from the receiver' (1953b, p. 155). So the transmitter can only transmit the message 'in an inverse form' (ibid.). Francisco Javier, for example, can only transmit a revolutionary message in the counter-revolutionary form of the receiving system of "our time" in which the message resounds. As in a mould, the message externally takes the 'inner form of language' (Humboldt, 1834, §21, p. 231). It takes the inverse form of the structure that articulates it. Thus, in general, the 'message' is 'articulated' by 'being constituted in the Other in an inverse form' (Lacan, 1958b, p. 167).

The discourse of the master takes its form in the Other, by the Other and from the Other. So its form turns out to be the Other's form. In this way, the *discourse of the master* takes an inverse form, as the *discourse of the Other*. The *subjective discourse of the conscious One* turns into the *predicative discourse of the unconscious Other*. The message of the transmitter is retroactively articulated by the receiver in an inverse form. This form is evidenced, within Francisco Javier's discourse, by his revolutionary "conviction" that inverts our suspect question in terms of conformist "obligations". It is also evidenced by his "revolutionary point of view", which is inverted in our revealing attribution of a "counter-revolutionary view".[13] These inversions reveal *truths* that relate not only to the interviewee, but also to the interviewer and especially to the analyst of their discourse, as each one of those subjects occupies a position in the signifying social structure. Although this *necessarily conventional* structure is not exactly the same for the different positions of those three subjects, it is nevertheless partly shared by them. Besides that, the structure is theoretically the same underlying structure in itself. In any case, whether in itself or for each one of us, the structure is only one, so that it constitutes a symbolic universe, or a language without a metalanguage, which determines my analysis and not only María Luisa's questions and Francisco Javier's answers.[14]

Even if all structural positions are determined by the structure, every position can become a dominant position that considers itself non-determined and thus different from all other positions. From the viewpoint of this unique position, we act as if we could objectively observe, analyze, and describe the exteriority of the structure, in itself, without being determined by it. This applies to Francisco Javier's "revolutionary point of view", but also to our Lacanian analytical point of view. From both points of view, the *discourse of the Other* seems to be our discourse, that is, the *discourse of the master*, of our master-signifier, with which we are identified. In a sense, that is the case. The fact remains that our master-signifier, just as any other signifier, is not only *the* signifier, but also *a* signifier among other signifiers. It is not only our position, but also one of the constituent positions of the structure. It is not only our voice, but also one of the voices of the system.

The signifier is not only One, but also Other. In the 'logic of the signifier', the signifier is 'internally' the One and the Other, 'One and Two' (Regnault, 2005a, 23.05.05). It functions thus as the 'primitive words' examined by Karl Abel, which logically attracted the attention of Freud (1910). Like these words, the signifier always has two 'antithetical' symbolic values, two 'opposite senses' (pp. 59–67). It is always expressed by us and articulated by the Other. As a master-signifier, it is simultaneously our power and the necessity of the system. It is both the representative of the enunciating subject ($\$\backslash S1$) and the enunciated subject of the predicative language ($S1 \rightarrow S2$).

In a symbolic system, any value depends on the opposing value. The obverse cannot exist without a reverse. The master 'cannot do without' the slave (Diderot, 1774, p. 664). The One implies the Other. *The* signifier (S1) implies *a* language (S2). 'The name implies a nomenclature' (Berger & Luckmann, 1966, p. 132). In the logic of the signifier, the element does not go anywhere alone. The word cannot do anything outside discourse. A "revolutionary" cannot make his revolution by himself. He is *not free* to make his revolution, but he is necessarily *chained* to the other signifiers in the signifying *chain*. In this chain, each component can only function as a link articulated with other links by the signifying structure. In this structure, each signifier is determined by all other signifiers. Thus, in a sense, *the* signifier is mastered by all other signifiers. The 'master' has countless 'masters' (Diderot, 1774, p. 538). The so-called slaves are the true masters of the so-called 'master' (p. 666). The mastery of the signifier obeys the functioning of a language. Actually, the conscious performance of the master-signifier forms part of the work of the unconscious discourse of language. The deeds of the "revolutionary" are deeds of "our time".

The subjective activity of the signifier is the predicative activity of a language. The 'operation of the master' is 'the operation of the slave' (Hegel, 1807, B, IV, A, p. 163). The purportedly conscious *discourse of the master* is the unavoidably unconscious *discourse of the Other*. The problem here lies in the insurmountable disparity between both discourses. In a sense, they have nothing to do the one with the other. And yet, they compose the same discourse, which can then be compared for a second time to the 'hybrid construction' of Bakhtin (1934). In this construction, even if the 'grammatical clues' indicate 'only one locutor', there are nevertheless 'two ways of speaking, two styles, two tongues, two semantic and sociological perspectives' (pp. 125–126). However, between those perspectives of the One and the Other, there is no 'formal frontier' (ibid.). The discourse 'belongs simultaneously to both perspectives' (ibid.). The discourse of the One is the discourse of the Other. The discourse of the "revolutionary point of view", for example, reveals at the same time the viewpoint of "our time", the thinking of a conformist cultural environment, the accepted wisdom of the signifying social structure particularized for the individual position of the "revolutionary".

As a particularization for *the* subjective signifier, the structure of *a* language is the predicative 'field of wisdom' in each discourse (Lacan, 1969–1970, 26.11.69, p. 12). It is the field of an 'unconscious entirely reducible to wisdom' (1975–1976, 13.04.76, p. 131). It is the 'field peculiar to wisdom, to the slave as the support of wisdom (*savoir*), as the one who has a know-how (*savoir-faire*), a wisdom totally transparent to itself' (1969–1970, 26.11.69, pp. 20–21). This transparency of wisdom confirms the intrinsic real emptiness of the structure. It gives us an idea about its unintelligible character. It is the transparency of the unconscious container, of its exteriority, of the outer world, as the translucent matrix of opaque ideology.[15]

The matrix of ideology does not have the impenetrable opacity of the articulated facts, but instead the invisible transparency of the articulating acts of the structure. As we know, these transparent ideological articulations constitute a pure know-how that determines the expression of the real subject. As practical wisdom, they are discursive techniques and not cognitive assumptions. They are signifying procedures and not signified knowledge. They must then be situated in the material work of the unconscious and not in the ideal commands of consciousness.

The transparent ideological articulations compose an *articulating expertise* in the work of the unconscious. Of course, this practical wisdom does not reside in the enunciating subject, but in the enunciating work itself, in this work of the unconscious, in this operation of the system, in this functioning of a language as articulating structure. As for the subject himself, he is just the workforce of the structure. He expresses what is articulated by the structure, but he does not know anything about this work of the unconscious. He is not conscious of anything. This is why the ideological articulations consist only of a purely practical wisdom, that is to say, a completely external wisdom, an unintelligible know-how, an unconscious corporeal expertise.[16]

As purely practical wisdom, the ideological articulations of the structure (S2) may be useful for the materialization of any kind of ideal (S1). The signifiers of language may be used by any master-signifier. The "family" and "society", for example, may serve the "revolution" as well as the "reaction". As noted by Stalin (1950a), 'languages' are 'means of production' that 'can equally serve capitalism and socialism' (p. 150). In other words, the unconscious enunciating acts of a language can *instrumentally* work for the "revolutionary", for the "nationalist", for the supporter of "marriage" and for any other purportedly conscious *operator.*[17] In any case, the 'unconscious works without thinking' (Lacan, 1973b, p. 556). And yet, 'the outcome is here: a wisdom that is not to be deciphered, since it just consists of ciphering' (ibid.).

As merely practical wisdom, the ideological articulations of the unconscious may cipher any kind of ideal. Any signifying operator (S1) may therefore employ their instrumental ciphering work (S2). At least in theory, this work of the unconscious is nothing more than a decompression and translation of the supposedly conscious master-signifier. It is a pure symbolization or signifierization. It only intends to give an account or explanation of the ideal. Thus, by ciphering the ideal, the ideological articulations ironically aim at deciphering it. Their predicative ciphering is an attempt to elucidate a subjective symbolic identity. In this attempt, the ideological discourse of the master construes the ideal of the master-signifier. *A* language reads *the* signifier.

By means of the enunciating workforce of the real subject ($), the enunciated slave-signifiers (S2) work hard to *interpret* the master-signifier (S1), its symbolic representativeness of the real subject ($\ S1), as well as the purpose of this representativeness, its intention, its ideal, its wish, its *desire* (*a*), which is not unrelated to the being of the represented real subject ($). In a sense, the discourse of the master is a predicative *interpretation* of the subjective master-signifier. Francisco Javier's discourse, for instance, *interprets* the "revolutionary" in terms of "marriage" and "monogamy". Now, as the awakening of class consciousness, this interpretation is necessary for the "revolutionary". To be supposedly conscious, the "revolutionary" needs to be interpreted by the unconscious. To signify something in the imaginary, *the* signifier needs a signifying interpretation in the symbolic.

As noted by Miller (1996c), 'the signifier alone is always an enigma, and this is why it is in a lack of interpretation' (p. 11). This is why it *needs* an interpretation. But 'this interpretation needs the implication of other signifiers' (ibid.). The interpretation of the ideal "revolutionary" needs the work of the ideological wisdom inherent in "marriage", the "monogamous family", the "moral conquest of our time", etc. In general, the interpretation of the supposedly conscious master-signifier needs the work of the unconscious, that is to say, the work of 'wisdom', the 'slave', the signifiers of language, which all use the same workforce of the 'proletarianized' real subject to do their work (Lacan, 1969–1970, 13.05.70, p. 173)

The working signifiers of language (S2) do not exploit the workforce of the real subject ($) merely for the purpose of interpreting his symbolic representative (S1). "Marriage" and the other signifiers enunciated by Francisco Javier, for example, do not employ the enunciating force of the proletarianized Eperrist with only the aim of *paying* or giving a symbolic value to his identification with the "revolutionary". *Besides the exchange value of the identification with a signifier, there is the use value of the alienation in language. The subject must accept the necessity of this alienation* (S2) *in return for his identitary symbolic wage* (S1). *In exchange for the payment of this symbolic exchange value, the signifying social structure can use the entire enunciating workforce of a subject* ($) *to reproduce a language, its economic system, or the cultural environment*. Now, by disposing of the entire use value or enjoyment value of the workforce of the proletarianized subject, the structure produces a surplus, a symbolic surplus-value, but also a real surplus-of-enjoyment (*plus-de-jouir*). The structure thus produces, respectively, something more ('surplus-value') than the 'exchange value' paid to the subject and something different ('surplus-enjoyment') than the 'use value' obtained from the workforce of the subject (Lacan, 1968–1969, 20.11.68, pp. 37–40).

Exchange value of the workforce: identitary symbolic wage for the subsistence of the subject within the system (S1)	Enjoyment value or *use value* (disposal) of the workforce: reproduction of the structure, system, language, culture (S2)
Enunciating workforce of the proletarianized subject ($)	Production, real *surplus*-of-enjoyment (*a*)

In my reading of the Lacanian reinterpretation of Marx (cf. Oliveira, 2004, p. 87), the 'exchange value' of the worker in the economic system becomes the 'representative' (S1) of the real subject ($) in the symbolic system, while the predicative 'discourse' expressed by the real subject corresponds to the 'use value' (S2) of his enunciating workforce exploited by the system of language (Lacan, 1967–1968, 12.04.67, 19.04.67; 1968–1969, 13.11.68, pp. 16–23; 20.11.68, pp. 37–40). As demonstrated by Marx (1867), this system *uses* the enunciating workforce of the subject ($) to such an extent that it produces more (S2) than the representative or identitary symbolic wage (S1) that it gives to the subject, for his subsistence inside the system, in exchange for the entire disposal of his workforce (S2). In the system, this product, as the 'non-paid' excess of the predicative 'use value' (S2) over the subjective 'exchange value' (S1), forms a symbolic 'surplus value' that gives a sense to 'discourse' and ensures its non-tautological nature (Lacan, 1968–1969, 20.11.68, p. 37). Furthermore, as demonstrated by Lacan (1968–1969), the symbolic system produces another excess, a real enjoyment (*a*) that cannot be used or assimilated by the symbolic (S2/*a*) and that coagulates as an object of desire, 'an object to be recovered, a lost enjoyment to be recovered as a surplus-enjoyment' (Oliveira, 2004, p. 86). Produced by the system, this object (*a*) causes a desire that leads the subject ($) to feed back into the system, alienate his workforce in it, and thus enable its work (S1→S2), the work of the unconscious, which produces the object of desire (*a*). By enabling the work of the system, the *desire of the subject* suits the system. It is *desirable* for the system. Therefore, it corresponds exactly to the *desire of the system*, as 'desire of the Other' (Lacan, 1969–1970, 18.02.70, p. 106).

Indistinguishable from the desire of the subject, the desire of the Other arises from the *wisdom* of the signifying social structure. This wisdom of the system determines any kind of desire, even the 'desire of the master', who logically 'desires' the 'working' of the system (Lacan, 1969–1970, 26.11.69, p. 24). Since the master belongs to the system, it is only natural that his desire depends on the wisdom of the system, the language, or the Other. Actually, without an Other of this Other, the wish or will of the master can only be a desire of the Other. As we know, the master himself is just a piece of the Other. The operator is a component of *his* instrument. His supposed consciousness forms part of the unconscious. As illustrated by Francisco Javier's discourse, even the "revolutionary" master-signifier is just a signifier among other signifiers of a fundamentally conventional language. As for the revolutionary message in itself, we must remember that it has been ciphered by the conformist wisdom of a code that may even be regarded as *bourgeois*. The revolutionary *discourse of the master* proves then to be a counter-revolutionary *discourse of the Other*, of the signifying social structure, of a 'language' that is 'itself' the symbolic universe of 'the bourgeoisie' (Marx, 1846, p. 1196).

Like Marx and Flaubert in the nineteenth century, Francisco Javier may understandably feel in "our time", in our symbolic universe, that 'everything is bourgeois': *everything*, including 'all humankind', and even 'the lower classes' (Flaubert, 1852, p. 52). Although the "revolutionary" claims to fight with his ideology against our bourgeois universe, we notice that his own "proletarian ideology", as an ideology *of the lower classes,* is included in the surrounding universal "bourgeois ideology" of "our time". Arising from the "moral conquest of our time", the ideology of the Eperrist cannot be regarded as a subversive ideology, but rather as a conformist one. Actually, from the Lacanian viewpoint, the opposition is not between the "proletarian ideology" of the "revolutionary" (S2) and his surrounding "bourgeois ideology" (S2), but it is rather between the "revolutionary" himself (S1) and his universe (S2), the signifier and a language, the ideal and a material ideology.

In a Lacanian Discourse Analysis, we must be able to detect clues of the assumed opposition between the structural position of the subject and the ideological articulation of the structure for his position.[18] The difficulty here lies in the same circumstance that makes analysis possible, namely, the problematic situation of the structural position within the opposite structure. Paradoxically, despite the opposition, the ideal forms part of the material ideology. The dominant master-signifier is integrated in the hegemonic language. Between the One and the Other, there is no 'organic distinction', but rather a 'methodical distinction' (Gramsci, 1934, §18, p. 386). Thus, in a sense, there is no real opposition between a "revolutionary" and his "counter-revolutionary" cultural environment. The opposition is purely symbolic. Since there is no Other of the Other, there is nothing really opposed to the Other, to language, or to its symbolic universe. In this universe that embraces everything, 'nothing' is really 'opposed to the symbolic, as the locus of the Other' (Lacan, 1975–1976, 16.12.75, pp. 55–56).

As evidenced by the ending of all revolutions, no revolutionary action can be really opposed to the reaction of the institutional system. No message can really resist its inversion. The real antagonism of the One is neutralized by the Other. The opposition to the symbolic universe has to be a symbolic opposition. It does not have to be anything more than the opposition of one signifier for another signifier. In this way, the "revolutionary" can only be a signifier opposed to another signifier. The "revolution" must be purely symbolic. Its movement must perform a function in the functioning of the system. Hence the scepticism of Lacan (1970a) with regard to political, and even scientific revolutions, which he compares to 'astral revolutions' (1970a, p. 420). Like the revolutions in the real universe, the human revolutions in the symbolic universe do not bring about a real 'overthrow' of the universe, the 'structure', or its economic system, which functions also as a 'turning machine' (p. 434).

In the rotational movement of the system, the centrifugal revolutionary action is inseparable from the centripetal conservative reaction. The decentring goes together with the re-centring. In the friction inside the engine, the activation already involves a deactivation. In the resistance of language, effort and courage imply fatigue and discouragement. Likewise, in the revolution, the 'political sequence' implies its own 'termination' because of the 'strictly immanent exhaustion of its capacities' (Badiou, 1998, p. 142). The Jacobin moment of 'virtue' and 'insurrection' cannot be separated from the Thermidorian moment of 'interest' and 'tranquillity' (p. 144). In Mexico, the *popular revolutions* of Villa and Zapata, that inspire Eperrists and Zapatistas at the present time, cannot be conceived apart from the *institutional revolutions* of Carranza and Obregón, that led first to the revolutionary authoritarianism of the PRI and then to the old-fashioned counter-revolutionary regime of the PAN.[19]

It must be granted that Francisco Javier is not well represented, in the current representative government of Mexico, by the institutional reaction of the PAN and its conservative ideology. But at the time of our interview, we might have already anticipated that Francisco Javier *would have become* the represented citizen of a "new society" ruled by the right-wing supporters of the symbolic values of "marriage", "faithfulness" and the "monogamous family". After all, Francisco Javier was himself a supporter of those values. His enunciating workforce was *used* to support them. Nevertheless, this unconscious conformist *use value* of his workforce (S2) must not be confused with his purportedly conscious revolutionary *exchange value* (S1). The revolutionary does not consciously act in collusion with the conformist system. The use of his expressing workforce does not belong to him, but it is the property of the articulating system that bought it in exchange for the signifier "revolutionary". Strictly speaking, the conformist work is not the work of the revolutionary, but the work of a reactionary unconscious, of a conventional articulating language, of a conservative signifying social structure that gives the power to the counter-revolutionary PAN. As a dominant representative of the hegemonic system, this party would have taken advantage of the *use value* of the expressing-voting workforce of real subjects, such as Francisco Javier. At any rate, these proletarianized real subjects are innocent of the way the system uses their workforce.

To achieve the symbolic identification with a "revolutionary", Francisco Javier was obliged to alienate his expressing workforce in a conventional articulating language. He was thus obliged to do the expressing work of this language. In that way, the revolutionary gave up all his speaking work to the counter-revolutionary symbolic system. In a sense, he sacrificed the entire *use value* of his expression in order to receive, as a symbolic wage, the *exchange value* of the signifier that represents him. In exchange for the supposed consciousness of the "revolutionary", the proletarianized subject had to do all the expressing work of the unconscious, of its conventional articulating language, of a cultural environment, and all this against him, against his "revolutionary" symbolic identity.

The product: Deprivation by discourse (a)

By doing the expressing work of a language, the speaking subject ($) permits the articulating language (S2) to *produce* something (*a*). This production is always involved in the work of a language. As Stalin (1950a) remarks, a 'language' is 'directly related to a productive activity' and 'cannot be distinguished from the instruments of production' (pp. 151, 153, 168). Actually, from the Lacanian viewpoint, the *reproductive* activity of the language is also a *productive* activity. Besides being a conservative instrument of reproduction, a language is an *instrument of production*. Besides reproducing the conventional symbolic values of words (→S2), a language produces a disrupting real surplus-of-enjoyment (→S2/*a*).

As the production of language, the Lacanian object *a* refers to a real surplus that is yielded or detached precisely because it cannot be symbolized by language. The surplus thus constitutes a real residue of symbolization. It is that which 'resists signifierization' (Lacan, 1962–1963, 13.03.63, p. 204). It is that which cannot be 'assimilated by the function of the signifier' (ibid.). Since it cannot be assimilated, the object *a* is expelled or excluded. It is a non-signifying remnant that is detached because it cannot be attached to the signifying chain. The production is a detachment, an expulsion, an exclusion, a leakage, a loss. It is the waste of a surplus-enjoyment (*a*) that cannot be enjoyed by the proletarianized subject ($) or by the system of production (S2). If this surplus-of-enjoyment had a symbolic value, it would be recovered by the symbolic system. However, unlike the Marxian surplus value, the surplus-enjoyment does not have a symbolic value. It has neither a use value nor an exchange value. Although its representatives have a symbolic value of enjoyment (S2), this value is not the real enjoyment itself (*a*), which cannot be really represented. Like the real subject, this real object can only be represented symbolically by the discursive representatives, whose cognitive representation would then be just imaginary.

Beyond the discursive psychology of symbolic representatives and the cognitive psychology of imaginary representations, the real presence of the object *a* is psychologically indefinable, indescribable, and unclassifiable.[20] It cannot be classified in any universal psychological inventory of emotions, attitudes, mental states, argumentative strategies, etc. Unlike objects of ordinary psychology, the object of psychoanalysis is 'impossible to universalize' (Soler, 1991, p. 62). It is radically individual. It is 'not collectivizable' (pp. 61–62). It is incommunicable. It is also 'incalculable' (Regnault, 2005a, 18.04.05). Unlike the Marxian symbolic surplus value, the Lacanian real surplus-enjoyment cannot be 'calculated' (ibid.). Nor can it be 'characterized' (ibid.). It escapes any rational quantitative calculation and any rational qualitative characterization. It escapes the immanent reason of discourse and cognition. The Lacanian object *a* can be then described as 'transcendental' and 'irrational', 'vanishing' and 'impossible' (Regnault, 2005b, pp. 4–5). In the mirror that reflects a cognitive signified reality, the object *a* appears as a 'hole' or a 'blind spot' (Lacan, 1968–1969, 30.04.69, p. 290). Behind the mirror, it corresponds to the vanishing point of intersection between the enunciating and enunciated parallels. It is a hypothetical point of impracticability at the axial end of the increasingly curved discursive signifying chain. It is, at this juncture, a conjectural 'point of inertia', an 'immobile core', a 'center of gravity' of a cyclical discourse that is not really 'centrifugal' (Soler, 1987, p. 146).[21]

In Lacanian Discourse Analysis, the analyzed symbolic elements may gravitate round a missing real being produced by the enunciated discourse and lost by the enunciating subject. As object *a*, this subjective being can be detected in the inexhaustible excessive residue of ontological overproduction, overexploitation, and overdetermination by the signifying social structure.[22] Now, as an 'object', the subjective real being must not be confused with the enunciating real 'subject' (Lacan, 1968–1969, 30.04.69, p. 292). This subject is torn to shreds by the structure of society, while his being is the 'shred of tongue' that permits the signifying 'relations' between 'subjects' in 'politics' (Milner, 1983, p. 82).

When analyzing the discursive materialization of politics and society, we must clearly distinguish between the real subject ($) identified with a master-signifier ($\S1) and his real being (*a*) alienated in all the other signifiers (S2/*a*). We must thus make a distinction, from an economic angle, between the enunciating workforce ($), represented by its exchange value ($\S1), and the real surplus extracted from the workforce (*a*), represented by the use value (S2/*a*) of this workforce ($\S1→S2/*a*).

By extracting the object *a* from the enunciating workforce, the discourse of the master 'conditions' the 'misery' of the proletarianized subject (Lacan, 1973a, pp. 517–518). In this misery, the subject lacks everything real, even his own body, which is totally symbolized and thereby becomes a simple device of the symbolic system, a letter of a language, a 'body lost by the slave only to become the place where signifiers are inscribed' (1969–1970, 18.02.70, p. 102). Here, the signifierization is an inscription that symbolizes the body by carving it, by emptying it of its real substance. This substance becomes an object (*a*) separated from the subject ($). The outcome is the corporeal presence of the symbol, a 'broken piece' (1975–1976, 18.11.75, p. 19), a divided literal subject ($) whose real being (*a*) divides from his alienated symbolized body ($\S1→S2/*a*).[23]

The object *a* arises from the same original division that gives rise to the subject. This division creates at once the subject and his object, the enunciating workforce and its missing product, the lack of enjoyment ($) and the lacking surplus-of-enjoyment (*a*). Here, logically, the origin of the lack is also the origin of the lacking surplus. This origin is the beginning of everything. Thus, unlike the Marxian surplus value, the Lacanian surplus-of-enjoyment is 'lost from the beginning' (Regnault, 2005a, 18.04.05). It is lost from 'the beginning' in which 'was the Word' (John, 1:1).

The Word is contemporary with that which is released by its emergence. The origin of the signifier coincides with the origin of that which resists signifierization. The symbolization at the same time creates the symbol and a remaining real that cannot be symbolized (*a*). This remainder is the price of symbolization. It is lost by the subject ($) transformed into the real support of the symbolic (S1–S2). More precisely, it is the difference between what he gains and what he loses by taking part in the symbolic system of discourse. All things considered, it is the qualitative difference between the gained symbolic and the lost real. However, from the viewpoint of this system, it is only the quantitative difference between the income (S1) and the outcome (S2) of the real subject ($), the cost and the productivity of his supporting function, the exchange value and the use value of his enunciating workforce. In any case, this difference exists from the beginning of civilization, since civilization itself is *the* symbolic system that thrives on this difference.

The symbolic system of discourse exploits the subject by using his entire real enunciating workforce in exchange for a purely symbolic enunciated identity. To receive this identity (S1), *the subject* ($) *accepts his alienation as the workforce of the system* ($\S1→S2), *a system whose work symbolizes everything, with the exception of a residual real surplus* (*a*), *which precisely underlies the use of the real workforce* ($) *by the symbolic system* ($\S1→S2/*a*). *Resisting symbolization, this real surplus cannot be either assimilated by the symbolic system or recovered by the real subject. Excluded and expelled, it appears simultaneously as the production of the symbolic system and the deprivation of the real subject.* However, this deprivation is logically proportional to the alienation of the real subject in the symbolic system. More alienation involves more symbolization, which involves, in turn, more deprivation of the real being that cannot be symbolized.

In the final analysis, the object *a* is that which is lost by a real subject, such as Francisco Javier, in order to become a symbolic subject, such as the "revolutionary". The object *a* corresponds to the *real price* of this *symbolic identification*. But this price has to be paid with an alienation in language. The price actually amounts to the difference between the purely symbolic advantage of the symbolic identification and the real disadvantage of the resulting alienation in the symbolic system, which exploits the subject, his life and energy, his real enunciating workforce.

S1	*S2*
Identification-oppression	Alienation-exploitation
$	*a*
Division-proletarianization	Production-deprivation

For the subject, his alienation in a language entails his exploitation by the language, by *the Other* (S2), which articulates its discourse (the discourse of the Other) by using the expressing workforce of the subject ($). Concurrently, for the same subject, his identification with a signifier entails his oppression by the signifier, by *the master* (S1), which dominates its discourse (the discourse of the master) by subjugating the subject identified with it ($). If this identification leads to alienation, the correlative oppression enables exploitation. Francisco Javier's oppression by his identification with the "revolutionary", for instance, enables his exploitation in the conventional language in which he is alienated. However, as we know, there is a contradiction between the two poles of identification-oppression (S1) and alienation-exploitation (S2). Both poles are even mutually exclusive, as evidenced by the tautological discourse (S1–S1), in which the sterile identification-oppression (S1) predominates and excludes the fertile alienation-exploitation (S2), as well as the division-proletarianization of the subject ($) and the production-deprivation of his object (*a*).

Leaving aside the tautological discourse, the subject is normally divided and proletarianized by a contradictory discourse (S1–S2) that alienates and exploits his enunciating workforce ($), depriving him of its production (*a*), which also has to be *marginalized* from the process of symbolization (S2/*a*). Thus, besides the deprivation of the subject, the production of the object *a* implies the marginalization of this real being that cannot be assimilated by the symbolic system. Now, to approach this real being, a Lacanian interviewer may push the interviewee to the margins of his discourse. For example, when the discourse is about the "revolution", we can always ask questions about the "family" of the "revolutionary". In this way, we move the discourse away from the tautological pole of identification-oppression and we stimulate a process of alienation-exploitation that arouses marginal proliferations and ramifications, which unsuccessfully try to surround and seize the real being that always escapes symbolization.[24] However marginal this symbolization may be, there is always *a margin of the margin*; there is always a remaining real; 'there is always a surplus', so that 'all attempts at totalization are doomed to failure' (Evans, 1996, p. 45). We are *never yet* in the "man's total fulfilment" of Francisco Javier. *Meanwhile*, the only successful totalization is the imaginary one. In the mirror, this totalization of the ego masks the contradiction in the enunciated discourse, the real division of the enunciating subject, and the lack of his object, which is separated from him.[25]

Mastery, university, hysteria and psychoanalysis

At the symbolic root of the imaginary totalization, the master discourse is not only reluctantly contradictory, but also willingly monolithic and despotic, oppressive and repressive, authoritarian and totalitarian. Besides determining the imaginary totalization of the ego, the master aims at a real totalization of the symbolic universe, as evidenced by the totalitarian symbolic systems that absorb everything real, including enunciating acts and missing beings, desires and drives, etc. This applies to any 'master discourse', even to the 'revolutionary' one (Lacan, 1972b), which is usually 'codified' and 'narrowed' in order to function as a 'point of reference and point of rallying' (Foucault, 1975, p. 1604).

According to Lacan (1969–1970), the 'master discourse' can 'be identified in a kind of purity on the political front', in which 'it embraces everything, even the so-called revolution' (18.02.70, p. 99). In actual fact, besides the revolutionary discourse, the master discourse embraces our two most influential political discourses, namely, the 'artful *capitalist discourse*' (Lacan, 1972d), which 'does not shield us from the master discourse' (Soueix, 1989, p. 144), and the *university discourse*, which is nothing more than a 'modern master discourse' (Lacan, 1969–1970, 17.12.69, p. 34).

As for the *university discourse*, we come across it in all socialist bureaucracies and liberal technocracies, in which it functions as a *master discourse* that disavows itself, claims to be merely rational and scientific, hides its own mastering functioning, 'denies its performative dimension' and its 'political decisions based on power' (Žižek, 2003, p. 26). If that is the way it is, then we can treat the *university discourse* as *a lie of the master discourse*, which passes itself off as another discourse, the university discourse, which is constituted by the lie. This 'constituent lie' of the 'university discourse' (ibid.) creates our free-thinking, our unprejudiced scientific inquiries, our psychological methodical analyses, our democratic liberal ideologies, our new orthodoxies in politics driven by the principles of the free market. Concealing their intransigence and their authoritarianism, these lying exercises point the finger at the intransigence and authoritarianism of the *other* discourses of the master, the more sincere and honest, such as the ones of Eperrist revolutionaries, committed Marxists, radical Islamists, dogmatic Lacanians, sectarian psychoanalysts and evangelists, etc. Now, if 'one of the telltale signs of university discourse is that the opponent is accused of being *dogmatic* and *sectarian*', it is because the 'university discourse cannot tolerate an engaged subjective stance' (Žižek, 2006). It cannot accept the choice of only one signifier to monopolize the commanding position of the enunciated subject. On the assumption that this position must be democratically shared by the wisdom of all signifiers, the university discourse revolts against the autocratic appropriation of the position by only one signifier.

As the professed discourse of all signifiers on an equal footing (S2), the university discourse (S2→*a*) 'cannot tolerate' the master discourse of an intolerant unique signifier, the master-signifier, in the committed 'stance' of Marxists or Islamists (Žižek, 2006). Thus, in a sense, the university discourse (S2→*a*) suffers from intolerance towards the intolerance of the master discourse (S1→S2). But we must not make a mistake on this point. Whether modern or traditional, intolerance is always intolerance. The university discourse itself proves to be an accomplished master discourse of an intolerant master-signifier called tolerance, liberty, impartiality, objectivity, political correctness, etc. Actually, at present, the master discourse remains the only discourse at our disposal. For the time being, our only discourse is this 'discourse of the mastering consciousness' (Lacan, 1969–1970, 11.02.70, p. 79), as 'the crystallization of the structure of the unconscious' (1973d, p. 187). Any other discourse constitutes, in a sense, somewhat of a master discourse. Despite most Lacanians, even their psychoanalytical discourse may be regarded, in practice, as a version of the master discourse.[26]

In an enlightened Lacanian Discourse Analysis, we must detect the master discourse in its four principal versions, namely, *classical*, *modern*, *psychoanalytical* and *hysterical*. As we shall see at once, these versions articulate the same discourse in completely different ways (Lacan, 1969–1970, 26.11.69, 17.12.69, 14.01.70, 21.01.70, 11.02.70, pp. 9–95):

- In the classical or obsessional version ($\S1→S2/*a*), the agent is *the* chosen signifier (S1→), whose power seems to dominate the instrumental wisdom of *a* language (→S2). This predicative wisdom apparently obeys the subjective signifier with which I identify ($\S1). Thus, as a "revolutionary", I must have some "conceptions of marriage". Proper to politics, tradition and civilization, this discourse dramatically produces a real scrap that cannot be seized by the symbolic system of wisdom (/*a*). Simultaneously, the consistent discourse masks the inconsistent truth of my division from this scrap ($\).

$$\frac{\mathrm{S1}}{\$} \longrightarrow \frac{\mathrm{S2}}{a}$$

- In the modern or university version (S1\S2→*a*/$), the agent is not *the* biased signifier, but all signifiers and their unbiased wisdom, the reasonable wisdom of *a* language (S2), whose neutral symbolic system seems to surround and grasp the real being (→*a*). This being appears to be enunciated in a wisdom that embraces it. For instance, if I am included in my "conceptions of marriage and the couple" (S2), then I can say what exactly is my real being (*a*). Suited to science, capitalism and modernity, this discourse automatically produces my division ($) from the enunciated real being (*a*/$), which cannot be at once real and enunciated. At the same time, the impartial discourse hides the partial truth of the master-signifier that masters it, predisposes it, and biases it (S1\).

$$\frac{\mathrm{S2}}{\mathrm{S1}} \longrightarrow \frac{a}{\$}$$

- In the post-modern or psychoanalytical version (S2*a*→$/S1), the agent is not something symbolic, but something real, the real being of the desiring subject, his object of desire (*a*), which explicitly governs his life (→$). As a desiring subject, I acknowledge being moved by this real scrap (*a*→$) that breaks away from discourse (S2*a*). Since this being arises from my own division, I joyfully and shamelessly assume all my dividing contradictions, as in a game, for instance by accepting to spend a lot of money to disguise myself as a miserable proletarian ($). My desire justifies everything. Fitted to publicity, adolescence, and post-modernity, this discourse artificially produces a master-signifier, such as the "revolutionary", with which I identify when I play at being a proletarian ($/S1). In concert, the discourse argues the simple real object of desire (*a*) to cover the complicated truth of the alienating symbolic system of wisdom whose desire is my desire $(S2\backslash a)$.

$$\frac{a}{S2} \longrightarrow \frac{\$}{S1}$$

- In the critical or hysterical version $(a\backslash\$\rightarrow S1/S2)$, the agent is the divided enunciating subject ($) who challenges the power of his enunciated master (→S1). Explicitly identified with this master-signifier, I pretend to submit its purely symbolic power to my real desire and capricious contradictions. My division between the revolution and social conventions ($), for example, cannot keep me from being a progressive writer who identifies himself with the "revolutionary" (→S1). Proper to femininity, art and authenticity, this discourse produces the conventional wisdom (S2) that implicitly grows away from the explicit original identification with the signifier (S1/S2). Concurrently, the discourse covers the ineffable truth of my real object of desire $(a\backslash)$ misrepresented by my own desire and by my own division from the object $(a\backslash\$)$.

$$\frac{\$}{a} \longrightarrow \frac{S1}{S2}$$

In spite of their common discursive nature and their shared mastering function, the four versions of the master discourse are *incommensurable*. There is just no translation or comparison between them. They do not say the same thing. They do not function in the same way. They do not use the same resources or the same strategies. We do not come across them in the same cultural environments. They do not configure the same individual, familial, social or political situations. In short, they do not refer to the same world.[27] Nevertheless, when we reduce them to their essence, we always find the same master discourse. This is why Lacan prioritizes this discourse over the others. He prioritizes it because it is *the* discourse that underlies any discourse. It is *the* discourse implied by language. It 'works just because there is a language' (Le Bihan, 2009, p. 58). In any discourse of language, we can detect 'the master discourse', which 'changes its style, mutates, but doesn't disappear' (p. 57).

In view of the fact that 'a discourse is a way of domination' (Miller, 2007–2008, 04.06.08, p. 8), we can regard any discourse as a *dominating discourse*, a *mastering discourse*, a *master discourse*. To be sure, any discourse is *control, command, mastery*. Since every discourse refers to something that it 'wants to master', every discourse can be 'classified in the family of the master discourse' (Lacan, 1969–1970, 11.02.70, p. 79). This family includes our quite modern university discourse as well as the classical one of Francisco Javier, the critical one of the hysteric and even the post-modern one of his psychoanalyst.

All discourses are master discourses because all discourses involve the mastery of the signifier. This signifier (S1) *exerts its power not only through the explicit subjective agency of the classical master discourse* (S1→S2), *but also in the hidden truth of the university discourse* (S1\S2→*a*), *in the anticipated production of the psychoanalytical discourse* (*a*→$/S1), *and in the challenged necessity of the hysterical discourse* ($→S1). *In any case, the signifier plays its role of mastery in discourse. The fact remains that this role is nothing but a myth. It is the myth of a real identity underlying the symbolic identification of the subject with the signifier.* It is the myth of the "consistent revolutionary" with his "individual sexual love", which comprises the "new society" and the "new man", the social and individual identity (S1), the non-dissociation and non-division of the proletarianized subject ($). It is thus the proletarian myth of socialist communism, as a constituent feature of the revolutionary mentality, and not only the 'bourgeois myth' of liberal 'individualism', as a 'constituent feature of the reactionary mentality' (Barthes, 1957, pp. 133–135).

According to Lacan, the master discourse 'begins' with the 'ultra-reduced myth' of a social or individual 'subject' who is 'identical to his own signifier' (Lacan, 1969–1970, p. 102). To subvert this myth and its master discourse, we must reveal its truth, the truth of the division or dissociation of the subject ($). This must be one of the chief purposes of a Lacanian Discourse Analysis. To achieve it, we must have recourse to the Freudian and Lacanian subversive analytical praxis, which demystifies any kind of individualism.[28] We may also resort to the Marxian and Marxist 'subversive' analytical praxis (Lacan, 1971, 16.06.71), which 'opposes the myth' (Barthes, 1957, p. 233), particularly the myth that gives rise to liberal individualism and utopian socialism. In that case, of course, we run the risk of relapsing into the myth of the "consistent revolutionary". But this 'left-wing myth', at least, is 'meagre' and 'indiscreet' (p. 236). It 'frankly shows' its *hood*, or 'its mask' (ibid.).

However awkward it may be, a revolutionary discourse is a mythical discourse. And yet, Barthes persuaded himself that 'revolutionary language cannot be a mythical language', but rather it 'excludes the myth', since it 'gives rise to a full speech, that is, an initially and finally political speech, contrary to the myth, whose speech is initially political and finally natural' (Barthes, 1957, p. 234). From this point of view, there would be a *mythical naturalization* of the political discourse that can be clearly observed in those versions of the master discourse, particularly the university one, in which discourse claims to be merely natural and hides its own mastering political artifices. Now, leaving aside the hysterical or critical discourse, this *mythical naturalization* can be attributed to any other version of the master discourse, even to the explicit classical version, in which the artificial symbolic identification with the social or individual signifier passes for a natural real identity. In Francisco Javier's revolutionary discourse, for example, there is an incontestable naturalization of "man" and "society", of "man's development and total fulfilment" and "sexual individual love as the foundation of the monogamous family". "Marriage" can thereby *naturally* amount to "the couple" and the "starting point for the establishment of family", which actually confirms the existence, 'in bourgeois society', of a 'left-wing myth concerning marriage' (Barthes, 1957, p. 235). Even if this 'myth' can be purely 'tactical' or 'accidental' (ibid.), it is an accomplished myth that demonstrates the mythical functioning of our revolutionary discourse. Just as any other revolutionary discourse, that of Francisco Javier proves to be a mythical discourse, as it presents all features of myths, namely the claims of naturality and causality, reality and totality, which lead to the religious totalization of the symbolic discursive connection (S1→S2) and the ensuing concealment of the real separation between the speaking subject and his missing being ($\$\lozenge a$).[29]

Notes

1. This complexity is not unrelated to the 'complex subjectivity' that Parker (1997b) considers equivalent, 'to some extent', to the 'psychoanalytic subjectivity' (p. 491). By 'taking seriously both the

intentions and desires of the individual and the operation of social structures and discursive forms' (Parker, 1994, p. 244), this complex subjectivity implicitly embraces the four elements of the discourse of the master: the *intentions* of consciousness (S1), the *desires* of the subject ($), the cause of these *desires* (*a*) and the unconscious *operation of social structures and discursive forms* (S2).

2. Here, in the Kleinian perspective of Hollway and Jefferson (2000), we might say that the protected enunciating subject is the 'defended subject', while the protecting enunciated subject corresponds to a *defensive* 'discursive subject' that materializes the 'defences' of the 'defended' one (p. 24).
3. In the Althusserian perspective of Pêcheux (1975b), we would say that Francisco Javier is taken by an 'identification-interpellation' that leads him to put on the hood of the "revolutionary", which functions as the 'evidence of identity' that 'hides the fact that identity results from an identification-interpellation of the subject' (pp. 139–140).
4. On this point, D'Unrug (1974) observes that 'the recurrence expresses in a discourse an attempt at mastery' that 'tries to neutralize' a 'conflict between a repeated idea and its contrary' (pp. 183–184). In this 'conflict between two antithetical elements', the 'eliminated notion *insists* through the enunciation, while the enunciated notion is repeated, as if trying to persuade' (p. 183).
5. As Parker (2005a) notes, 'a speaker adopting the position of S1 here makes a claim to authority that is maintained by repetition of the claim rather than reasoned argument' (p. 170).
6. Here is the symbolic discursive substratum of the imaginary 'cognitive dissonance', classically defined, by Festinger and Aronson (1960), as the 'simultaneous existence of elements of knowledge that do not agree' (p. 107). Besides their imaginary appearance, these *dissonant elements of knowledge* are nothing more than *different signifiers of wisdom*. As for the master-signifier, it can be regarded as the symbolic substratum of that which 'reduces the dissonance' (ibid.).
7. Thus, in social psychology, this univocal attribute of discourse might hypothetically account for the 'inter-personal consistency' that would, in turn, 'account' for the 'influence of minorities' (Moscovici, Lage & Naffrechoux, 1969, p. 541). If this were the case, the influence would be an effect of the purely symbolic mastery of discourse.
8. This is what enables Parker (1997a) to 'move from the level of the individual to a conception of the ego as an institutional apparatus which ties together particular senses of self and social organization, senses which warrant and reinforce the state' (p. 166). On the

assumption of a *fundamental fusion and confusion between the political state and the psychological ego*, we understand that 'psychology and social psychology' might become 'forms of state apparatus which can only be comprehended with a properly collective analysis of subjectivity' (ibid.). Along with us, Parker finds this analysis in psychoanalysis and especially in Lacanian psychoanalysis.

9. For instance, when the enunciating subject is represented by the enunciated "scientist", he should be ideally submitted to the "scientific" master-signifier and dominated by its "scientific" discourse. In this discourse, the subject must be nothing more than a workforce for organizing "scientific" meetings of "scientific" societies, writing "scientific" papers in "scientific" journals, making "scientific" quotations in "scientific" papers, etc. As a proletarianized workforce of the "scientific" master, the enunciating subject cannot take the liberty of a 'contemptuous attitude' for which the undisciplined Lacan is reasonably reprimanded by Billig (2006a, p. 22).
10. For 'the laws to be operative, there must be a One', a 'master', a 'person' with an 'external unlimited power that is precisely the *reflexive determination* of my egotist subjective stance' (Žižek, 2000). What really matters here for us is the *collective* character of this *reflexive determination*. This collective character results from the common identification of many subjects with the same master-signifier. Because of this common identification, the subjects partly share the same structural position. Therefore, they must relatively obey the same laws of the structure for this position. *By law*, for example, the Mexican "revolutionaries" must resign themselves to the risk of being incarcerated, tortured, killed, etc. Without the power of the master, it would be hard to ensure this resignation and the obedience to other merciless laws that govern all signifying social structures. Now, by virtue of a shared political identity such as the one of the "revolutionary", we would sacrifice our despicable earthly life in order to conserve our existence in discourse. In this way, to avoid a symbolic 'second death', we would rush towards our real 'first death' (Lacan, 1959–1960, 22.06.60, pp. 291–301).
11. This would be how 'the emptiness' or 'the virtuality of the Other enables it to act as a master-signifier', which would be 'thus able' to 'consolidate the social field' (Hook, 2008, p. 63).
12. Supposing that 'critical and social psychological analyses should focus on the vicissitudes of symbolic modes of identification', Hook (2008) suitably situates these modes here, in this *socialization through individualization*, in this 'precipitate identification' that 'involves' a

'relation with an inconclusive (Master) signifier that others have also taken on' and 'have done so as a means of avoiding the uncertainty of their (our) social being' (pp. 64–65).

13. This is how the Lacanian idea of the inversion 'leads us to look for the way modes of speech in a text call upon a response, and the way a response may send the message back to the speaker as if in reverse, thereby revealing some truth that was concealed in the original message' (Parker, 2005a, pp. 174–175).
14. By acknowledging this, the analyst takes up an *'ethical position'*, in which he 'speaks not from within a *metalanguage*, but as reflexively positioned in relation to the text' (Parker, 2005a, p. 175).
15. Pêcheux (1975b) would see here the 'transparency of sense' that 'conceals', in a 'discursive formation', its 'dependence' on a 'complex of discursive formations inherent in a complex of ideological formations' (p. 146). Now, in a Lacanian perspective, the *ideological formations* are nothing more than *discursive formations*. As for the *transparency of sense*, it prevents us from thinking about the *formations* themselves and not only their *dependence on the complex*. In other words, the transparency keeps the subject from being conscious of the *structure for his position* and not only of the *structure in itself*. This is why the structure for his position amounts to his unconscious. This 'unconscious' functions as an 'ideology' that 'conceals its existence inside its functioning by producing a tissue of subjective evidences' (cf. Pêcheux, 1975b, p. 136).
16. Pêcheux (1975b) would observe here that 'ideologies do not consist of ideas, but of practices' (p. 128). Among those practices, there would be the 'discursive process' (pp. 145–146). As a method to approach this process, the Althusserian-Lacanian Discourse Analysis of Pêcheux allows us to analyze a 'discursive formation' in an 'ideological formation' (pp. 144–145). As for our Lacanian Discourse Analysis, it enables us to analyze an *ideological formation* in a *discursive formation* (or *discursive process*) that embraces every *ideological practice*.
17. Perhaps we may hazard the conjecture that an operator in one discourse can become an instrument of another operator in another discourse expressed by the same subject at any time, even at the same time as the first discourse. If this were the case, both discourses would be expressed by the same subject represented simultaneously by two different master-signifiers. Francisco Javier, for example, might be simultaneously represented by "marriage" and the "revolution". On that assumption, the "revolution" could be useful to the supporter of "marriage" just as "marriage" is used by the "revolutionary".

This would be a plausible reason for why the 'operating motives' of the 'psychological level' might be 'instrumental motives' of the 'sociological level', and vice versa (cf. Doise, 1982, pp. 191–192). Both levels would explain, in the same text, two different discourses of two different master-signifiers, the one rather *social*, the other rather *individual*, so to speak. Since the real subject would not be anything more than the enunciating workforce of both discourses, he might certainly express both of them at the same time.

18. It would seem that our analytical assumption runs counter to the 'theory of rationalization' of Beauvois and Joule (1981), which assumes that 'social actors have an ideology that is adequate to their positions' (p. 158). Nevertheless, in a Lacanian perspective, this theory can be accepted, provided that the *adequacy* does not exclude a *perfectly adequate opposition* between the ideology and the position of the subject. After all, this *opposition* functions as the intrinsic *structural adequacy* between each position and the other positions in the structure.
19. At all times, revolutions result in the 'return to the master who makes them useful' (Lacan, 1970a, p. 424). In this way, 'revolutions always end up being quickly reinserted into the generally accepted normality' (Gross, 1913a, p. 47). In Francisco Javier's discourse, for instance, the revolutionary "construction of the new society" ends up in a reconstruction of the "moral conquest of our time", including "marriage" and the "monogamous family". In the terms of Gross (1919), the 'revolutionary psyche' of *the* signifier ends in its reintegration into the 'adapted psyche' of the signifying social structure (p. 106). Gross (1913a) would explain this reintegration through the fact that 'the revolutionary carries authority in himself', in the form of his 'family' (p. 47), which makes us think of Francisco Javier's "monogamous family". Now, as the "pillar" of "society", this "monogamous family" may be a metonymical-metaphorical translation of the *monogamous father* as the *pillar of the family*. If this were the case, the "monogamous family" of the Eperrist would not be unrelated, in Gross, to the hypothetical 'patriarchal right' of a *monogamous father* who would 'enslave individuality' (ibid.). Anyway, Francisco Javier would be still far away from the 'liberation' that Gross (1913b) situates in the 'destruction of monogamy and its more pathological form, polygamy' (p. 56).
20. Understandably, as Parker (2003) notices, such a concept would be 'anathema to the discipline of psychology, and it is important that psychologists who may be attracted to Lacan's work recognize this' (pp. 108–109).

21. In a Lacanian Discourse Analysis, we can encounter this object in the form of 'a cause around which a speaker circles' (Parker, 2005a, p. 171). In this form, 'the object is not empirically real, but is an analytically fruitful device to explore the orientation of a speaker' (ibid.).
22. With the aim of serving 'the aspirations of qualitative work', this is how we can 'adopt', in our Lacanian perspective, 'the notion of an over-determined subject, of a way of being that is *excessive*, too much' (Frosh, 2007, p. 639).
23. Unlike the individual master-signifier (S1), its literal support is divided ($). In spite of Derrida (1975), the Lacanian 'letter' is *not* an 'indivisible singularity' (p. 492). The 'indivisibility' of the 'letter' cannot be 'found anywhere', except in the imagination of Derrida (1992, p. 78), who inexplicably ascribes this idea to Lacan (Miller, 2005, p. 232).
24. By definition, this real being must escape any kind of symbolization, even the most marginal kind. This is why 'the margins are not places for some truer essence of the human subject, and certainly not just for a technology for the recovery of something that the centre (e.g., in the form of mainstream empiricism) has left out' (Frosh, 2007, p. 642). If the real being could be recovered, it would not be what it is, what must be marginalized, what cannot be exploited. Here lies the difference between the Lacanian marginalized surplus of enjoyment and the Marxian exploited surplus of value.
25. As Frosh, Phoenix and Pattman (2003) remark, 'the ego is created only in relation to something outside of itself, coming into being as an imaginary capture, a moment of mistaken self-identification that is the beginning of a permanent tendency whereby the subject seeks imaginary wholeness to paper over conflict, lack and absence' (p. 40).
26. In my opinion, the psychoanalytical discourse, like the university one, is just a dominating discourse that *unsuccessfully* 'excludes domination' (cf. Miller, 2007–2008, 04.06.08, pp. 7–8). Of course, psychoanalysis 'is opposed to any will, at least confessed, of mastering', but the *unconfessed or unwilling mastering* is practically *always* at work, as 'it is simple, after all, to *always* fall back into the discourse of mastery' (Lacan, 1969–1970, 11.02.70, p. 79).
27. So, with good reason, Parker (2005a) considers that 'the delimiting' of those versions 'as rhetorical strategies and social bonds in a form of critical discourse analysis would also require an analysis of the *political* projects and suppositions about the nature of the world that each calls upon' (p. 173).

28. Together with Pichonian social psychology, this praxis is diametrically opposed to the 'individualism' of a 'psychoanalytical praxis' that 'provides a service to passive adaptation' (Pichon-Rivière & Quiroga, 1972).
29. In this twofold religious movement of *concealment* and *totalization*, the mythical *master discourse* is not unrelated to the 'profane religion' of Moscovici (1985), which simultaneously 'conceals a mystery' and involves a 'total vision of the world' (pp. 462–463). Like our master discourse, this 'profane religion' is attributed, as if by chance, to the revolutionary discourses of 'socialist visions' that 'have fired and roused the oppressed masses of the world' (ibid.).

CHAPTER NINE

The being of speech

We now turn in this chapter to the mechanism whereby a supposedly social being appears and fleshes out in discourse. At an ontogenetic level, this infra-structural mechanism of symbolic signifierization is contrasted with the super-structural process of imaginary signification. Following the last teaching of Lacan, the mechanism is also contrasted with the correlative elimination of a real being that therefore becomes insignificant. This leads us to review in more depth the Lacanian differentiation between the real, the imaginary and the symbolic. Such differentiation enables us to shed new light upon topical issues in current social sciences. In a Lacanian perspective, we reassess ideas of Taguieff, Touraine and Wieviorka. With the background of a real kind of violent acting out, we go over the contradiction between symbolic violence and imaginary aggressivity, universalistic discrimination and particularistic segregation, intra-discursive class struggle and extra-discursive clash of civilizations, etc.

Individual speaking being, socializing spoken being, social speech-being

The symbolic discursive connection (S1→S2) between the subjective signifier (S1) and its predicative explanation (S2) conceals the real separation ($◊*a*) between the speaking subject ($) and his missing being (*a*). Here, behind the screen of the enunciated fact, the real being is missing precisely because of the enunciating act. If the enunciation involves a symbolization of the subject as a support of the symbol, this symbolization also entails a separation of the symbolized subject from his own real being. This being cannot be symbolized. It emerges then as a residue of symbolization. It is that which resists the total symbolization of the subject. It appears thus as a difference between the real subject ($) and his symbolic identity (S1). It *is* this difference (*a*) between the real enunciating workforce ($) used by the symbolic system ($\S1→S2) and the enunciated symbolic exchange value (S1) of this workforce in the system (S1→S2).

S1: exchange value of the real subject in the symbolic system	S2: use value of the real subject in the symbolic system
$: proletarianized real subject (enunciating workforce)	*a*: difference between the used real subject and his exchange value

As a difference between the proletarianized real subject with his use value and his exchange value in the symbolic system, the *missing being* of the subject (*a*) can be regarded as the *missing link* between the real subject ($) and the exteriority of the symbolic system (S1→S2). Since the real being is missing in the symbolic system, it causes the desire of the subject, who is detained in the system by his desire for that which is missing in the system. In this way, by causing the desire that keeps the subject in the system, the missing being ironically functions as the 'point' in which the subject is 'articulated' with the system (Milner, 1978, p. 66). Thus, in relation to 'the symbolic order', the subject is 'caught in it in his being' (Lacan, 1956a, p. 53). After 'making his entrance' in the symbolic system 'by passing through the radical defile of speech' (ibid.), the real subject cannot leave without his missing real being. He cannot get out of the exteriority of language in which he lost himself. He cannot break away from this 'geometrical place' in which he got lost (1953b, p. 147).

The real subject must logically stay in the symbolic system in which his real being is missing. In this symbolic system, the real being can be sought, of course, but it cannot be recovered. Nevertheless, as compensation for the lack of the real being, the subject finds all sorts of symbolic beings. Once cleared from the unspeakable real being of the speaking subject, the locus of speech is invaded by 'speech-beings' (*parlêtres*) whose symbolic 'beings' come from 'speech' (Lacan, 1974–1975, 17.12.74). In our locus of speech, all things *are* these speech-beings. As symbolic beings, they are the only constituent elements of our symbolic universe. They entirely compose our exteriority. We must know our world through them. In our world, they *are* everything, including us.[1]

In our world, the 'speech-beings' are not only 'spoken' facts, but also 'speaking' acts (Miller, 2003, p. 113). They are not only symbolic *spoken-beings*, but also real *'speaking-beings'* that 'get their being from speech' (Lacan, 1972c, p. 549). The "revolutionary", for example, is not only symbolically *spoken,* but is also really *speaking* through the mouth, the arms, the body of Francisco Javier. Unlike the Aristotelian man, as thinking-being that thinks with his soul, the Lacanian 'man' is a 'speech-being' that 'speaks with his body' (1979, p. 566). Now, besides speaking, this body 'enjoys while speaking' (1972–1973, 08.05.73, pp. 134–146). It is a 'living body of enjoying substance' (Soler, 2005, p. 15). Far from the thinking spiritual substances of Aristotle and Descartes, the Lacanian speech-being is a speaking and enjoying corporeal being. Its body enjoys its speech that consumes its body. This speaking *consumption* is the same thing as the corporeal *enjoyment*. Speech becomes the same thing as the body. The body melts into speech.

In the corporeal speech-being, 'the being and speech are tied and reciprocally corrupted' (Milner, 1978, p. 98). By 'affecting the body of the being that makes itself a being of speech', the 'wisdom' of language creates the *literal support of the signifier*, the *speech-being*, which functions as a *speaking-spoken being* ($\\S1) in which the speaking real act ($) and the spoken symbolic fact (S1) cannot be easily differentiated (Lacan, 1972c, p. 550). *The symbolization of the real* generates *the real of the symbolic*. In this symbolization, however, there is no recovery of the real being of the subject. Far from it, the symbolization 'carves up' the subject and 'produces the scraps' of his real being (ibid.).

In the symbolization, the real being is not recovered, but rather it is just lost again. It is replaced anew by a *literal, speaking-spoken* or *real-symbolic* being. Actually, each *literal being* can be treated as a *real symbol* of the loss of the *real being*. In the origin of each literal being, there is a loss of the real being that results from the corruption of the real by the symbolic. To be sure, this corruption is a denaturalization that produces the detachment of the real being, the object of drives and desires, which entails, in turn, an evolution from nature to culture, from the prehistoric real ecosystem to the historical symbolic system, from the herd animal to the political animal, from need to desire, from instinct to drive, from satisfaction to enjoyment, from the sexual relation to the signifying relation.[2] In this evolution, "individual sexual love" turns into "mutual respect and faithfulness from conviction". As for "the couple", it is replaced by "marriage" with its "importance and significance for the revolutionaries".

"Marriage" seems to make up for the real separation between the subject and his object. Compensating for this lack of a *sexual relation*, "marriage" ostensibly functions as a *civic bond* theoretically established by the *signifying relation* between the One and the Other, the signifier and the signifying social structure, the "revolutionary" and the "familiar obligations" of his cultural environment. Because of the 'belief in this bond' that 'structures his animality' (Milner, 1983, pp. 132–142), the subject *speaks himself* and becomes thus a *political animal*, a *symbolized real*, a *speech-being*. Through his speech, the subject develops into 'a political animal because he is a speaking and spoken being, a speech-being, a subject of the unconscious' (Miller, 2003, p. 113). His political animality resides in his functioning as an animal of the symbolic body of people, an element of the signifying social structure, the subject of the predicate, the One of the Other, the revolutionary of the political system. This belonging to the system obliges the subject to 'receive from the Other the signifiers that master him, represent him and denaturalize him' (ibid.).

Unable to *denote* the missing real being (*a*) of the enunciating subject ($), the speech-being *connotes* the available symbolic being (S2) of the enunciated subject (S1). Actually, the speech-being *is* this *connoted-being*. It *is* this *predicated-subject* or *political-animal* (S2–S1). It *is* this symbolic being immanent *in* speech, and not a transcendent real being produced *by* speech. Now, unlike this real missing being (*a*) that belongs exclusively to one unique subject ($◊*a*), the speech-being can be socialized, at least to a certain extent, in the form of a subjective signifier (S1), which represents several subjects within the predicative symbolic system (S1→S2). Within the exteriority of this system, the Lacanian speech-being may function as a partially transindividual subjective being. It may thus function as a partly shared individual position within the signifying social structure in itself.[3]

Within the real structure of the symbolic system, a number of real individual speaking beings may be partly positioned in the same symbolic spoken being. This being turns out to be real as a relatively social speech-being. Its symbolic value is simultaneously realized and socialized by its literal embodiment in the meeting or common positioning of several subjects. The realization is a relative socialization. The "revolutionary" and the "married", for example, become real as relatively social speech-beings in which the symbolic spoken-beings are literally embodied by countless real speaking-beings that take up the positions of "marriage" and "revolution". Now, however real they may be, these speaking-beings 'are nothing but speech-beings', as they must 'speak' in order to 'be' (Lacan, 1974–1975, 18.02.75). Even their real speaking-being is thus a speech-being 'imposed' by the 'language' that articulates their speech and makes them 'speak' (1972–1973, 16.01.73, p. 59).

Accessible to our Lacanian Discourse Analysis, the speech-being can be analyzed in the *discourse of the Other*. It completely resides in this *spoken discourse of a speaking language*. In this *spoken-being of a speaking-being*, the 'speech-being is only made of that which speaks' (Lacan, 1976–1977, 15.02.77). That which speaks is the articulating language, of course, but also its embodiment by the expressing subjects, the real speaking subjects, as the real enunciating workforce of the language, the structure, the Other. Expressing the discourse of the Other, this workforce does the speaking work of the unconscious. By doing this work, the real subject becomes the real support through which the unconscious speaks. At the same time, without its missing real being, the 'subject' is also symbolically 'supported' by the 'speech-being' of the unconscious (1975–1976, 16.12.75, p. 56). In this, the subject is not only the workforce of the unconscious, but he 'is the unconscious' (ibid.). He *is* the discourse of the Other. He is alienated in the Other to such a point that his being does not belong to him, but it instead belongs to the Other. Actually, this Other 'obliges' the subject, in his proletarian condition, to 'admit that he will not have anything of the being' (Lacan, 1972–1973, 16.01.73, p. 59). He will not *be* his speech-being, which will always be Other than he.

Unlike the subject in the flesh, the speech-being will be always *nothing more than words*. These words cannot become identical to the missing real being of the subject. They cannot become the real being of the subject. They are purely symbolic. The 'speech-beings' (*parlêtres*) are merely 'seeming beings', 'apparent beings', or 'appar-beings' (*parêtres*), which always stay only 'next to (*appar-*)' the real being (Lacan, 1972–1973, 16.01.73, p. 59). Even in the speaking act, the real appearance of the speech-being of words always leads to the words themselves, to their petrified appearance-of-being, to their symbolic spoken-being that has nothing to do with the missing real being of the speaking act.[4]

The master-being signifier and the reduction to the slavery of language

When the appearance-of-being explicitly passes itself off as the speaking subject ($), its being corresponds to the symbolic spoken-being of the master-signifier (S1). This signifier can be then called a 'master-being signifier' (*signifiant m'être*), as it constitutes the mastering signifying being that 'I am myself to myself' (*m'être à moi même*) in the spoken discourse in which *I speak, therefore I am* (Lacan, 1969–1970, 20.05.70, p. 178). Here, as discussed before, *I am* as *I am spoken* (symbolic spoken-being) in that which *I speak* as *I am speaking* (real speaking-thing). In any case, this *I* is the elementary symbolic form of any master-signifier. It is the "consistent revolutionary" *I* am when *I* express my "conceptions of marriage". As the speech-being, it is the *spoken One I am* when *I am speaking*. It is already a *master-being-signifier* that 'asserts itself first through the mark of a 1' (p. 183).

Through the mark of *a One*, the master-being-signifier cannot assert itself as *One* without commanding the subject *to be One*. Under the mastery of *the* signifier, the subject *must be One*. He *must be*. He *is* at the signifier's command. It is a *word of command*. By virtue of this word (S1), the subject must constantly assume that he *is One*. In spite of the lack of his missing being, he must have *One being*. He must carry on this *transcendental consciousness* that underpins the conscious imaginary. He must keep a feeling of ontological consistency, continuity and stability, unity or community, society or individuality, notwithstanding his division and dissociation ($) between his identification with the One (S1) and his alienation in the multiple speech-beings of the Other (S2).[5] In this way, "consistent revolutionaries" such as Francisco Javier, together with "inconsistent revolutionaries" such as the members of the Mexican Institutional Revolutionary Party (PRI), do not have permission to lose their conscious revolutionary identity even when they cross oppression and repression, authoritarianism and conformism, traditionalism and loyalism, faithfulness and monogamy, and all other values that flagrantly betray the same "revolutionary consistency" that they imperiously affirm and reaffirm.

Imperiously affirmed and reaffirmed, the being of the master-signifier is not only *a being commanding the subject*, but also *the being commanded to the subject*. As the commanded and commanding being of the subject, the 'master-being' (*m'être*) is 'the being of command' in the subject (Lacan, 1972–1973, 16.01.73, p. 53). It *is* actually a command for the subject. It is a *command of being*, a 'command' given by the 'master discourse', which 'puts the accent on the verb *to be*' (09.01.73, p. 43).

As we are under the command of the master discourse, we must *be*. We must *be something, someone, One*. We do not have the right to be *no one* or *nothing*. Since the 'master discourse' is a 'discourse of being' that needs our being, we *have to be* (Lacan, 1972–1973, 09.01.73, pp. 42–43). We have to be for the symbolic system of the master discourse. We are not authorized to deprive it of our being. We are not allowed to assume the lack of our missing real being. We must be a piece of the system, just one piece, any piece, even a "revolutionary" one. Even if we are against the system, we must be in it, as we are necessary for it.

The symbolic system of the enunciated discourse (S1→S2) cannot work without our enunciating workforce ($). Accordingly, for the working of the system, we must be a part of the system. We must have a being in it. We must have a symbolic being. We must *be* this 'master-being', this 'imperative signifier', that precisely 'commands' us 'to be', to be with it, to be precisely what it is, 'a signifier' (Lacan, 1972–1973, 09.01.73, pp. 43–44). Once we are this exchange being ($\S1), we can be incorporated into the symbolic system of language ($\S1→S2), which can then make use of our entire speaking workforce ($). Our useful alienation in language, as speaking-beings, is permitted by our identification with the spoken-being of the signifier. This is why we must be identified with this being. We must *be* 'the signifier' in order to *be* 'collectively' used by 'a language' (pp. 44–47). *Thanks to our identification with a master-being signifier, we can usefully reduce ourselves to the slavery of language. Our identification with the symbolic spoken-being enables the utilization of our real speaking-being by the symbolic system. Our being, the speech-being, makes our utilization possible. This is why we must be. We must be to be at language's disposal. We must be to be exploited by the symbolic system of culture and civilization. In this symbolic universe, I must be exploited, therefore I am.*

The real beings as litter and letters

In the symbolic system, the subject must be to be exploited. He must have a symbolic being to be an exploited being. Now, even if his symbolic being enables his exploitation, his symbolic being *is not* his exploited being. Of course, the symbolic being is exploited to exploit the subject, but its exploitation is not the exploitation of the subject.

S1: symbolic subjective being (identitary exchange value of the workforce)	S2: symbolic predicative exploitation of the real being (use value of the workforce)
$: real subject as enunciating workforce	*a*: real being of the subject, of his workforce, of his body

When we say *the exploitation of the subject*, we refer to the exploitation of his real speaking-being. To be sure, the exploited being is the real being. Now, in the symbolic system (S1→S2), the subject ($) must have a symbolic spoken-being (S1) in order to provide an exploited real speaking-being ($\S1→S2/*a*). In exchange for the symbolic predicative exploitation of this real being (alienated use value of the enunciating workforce), the subject receives, in anticipation, his identitary symbolic subjective being (identitary exchange value of the enunciating workforce). This symbolic being constitutes a wage to buy the real being of the subject, his workforce, or his body. Absurdly, the subject ($) sells his real being (*a*) in exchange for a symbolic being (S1) with the aim of recovering his real being (*a*). The subject sells what he wants to buy. This is how the real being will have been missing. It will have been missing because he must have been already missing to become the real of the symbolic.

The missing real being of the subject is the speaking-being of the spoken-being. It forms the only real support of the symbolic system. It composes the body of the Other. It makes up the literal 'materiality of the signifier' (Lacan, 1956a, p. 24). The real 'being' is missing for the subject precisely because it becomes, as 'the letter', the 'being of wisdom' (1972–1973, 20.03.73, p. 124). In this 'wisdom' of language, the real 'being' of the subject 'makes itself the letter of the Other', but it does this 'at the expense of itself', since it has to be neutralized in itself to become the literal being of language (p. 125). As a piece of the symbolic system, the real being of the subject is missing in itself (*a*). In itself, the real being must be excluded from discourse (S1–S2/*a*). It must be rejected in itself to be exploited as a letter of discourse.

The exploitation of the 'letter' of discourse turns its own being, the real being of the subject, into 'litter' (Lacan, 1971, p. 11). Actually, the 'letter' of discourse is already a being that 'kills' the 'being' of the subject (1972–1973, 20.03.73, p. 124). This must be understood literally. By now, the literality of the "revolutionary" has already killed several Eperrists in the fight against the Mexican Army. Similarly, the real beings of the kamikazes are killed every day by their literal presence as signifiers. This also applies to any other voluntary hero, but also to involuntary heroes, such as those killed by their "Mexican" literal signifying presence on the border with the United States. In any case, as a 'letter' of language, 'the signifier materializes the instance of death' for the subject (1956a, p. 24).

By killing the real being of the subject, the letter becomes the real being of the Other, the real support of the signifier, the real of the symbolic universe. In this universe, the 'letters' compose a 'semblance' of 'the real', of course, but they are also the only accessible beings in which we can find 'something real' (Lacan, 1970–1971, 20.01.71, p. 28). Around us, the letters are the only *sign* of the real being. They can then be treated as *the real being*. In Lacan (1972–1973), this real being, 'the being' (*l'être*), is inseparable from the 'letter' (*lettre*), which is 'conveyed' by 'the being' (20.03.73, p. 124). According to Miller (1988), this homophony between the two terms (*l'être* and *lettre*) indicates two successive ideas in the evolution of Lacanian theory, namely, the 'signifying' character of any 'being', whose *Dasein* can only be a 'being-in-language', and the fact that our 'being' is 'made' by 'something' as concrete as a 'letter' (p. 12). In any case, within our symbolic universe, the real being may only be accessible as a real being of the symbolic, as 'a letter', as a 'material medium that concrete discourse borrows from language' (Lacan, 1957b, p. 492). In our universe organized by this language, the 'letter' proves to be *the* real 'being', the only one, which 'appears' in 'the emptiness of the verb *to be*' (p. 517). Here, in this real emptiness of the structure, something cannot *really be* without being a perceptible support of the symbolic, whether visible or audible, wearable or habitable, etc.

In the real emptiness that surrounds us, the only present real being supports the symbolic representatives of the absent real being whose absence opens the real emptiness. As for this absent real being, it cannot be recovered in itself, since it has been entirely excluded in itself in order to become the real being of the literal presence of the signifiers that symbolically represent it. *Paradoxically, the real being disappears in itself, as litter, to reappear, as the letter, in the real support of its own symbolic representatives. Thus, in civilization, the human creature loses his body, which then becomes the body of that which represents him, namely, a signifier, a piece of civilization, a limb of the Other*. Composing the Other, this body of the symbolic representative cannot be regarded as the body of the subject anymore. Actually, despite its real presence, the alienated body cannot even be regarded as a real representative of the real body of the subject. Whatever it may be, this real body cannot really be represented. This is why its representatives are purely symbolic. This is also why its representations are merely imaginary. The real body stays always away from its literal or figurative embodiments. In all these representative or representational presences, the only presence of the real body is *its lacking presence in its noticeable absence.*[6] This *presence* is its only real presence, a presence of misery and dispossession, privation and frustration, drives and desires. These negative manifestations of the traumatic structural emptiness constitute the only presence of the real being of the subject. They are his marks. In a concrete discourse, they can only be revealed in gaps, fissures or openings in the signifying chain, as well as in zones of transparency in the mirror signified surface of the imaginary.

In Francisco Javier's discourse, for instance, a real being of the subject might be showing through beneath the "individual sexual love" that "leads" to "a dissolution of the couple, when the feeling disappears". In this unexpected "dissolution" to which love "leads", a Lacanian Discourse Analysis might eventually detect a real being that is not unrelated to the dissolution of some Eperrists dead in combat. Like the "dissolution" of the "individual sexual love", the heroic first death of an *individual sexed body* reveals not only the *vanishing point* of the second death, but also the *vanishing* of the mortal real being of the body, which will have been transformed into the immortal real being of the literal support of the signifier. In any case, the real being of the subject must be ejected from the symbolic in order to develop into the real of the symbolic. To be converted into the literal support of our entire symbolic universe, our real body must be excluded from the supported universe.[7]

Lacking-of-being and lacking-to-be, real being and symbolic being, surplus-enjoyment and surplus value

In the symbolic universe, our real body may turn into the literal support of each human being and its ramifications, for instance a model and her clothes, a weightlifter and his dumbbells, a bricklayer and his bricks, an architect and his buildings, an operator and his machines, a researcher and his papers, a fighter and his guns. But all these things are no longer the real body excluded from them. Of course, the fighter and his guns are not less real than a corpse riddled with bullets. Yet the real being is not the same in both cases. On the one hand, there is the *teleological real being* of the fighter and his guns, as the literal 'support of the message', which fulfils the 'function of the signifier' (Miller, 1988, p. 12). On the other hand, there is the *scatological real being* of the corpse, which 'does not have a function, but a fate', a 'fate of waste' (ibid.). Now, as evidenced by a picture of Che Guevara or the mummy of Lenin, the corpse can also become the literal support of a message. However, in that case, the teleological being of the symbolic revolutionary is still preserved. We see it before its death, the second death, and after the consummation of the first death, the death of the scatological being of his real body. In the interstice between both deaths, the revolutionary's corpse may still function as the teleological real support of a symbolic being that 'becomes an eternal sign for the others' (Lacan, 1957–1958, 12.02.58, p. 245). But this literal support of the symbolic being (the mummy of a "revolutionary") is the effect of the first death, the death of the real being, which begins with the *birth* of the symbolic being (the transformation into a "revolutionary"). To be sure, the teleological real being (the support of the "revolutionary") can only exist through the lethal sacrifice of the scatological real being (his own body sacrificed in the revolutionary action). This applies to all human beings. This is why their real being is a mortal being, a permanently dying being, a scatological being that is always coming away from the symbolic.

Whether as a scatological being or as a teleological being, the real being always appears *at the end*. It arises as a 'consequence' (Lacan, 1971, p. 15). It is the real consequence of symbolization. As we know, it composes the real of the symbolic. However, even symbolized, this real of the symbolic is not the same thing as the symbolic. The symbolic being *is not* the real being. Actually, by definition, the symbolic being is a *real nonbeing*. In Lacan's terms, 'the being of language is the nonbeing of objects' (Lacan, 1958d, p. 105). It is the nonbeing of objects because it is the nonbeing of *the* object that underpins any object, namely, the object *a* defined as the real being of the subject.

The real being (*a*) of the subject ($) is a nonbeing in the discourse of language (S1→S2). This is why the enunciated discourse is not recognized by the enunciating subject. Without his real being, his discourse appears to him as the discourse of an Other. In 'this discourse of the Other, which is the unconscious, something is lacking, something that would enable the subject to be identified as the subject of this discourse' (Lacan, 1958–1959, 13.05.59). What is lacking is the real being of the subject. It is his object *a*. It is this object that functions as a symbolic nonbeing of the real in the symbolic system of discourse.

Indicated by the phallic symbol Φ in the Lacanian formulation, the symbolic nonbeing of the real is a negative signifier 'excluded from the signifier' (Lacan, 1960–1961, 26.04.61, p. 306). If this negative signifier were not excluded from the signifier, it would be the only signifier that would really represent the real being of the subject. But, after all, the Φ does not need to *represent* this being, since it *presents* it. It presents the real 'speaking being of discourse' (1969–1970, 20.05.70, p. 177). More precisely, it *is* the symbolic nonbeing that presents this real speaking being as an absence, a nonappearance, a lack in the spoken discourse.

In Lacan (1960–1961), the symbolic nonbeing of the real being is described with an ambiguous expression, *manque-à-être*, that may simultaneously mean 'lacking-of-being' and 'lacking-to-be' (14.06.61, p. 427). This lacking of the real being enables it to be the 'complementary' symbolic being, a 'being of lacking', of 'lacking-of-being' (Soler, 2006, p. 33). Thus, as the *lacking of the real being* that enables it *to be a symbolic being* in discourse, the *manque-à-être* 'arises' from a 'certain' double 'relationship to discourse' (Lacan, 1960–1961, 14.06.61, p. 427). In this relationship, the lacking is at the same time a positive 'lacking-to-be' that generates a symbolic 'effect of being' in the enunciated discourse, and a negative 'lacking-of-being' for the enunciating subject, whose real being is produced 'as an object' (1969–1970, 20.05.70, p. 177). Once the symbolic being is *generated* in discourse, the real being is *produced by discourse*, in the sense that it is *turned out* or *removed from discourse*. This production of an object removed from discourse always accompanies the generation of the signifier that is a constituent of discourse. *In order to be, the symbolic needs a lacking of the real being. This lacking-of-being is a necessary lacking-to-be. The generation of a symbolic surplus value implies the production of a real surplus-enjoyment. The non-tautological nature of discourse is conditioned by the former, while the mere existence of the symbolic being of discourse is conditioned by the latter. This is why both processes must interest a Lacanian Discourse Analysis.*

In a Lacanian Discourse Analysis, the real being lacking in discourse may be treated as a surplus-enjoyment that has to be produced by words, since words cannot absorb it.[8] This surplus-enjoyment amounts to that which is earned and lost by speaking. It forms the real being removed or produced by the work of the unconscious symbolic system that exploits the enunciating workforce of the subject. It is concurrently the enjoyment of this work and the renunciation of this enjoyment, a sacrifice inherent in any kind of work, a discontent inseparable from civilization. Unlike the surplus value of Marx, this surplus-enjoyment of Lacan is not a symbolic value that can be reinvested in the symbolic system. Far from it. The surplus-enjoyment is a real being that must be lost by the system, which can only deploy its own symbolic being in the emptiness of the lost real being.

Discourse and silence, use and enjoyment of the real being

During the course of the enunciating work, the enjoyment of work is always lost. *It has to be lost*. Otherwise, this real experience would obstruct the functioning of the symbolic system. It would even involve a sort of work stoppage. Accordingly, the subject must renounce the enjoyment of his real being at work. He must renounce it as it involves a sort of consumption of the real being, of its raw material, that must be 'used' (*uti*) by the system instead of being 'enjoyed' (*frui*) by the subject (cf. Augustine, 400, XIII, pp. 340–349). The renunciation of enjoyment thus amounts to a renunciation of the enjoyable real being. It is this renunciation that enables the transformation of the real being into the literal support of the symbolic system of civilization. However, this literal support is no longer its raw material. It is no longer the real being in itself, the real body of the subject, or the real experience of it. This living matter is lost. Even if the subject renounces all thought of consuming his real being, this being cannot be preserved in his symbolic universe. In this universe generated by the work of symbolization, the real being of the subject is necessarily excluded. It has to be removed from the symbol. It has to be thus *produced* by the symbolic system. But it is produced as waste. It is produced by being lost and in order to be lost.

The production (*a*) breaks away from the production line (S1→S2/*a*). Although this enunciated signifying chain (S1→S2) can use an enunciating workforce ($\S1→S2), it cannot do anything with the real being (*a*) of the proletarianized subject whose workforce is used ($). This intemporal real being continuously slides out from the symbolic metonymical slide of temporality. Now, as a slide in a slide, the real being of the subject appears to him in a sort of stillness that 'fixes' and thereby 'revalues the slide' (Lacan, 1960–1961, 01.03.61, p. 202). Thus, the real being 'gets the value of a privileged object' that permits the subject to 'recognize' his own being as 'fixed' (ibid.). This object of recognition *is* the Lacanian object *a*. It is an 'overvalued object' that 'saves our dignity as subjects' (p. 203). It saves this dignity by allowing us to *really be* something more than a *symbolic being* 'submitted to the slide of the signifier' (p. 203).

Like any one of us, Francisco Javier cannot resign himself to wandering in the alienating discourse of "our time". The subject cannot be satisfied with this purely symbolic existence as a signifier of "our time". He needs to be something more, something intemporal, something real. He needs to be a real being outside the symbolic system. In Lacan, this real being is indicated by the object *a*, which fixes the subject outside his metonymical slide, in the impossible exterior of his symbolic universe, in the exteriority of his unconscious exteriority. Through this object, the subject may be without being in the history that determines him. He may be without being in the factory that exploits him. He may really be without being a simple device in the machine, a literal support of the symbol, a little piece of the system. He may *really be*, for instance, in a totally irrational violence that cannot be used or exchanged. Since this violence cannot be incorporated into the system, it may stand for the real being that has been rejected from the system.[9] This allows the one responsible for this violence to *really be* through the violence. Nevertheless, through this violence, the subject can only *really be* out of the system, out of the symbolic universe, *out of everything*. He can only *really be* in this impossible place, in this useless and non-exploitable situation, in this totally segregated non-structural position. This marginalized position is the only one in which the violent subject can *really be*. His real being thus presupposes a 'marginalization' from the signifying social structure in which 'he learns' to reject 'violence' (Foucault, 1972, p. 1205).

To recover the real being that is lost in the signifying social structure, the subject has to marginalize himself from this structure. In this structure, the subject cannot *really be*. Through the signifying chain, the subject cannot reach his real being that continuously slides out of the chain. Understandably, the subject cannot use the chain to get out of the chain. As noted by Lacan (1957–1958), 'the more the subject employs the signifier to get out of the signifying chain, the more he is integrated into the chain, and the more he becomes a sign of the chain' (12.02.58, p. 245). Francisco Javier, for example, is progressively implicated in the conformist and regressive system of "our time" as he progresses in his revolutionary discourse "for the construction of the new society and the new man". Similarly, any discourse implicates the subject in the system. *Any spoken discourse confines the speaking subject to the symbolic system in which he is used by language. To get out of this system, it would be better for the speaking subject to stop speaking, which is impossible for him as a speaking subject. But only a break in speech may allow him to come back to a real speaking being that is missing in the symbolic spoken being. By bringing the subject back to his expressing act, the inexpressiveness may involve a real experience of this act, an enjoyment of its real being, before the privation of this being, which is excluded from the expressed fact.*[10]

In discourse, only inexpressiveness may really represent the real being (*a*) without excluding it, nullifying it, betraying it (S2/*a*). In practice, of course, inexpressiveness is impossible for the expressing subject. However, in theory, this subject ($) may always withdraw into silence, as an absolutely "consistent revolutionary", behind the hood of the master-signifier ($\S1). He may also have the perverse idea of taking the hood off, forgetting the revolution and giving up his life to silently fantasize or act out the fantasy of his real being ($◊*a*). Otherwise, if the theoretical silent subject does not have a propensity for perversion, he will probably prefer the heroic suicide of the melancholic martyr of the revolution. In that case, at least, he will permanently reduce to silence the inconsistent mouth of the structure that pleads for "marriage" and "monogamy". In other words, he will suppress his alienation in the system by allowing himself to be led by the object *a*, which is excluded from the system. Led out of the inconsistent signifying chain (S1→S2), the subject ($) may then become the kamikaze that immolates himself, with his real being (*a*), for the symbolic being of the consistent signifier (S1).

Diametrically opposed to Francisco Javier and to any theoretical silent revolutionary, there is a rather noisy protester who shows great tolerance for his own inconsistency and intermittently stays in the signifying chain of the system. In a classic trade union strategy, this militant may refuse from time to time to continue working in the production line. He may stop negotiations, go on strike, and say: "No, I will be consistent, I will not work for the conformist system". But in due course, the strike ends and the subject is reincorporated into the system. Actually, 'his successive refusals reinforce the chain, to which he is progressively attached' (Lacan, 1957–1958, 12.02.58, p. 246).

To detach oneself from the discourse of the Other (S1→S2), one must renounce the symbolic being of the Other (S2) instead of renouncing the real being of oneself (*a*). Instead of going on strike to prevent the reduction to the marginalization of one's real being in the symbolic system, one must willingly reduce oneself to one's marginalized real being, for instance through the real experience of a pure enunciating act, such as the impulsive, blind and useless violent acting-out of the Eperrists in some exceptional circumstances. Thanks to the real experience of this elementary violent enunciating act, any kind of violence, and not only the 'violence of the disseminating writing' of Derrida (1972), can ultimately 'unpick the symbolic' and 'disrupt' it 'with the force of a certain exterior' (pp. 112–119). Unlike the enunciating workforce alienated in the symbolic system, this subversive force acts from the exterior of the symbolic system, so that it may enable the subject to assert his real being, which is excluded from the interior of the system. But this assertion of the real being leads again to its symbolization, its transformation into the real support of the symbol, and its incorporation into the symbolic system. In this way, the experience of the violent acting-out again turns into the enunciated fact of the enunciating act. The real being of the subject is thereby reabsorbed into the symbolic being of the signifier. The circular movement of the revolution is accomplished. We return to the starting point, except for one detail, the reinforcement of the system. This reinforcement can be observed in most post-revolutionary governments, such as the Napoleonic Empire after the French Revolution, the Stalinist regime after the Soviet Revolution, or the PRI System after the Mexican Revolution. In any case, after the tear, the symbolic fabric is not only sewn up again, but it is also strengthened. Paradoxically, the disruption of the system underlies the rational strengthening of the system. The reactive and reactionary strength of the enunciated fact is reflexively founded on the violent force of its revolutionary enunciating act. This pre-reflexive violence ($) underpins the reflexive establishment (S1). This peaceful and powerful establishment is established, enforced and reinforced by an irrational violence ($\S1) that may always weaken, undermine and again subvert the rational establishment.[11]

Imaginary aggressivity, symbolic hostility and real violence

Against the irrational violence that underpins and may subvert the establishment, there is a rational violence that serves and obeys the conventional rationality of this establishment. Since the rational violence forms part of this political rationality, we may say that this rationality is protected by its own rational violence. It is protected against its underlying irrational real violence, but also against the rational violence of other symbolic rationalities. In any case, we may paraphrase Karl Von Clausewitz and assume that *rational violence is the continuation of the political symbolic rationality by other means*. It is a rational argument among other rational arguments. It is just one link between the other links in the signifying chain. When Francisco Javier deliberately and strategically shoots at a Mexican soldier, for example, his shot is nothing but an incisive signifier of his revolutionary discourse. It thus functions as a piece of the symbolic system.

The violence of the system fights the violence against the system. In both sides, the violence refers to the system. Whether in favour of it or in opposition to it, human violence is related to the symbolic system. It is determined by the symbol. It is fundamentally *engendered* by the signifier. The signifier actually provokes human violence in contexts in which there would be no violence between non-humans. Between 'one lion' and 'three marvellous lionesses', for example, there would be 'peace' and 'harmony', since 'the lion does not know how to count up to three' (Lacan, 1956–1957, 20.03.57, p. 237). Instead, by virtue of the signifier, the human subject knows how to count up to three. This may unsurprisingly create a hell of violence between *one man and three marvellous women*. In this 'hell' composed of 'the others' (Sartre, 1944, p. 93), there is inevitably the signifier, the 'word', and no one can 'remain silent', so that each one becomes the literal support of the symbolic system, the instrument of the Other, or a 'tormentor of the others' (p. 42). Between the tormentors, the conflict is unavoidable. Logically, to 'understand' this kind of 'interhuman conflict', we must take 'the signifier' into account (Lacan, 1956–1957, 20.03.57, p. 237).

Human violence is fundamentally engendered by the signifier. Nevertheless, it is also fundamentally prevented by the signifier.[12] This can be illustrated by considering the dangerous meeting between one man and three marvellous women. On the one hand, the signifier may engender violence between them, since *one* is brutally challenged by *three*, and *two* can only be ferociously opposed to *one*, besides the fact that *one* is perfidiously identical to *one*, so that each *one* must be cruelly excluded by another *one*. On the other hand, the signifier may prevent violence between all these signifiers, since *three* can be reduced to *one* and *two*, and *two* may be treated as *one* and *one*, while each *one* can be assimilated to another *one*, in such a way that *two* will not be opposed to *one* any more. If the man and the three marvellous women considered all this, there would certainly be the same peace and harmony among them that Lacan observed between the lion and the three lionesses in the zoo. Therefore, the man and the women are not only violent among themselves because they count up to three, but also because they 'do not count very much better than the lions', and the 'number three is not completely integrated, but only articulated' (Lacan, 1956–1957, 20.03.57, p. 237).

Articulated by the structure, the signifier cannot be completely integrated *for* the proletarianized subject who only expresses it. Nor can it be completely integrated *into* him. In relation to him, the signifier can be just an unintelligible external element that functions as a constituent element of the unconscious. Even literally supported by the real being of the subject, the signifier is an unintelligible external element for the subject, whose real being is lost for him when it becomes the literal support of the signifier. Under these circumstances, the subject must resort to violence with the purpose of recovering his real being, turning it into a non-alienated literal support of the signifier, and by this means, in return, reintegrating the unconscious unintelligible external signifier into himself and transforming it thereby into a conscious intelligible internal sign. In a sense, we are violent to become conscious. We are thus violent because of the unconscious, or, more precisely, because of all troubles involved in the unconscious, namely, the frustrating exteriority of everything from ourselves, the annoying absence of our real being in the symbolic universe, the infuriating non-integration of the signifiers for all of us, the aggravating lack of a shared real signification, the individual and incommunicable character of all conscious imaginary significations, which are thus controversial, contentious, and conflicting. Because of these troubles, there is understandably a violent struggle between different subjects who cannot consciously communicate, agree, and reconcile their unconscious points of view.

If the *troubles of the unconscious* provoke the *violent struggle between different subjects*, then this struggle can be regarded as a *conflict of the unconscious*, in view of the fact that its causes reside in the unconscious, in the discourse of the Other, of language, of the signifying social structure for each position in the structure.[13] In some way, the struggle between different subjects is also friction between differing unconsciouses. It is also a clash between divergent ways in which the same structure in itself manifests for different subjects.

In the signifying social structure in itself, the unique multifaceted position of each signifier can be described as the intricate combination of its diverse positions in the divergent manifestations of the structure for different structural positions. Now, leaving aside the theoretical structure in itself, each signifier is fragmented between its diverse positions in the divergent manifestations of the structure. Each signifier is thus disintegrated into its diverse symbolic values in divergent languages of different subjects. The "revolutionary" is objectively disintegrated, for example, into its positions in the divergent languages that articulate the discourses of Danton and Robespierre, Blanc and Lamartine, Lenin and Kerensky, Trotsky and Stalin, Chian Kai-Shek and Mao Zedong, Zapata and Carranza, Villa and Obregón, Lucio Cabañas and Luis Echeverría, Francisco Javier and Ernesto Zedillo, etc. This disintegration provokes contrasting imaginary significations, misunderstandings and communication gaps between the "revolutionaries", as well as violent struggles between them. But these violent struggles between the "revolutionaries" (S1) are brutal clashes between their languages (S2). In any case, once reabsorbed by the symbolic system, the violent acting-out of the real being ($\$\lozenge a$) turns into a violent assertion of a symbolic being (S1→S2). The real violence of the expressing subject becomes a symbolic hostility of the articulating language. This symbolic hostility is a structural violence inherent in the signifying social structure. Now, like everything in this structure, this violence is perceptible, but unintelligible. The structural violence is an unconscious violence. To be sure, it is 'repressed', since it is incorporated into the 'structure of speech, that is to say, the signifying articulation' (Lacan, 1957–1958, 18.06.58, p. 460). In this articulation of discourse, 'the aggressiveness is symbolized and taken by the mechanism of repression' (ibid.). Taken by this 'mechanism of the unconscious', it becomes a symbolic structural hostility that 'can be analyzed' (ibid.).

In a Lacanian Discourse Analysis, we can only analyze the symbolic structural hostility between divergent languages, discourses, manifestations of the structure, signifiers, and fractions of disintegrated signifiers.

Accordingly, the real impulsive anti-structural violence against the symbolic system can only be analyzed after its symbolization by the system. As for the imaginary aggressivity aroused by misunderstandings, communication gaps, and contrasting significations, it can only be analyzed when it is reduced to its symbolic foundation. In this analytical reduction, the aggressivity may be explained by the necessity of the incomprehensible signifying difference and the merely imaginary character of any kind of signification, understanding, and communication. To be sure, if signification, understanding, and communication are merely imaginary things, then misunderstandings, communication gaps, and contrasting significations are as unavoidable as the resulting aggressivity between those fellow men who aspire to signification, understanding, and communication. After the elimination of the 'fellow man latent in this imaginary relation', we can reduce the imaginary 'aggressiveness' against the fellow man in the mirror to the symbolic hostility between positions in the 'structure' (Lacan, 1957–1958, 18.06.58, p. 460). Between these different positions, the difference may intrinsically imply inequality, contradiction, opposition, and even conflict, as well as violence. This violence can be treated as a structural hostility inherent in the structural difference. Instead, the imaginary aggression, aggressivity, would result from the discrepancy between this difference in the structure and the imaginary identification in the mirror. In contrast to this illusory identification or equalization, the evident difference or inequality seems to be intolerably unjust and unjustified. Faced with the symbolic inequality, the subject would have a feeling of injustice that fully justifies his aggressiveness, but only in the imaginary sphere.[14]

In the imaginary sphere, there is a comprehensive confusion that merges the subject, his missing real being, the literal support of the symbol, *the* symbol itself, and all other symbols. This imaginary amalgamation permits the subject to imagine that he can retain his real being through his own identification and equalization with the fellow man in the mirror. Instead of the impulsive violence aimed at recovering the real being, such an illusion constitutes an imaginary recovery of it. But this recovery is doomed to failure. Sooner or later, the subject must acknowledge the manifest lack of his real being, the unreality of his image in the mirror, the imaginary character of his equalization or identification with his fellow men, and the inevitable symbolic difference or inequality not only between himself and others, but also between himself and himself. When the subject acknowledges all this, his frustration may result in an aggressivity whose force can only come from the impulsive anti-structural violence aimed at recovering the real being.

Exclusion of the real surplus-enjoyment and assimilation of a symbolic surplus value

We may draw a distinction between the *automatic structural violence*, which is inherent in the symbolic opposition and inequality (S1–S2), and *impulsive anti-structural violence* ($◊*a*), which may develop into the aggressiveness resulting from a frustrated imaginary identification or equalization [*ego* | i(*a*)]. This distinction may conceivably not be unrelated to the sociological distinction, in social conflict, between the two sides of 'inequality' and 'difference' (Touraine, 1993, pp. 24–27), 'discrimination' and 'segregation' (Wieviorka, 1991, pp. 107–142), 'assimilation' and 'exclusion', modern 'universalist' social struggle and 'traditional ethnic' confrontation (Taguieff, 1987, pp. 393–410). To be sure, the structural violence within the symbolic universe can be distinguished from the anti-structural violence that comes from outside this universe. A revolution inside a civilization cannot be compared to a clash of civilizations. The castes war in Chiapas is not the same thing as the class struggle in Mexico. In any case, the two distinguished poles seem to be mutually dependent. In Mexico, for instance, we exclude Indians as Indians (*a*) with the intention of assimilating them as slave workers (S2/*a*). We reduce them to 'dregs of the human race' with the purpose of 'recycling' them as 'industrial scraps' (Rouzel, 2003). By marginalizing them from the enjoyment of the wealth they generate, we keep them from recovering this wealth, so that we can obtain the wealth they generate for us, here in the centre of modernity, which becomes the centre precisely because of the wealth that we obtain from the margins.[15] Even if we cannot really *enjoy* this wealth that we *obtain*, we deprive the others of its enjoyment (*a*) with the purpose of exploiting them ($) by transforming the enjoyable real being of their workforce ($◊*a*) into the literal support of our symbolic being ($\S1–S2/*a*). This also applies to the relation between developed and underdeveloped countries. In general, by segregating the real being of other subjects (*a*), that which remains of them ($) can be discriminated as inferior or underdeveloped and thereby used as a cheap proletarianized workforce in our developed symbolic system ($\S1–S2).[16]

Exploitation of the proletarianized workforce ($) in the system ($\S1–S2)	Marginalization from the enjoyment (*a*) of the system (S1–S2/*a*)
Assimilation of a symbolic surplus value	Exclusion of the real surplus-enjoyment
Discrimination of the subject as inferior or underdeveloped	Segregation of the real being of the subject
Structural violence	Anti-structural violence

Between marginalization and exploitation, there is not a mutual exclusion, but a dependence of the latter on the former. In this dependence, the marginalization of the other from the real enjoyment of the symbolic system enables the exploitation of the other in the same system. In other words, the exclusion or production of the real surplus-enjoyment of the other permits the assimilation or generation of a symbolic surplus value for us. In this exclusion, contrary to widespread opinion, we do not exclude the other with his enjoyment, but we exclude his enjoyment (/*a*) in order to assimilate and exploit his workforce ($) in our system ($\S1→S2). It does not matter that we also have to renounce the enjoyment of his work. What really matters is that we use his workforce for the work of our symbolic system. The fact is that we 'do not let the Other' preserve his symbolic system or 'way of enjoyment', but we 'impose' on him our own system, in which we can treat him as 'underdeveloped' (Lacan, 1973a, p. 534). Then, as underdeveloped, he can function as an inexpensive supplementary enunciating workforce ($) for our expensive enunciated discourses ($\S1–S2). He can thus generate a predicative surplus value (S2) that prevents these discourses from becoming poorly tautological (S1–S1). All of this can be illustrated by considering the luxury of the words I am writing, and their conditioning, not only by my workforce used here in Europe, but also by the low-cost workforces exploited in Asian factories or African mines.

Notes

1. In the terms of Branney (2008), 'we are symbolic beings who draw upon language to understand our world and ourselves, which means that self-knowledge is always socially mediated and full self-consciousness is impossible' (p. 585).

2. Here is the threshold where begins the field of social psychology. As the symbolic universe of the signifying 'socio-economic structure', this field is also that of Lacanian Discourse Analysis, whose position, Lacan's position, is diametrically opposed to any kind of 'instinctivist theory', 'biological model', or 'metaphysical illusion of a *human nature*' (cf. Pichon-Rivière & Quiroga, 1972).
3. This is what permits Georgaca (2003) to properly appreciate 'Lacanian theory as a view of subjectivity that respects its social and linguistic properties' (p. 542). In this *view of subjectivity*, 'the psyche is made of the same material as that of the social world, the material of the signifier' (ibid.). This remark is true and crucial. We must face the *fact* of a signifierization that also involves a socialization and externalization of everything in our symbolic universe. However, in my opinion, this *fact* does not necessarily imply a 'collapse' of 'the distinction between the individual and the social, the internal and the external' (ibid.). Instead of a collapse, I would rather see here a redistribution of the places. As a being inherent in the 'Other of language' (ibid.), the speech-being stays in an exterior structure that is essentially social in itself and even in its particularization for each individual position. As for the imaginary being as a 'reflection of the other' (ibid.), it still resides in the conjectural interiority of cognitive psychology. Finally, this imagined individual interiority must not be confused with the real individual interiority of the 'Other's object' (ibid.). If we do not want to contribute to the generalized conceptual impoverishment of psychology, we should not 'refuse' oppositions such as the ones between 'exteriority and interiority', society and individuality, or 'objectivity and subjectivity' (cf. Dunker & Parker, 2009). Rather than refuse these oppositions, we need to use them in a new way. After all, we are already doing this when we consider such monstrous things as an exterior unconscious, a divided individual subject, or an object as the real being of the subject.
4. As demonstrated by the difference (*a*) between the enunciated words (S1–S2) and the enunciating acts ($\S1–S2) of hoteliers towards Oriental people, in the classical experiment of LaPiere (1934), the real being of the enunciating act is 'a great deal more than a series of words' (p. 101). The real surplus (*a*) is *more* than the discursive statement, which does not necessarily mean that it involves a cognitive attitude. The mental existence of this attitude is purely conjectural and questionable, while the real being of the enunciating act can be easily confirmed.
5. Therefore, despite its purely symbolic discursive character, the One of the master-being-signifier might function as a 'core of personal

identity' that would give us 'a sense of a unified, trans-situational personal identity' when crossing the exterior speech-beings of the Other (cf. Hitlin, 2003, pp. 121–122).

6. In consequence, as Hook (2003) remarks, the 'unfathomable figure' (p. 2) of the real body constitutes a 'problem to representation' (p. 1). It exists as 'an absolute rival to representation' (p. 27). It 'shatters meaning and destroys representability' (p. 23). It offers 'resistance to any form of symbolic mediation or representation' (p. 20).
7. This is how we may explain, in a Lacanian perspective, the 'exclusion' inherent in 'the symbolic', that 'actively rejects what cannot be borne, what stands outside language as its radical other' (Frosh, 2007, p. 641). From our viewpoint, this *radical other* cannot be borne by language precisely because it has to *bear* language. Once it bears language, of course, the real being is not the *radical other* any more. The structure is no longer its real emptiness. Nevertheless, it is a transformation of this emptiness, which coagulates in the form of the signifying social structure.
8. Here is our negative explanation of some kind of 'pleasure' that we may still regard, together with Frosh (2002), as a 'realm' in which 'psychoanalytic thinking of a non-discursive reduced kind might have something to offer' to social psychology (p. 191). Like Frosh, we are convinced that an abstract discursive psychology is exceeded by 'this astonishing psychic energy' (pp. 192–193).
9. Hélène Chauchat (1999) rightly notes, in her social psychological theory of subjective identity, that 'what is not named, spoken, taken in the symbolic', may still 'exist precisely because of the fact of not being taken', and 'it may eventually appear in another form, such as violence' (p. 17).
10. Therefore, as Frosh (2002) notices, 'avoiding words—staying outside discourse—can be driven by something that, for want of a better term, one might call *emotion*, fuelled by the (possibly non-cognitive, even non-discursive) understanding that words would not do justice to the fullness of the experience' (p. 191). The silence thus functions as *the only alternative* to 'multiple possible discourses on anything and everything' (ibid.). In these discourses, 'whenever something precious is put into words, some other aspect is lost' (ibid.). This *lost aspect* is not unrelated to the Lacanian object *a*. To preserve this real being of the enunciating act, we must certainly not put it into the enunciated fact.
11. It is 'as if our reflexive power can flourish only insofar as it draws its strength and relies on some minimal *prereflexive* substantial support that eludes its grasp, so that its universalization comes at

the price of its inefficiency, that is, by the paradoxical re-emergence of the brute real of *irrational* violence, impermeable and insensitive to reflexive interpretation' (Žižek, 2006).

12. Hobbes (1651) was not wrong when he remarked that 'without' language, 'there had been amongst men, neither Common-wealth, nor society, nor Contract, nor Peace, no more than amongst Lyons, Bears, and Wolves' (I, §4, p. 24). The fact remains that man is still a wolf for man. However, thanks to the signifier, man's violence is not identical to wolf's violence. It may be worse, of course, but it is not identical. Unlike animal violence, human violence cannot be completely independent from the signifier.
13. Here is a radicalization and inversion of the idea that 'the unconscious is both generated by this struggle and generative of its consequences' (Frosh, Phoenix & Pattman, 2003, p. 42). If the unconscious is generative of the struggle's consequences, it is because the unconscious includes the struggle as the cause generative of its own consequences. In the Lacanian perspective, the unconscious is not only a mediation between the cause and its consequences, but it embraces the cause, as well as the consequences, which cannot be more conscious than the struggle that causes them.
14. In this sphere, which concerns cognitive social psychology, the aggressiveness can thus be justified by a 'feeling of suffered injustice' that has an 'influence' on 'beliefs about the legitimacy of violence and aggressive behaviours' (Goutas, Girandola & Minary, 2003, p. 141). If beliefs and behaviours are influenced by the feeling of injustice, this feeling seems to be determined by the contrast between an imaginary equalization and a symbolic inequality. Fortunately, this inequality would intrinsically imply a *violent potential* that can produce any kind of struggle, including class struggles, without ingenuous dreams of equality, vain feelings of injustice, and hazardous episodes of clumsy aggressiveness.
15. Therefore, in general, 'the central subjects of modernity cannot be understood outside their dialectical link to the marginal(-ized) subjects of modernity' (Hayes, 2003).
16. The question is not whether 'the other possesses the object-treasure, having snatched it away from us (which is why we do not have it), or he poses a threat to our possession of the object' (cf. Žižek, 2006). In his 'privileged relationship to the object' (ibid.), the other is marginalized from his real being as an object (*a*) because this real being *poses a threat to our possession* and exploitation of the subject ($). Actually, we possess the subject, but nobody possesses the object. Even if we snatch the object away from the subject, we cannot possess the object, which is necessarily missing.

CHAPTER TEN

The interpretation of wisdom

This last chapter deals with the problem of the scope for interpretation. In line with Lacan, I maintain that interpretative means and results must always be related to both the symbolic sphere of analyzable discursive data and the real material of corporeal or literal signifiers. I also explain why interpretation, from a Lacanian point of view, should not make sense, but should rather look for the nonsensical, the enigmatic, the unbelievable and the incomprehensible. As we will see, this Lacanian psychoanalytical idea of interpretation is diametrically opposed to a Ricœurian hermeneutic reading of text.

Observable signifiers without a comprehensible signification

When we analyze a discourse, we must be aware that it is not only conditioned by the *individual expressing workforce* of the one who states it, but also by the *collective sustaining workforce* of those who create the conditions for his expression. Now, besides these *real workforces*, the discourse primarily arises from the *symbolic system* whose work uses the workforces in order to articulate the discourse. In fact, the analyzed discourse *is* the discourse of this system. It is the discourse of this Other, of this signifying social structure, of this *articulating and repressing language*. Therefore, in relation to its *expressing subject*, the analyzed discourse may be described as *the unconscious*.

In a Lacanian Discourse Analysis, we must deal with the unconscious. Even when we dare to interpret what we analyze, we must carefully tackle unconscious words without a conscious meaning, perceptible discourses without an intelligible cognition, observable signifiers without a comprehensible signification. As an alternative to the 'understanding' of the 'signification', our 'interpretation' must proceed through 'the handling of the signifier' (Lacan, 1957–1958, 11.06.58, p. 444). Therefore, it must avoid any kind of 'significative' or 'comprehensive intervention' (ibid.). It must not try to comprehend. In 'a reversal' of the 'ordinary sense' of the word 'interpretation', the Lacanian 'analytical interpretation' is diametrically opposed to a supposed comprehension of the analyzed discourse (1969–1970, 26.11.69, pp. 15–17). When we interpret, we must concentrate on the words, as perceptible symbolic representatives, and not on an understandable meaning that is nothing more than its own intelligible imaginary representation.

The understanding is an understanding of the imaginary. When we 'understand' a 'word', there is a sort of 'image' that 'enters our head' (Wittgenstein, 1949, §139, p. 93). However, given that the material word remains outside our head, the ideal image seems to be the only understood thing. It is actually the only understandable thing. Somehow or other we understand an image. We do not know what this image is exactly, of course, but we know that it is something imaginary. We recognize that it is something merely internal, intelligible and imperceptible. In view of the fact that we cannot externalize the image in a perceptible form, we must also grant that it is an unapproachable thing. Funnily enough, this *indemonstrable thing* is the only *understandable thing*. When we understand, we imagine this imaginary thing and not the material word itself, the demonstrable symbolic thing, which is perceived, of course, but cannot really be imagined, comprehended or comprehensibly interpreted.

Between the incomprehensible 'symbolic' and a comprehensive 'interpretation', there is a *mutual exclusion* and not a mutual 'solidarity' (cf. Todorov, 1978, p. 18). Now, in a Lacanian Discourse Analysis, our interpretation must be focused on the symbolic. For this reason, our interpretation cannot be a comprehensive interpretation.

When we interpret "the foundation of the monogamous family", for example, we may ask ourselves what this "foundation" *consists of* and *involves* (such as "love" and "our time"), but we must not wonder what the "foundation" *means* (such as a romantic belief or an idealistic representation of the family). Instead of understanding a meaning, we must interpret the words of discourse. We must construe the discursive construction of interwoven words, but we are not supposed to erect our own cognitive construction composed of the associated mental meanings that we assign to the words.[1]

In a Lacanian interpretation, we are not expected to add an interpretative cognitive construction to the interpreted discursive construction. Nevertheless, on the basis of our analysis, we may interpret the discursive construction built of the analyzed literal words. Since these real 'building materials are not the building itself' (Stalin, 1950a, p. 167), we may piece together the building, or the symbolic system, by inferring the symbolic values of the analyzed literal supports. Thus, by situating these words in their structural positions, we may reconstruct the structure. We may reconstruct Francisco Javier's discursive building, for instance, by locating the lower "individual sexual love" of "our time" in relation to the upper "construction of the new society and the new man", the former as "the foundation of the monogamous family" and the latter as that which is sustained by the "family" as a "fundamental pillar", so that *the novelty of man and society* rests on *the monogamy of the familiar pillar* that rests in turn on *the individuality of current sexual love*. In this quick outline of interpretation, we do not understand a cognitive content, but we simply have another look at the analyzed discursive containing form of the structure. This structure is not only assessed through its literal elements, but is totally reassessed through their structural relations, in this case from an altered viewpoint that imposes a substance on the adjectives. Thus, after the analytical decomposition of the adjectives, there is a synthetic recomposition or reconfiguration of their structure. But *the* structure is always here, at hand, under our regard. We do not need to understand it in order to perceive it in a new way. At least at this first stage, our interpretation is just an experimental observation. It is not a speculation. It is not even open to discussion. There is nothing essentially questionable about it. Unlike comprehension, our interpretation is not intrinsically debatable.

Lacanian psychoanalytic explanation and Ricœurian hermeneutic comprehension

As an 'interpretation' that involves 'comprehension', the comprehensive interpretation is intrinsically debatable (Lacan, 1966b, p. 211). We can always debate it, given that 'any comprehension is also a non-comprehension', and 'any convergence between thoughts and feelings is at the same time a divergence' (Humboldt, 1834, §14, p. 203). Put differently, any analogical similarity between images is at the same time a dissimilarity that involves discrete differences besides identities. This is why comprehension is also non-comprehension. It is only an apparent understanding because its likelihood only depends on the likeness of the imaginary similarity.

Of course, when I understand the meaning of "love" in Francisco Javier's discourse, the imaginary content of my understanding is based on the symbolic value of the word "love", so it may be similar or equivalent to the image of love that crossed the mind of the Eperrist while he expressed his discourse. However, as discussed in the first chapter, this similarity or equivalence is not the same thing as an identity. At the heart of our Lacanian interpretation, the discrete symbolic identity can only be regarded as itself ("love" = "love"), while the analogical imaginary similarity of comprehensive interpretation (love ú omanticism) can be also regarded as a dissimilarity, since it implies a discrete difference ("love" ≅ "romanticism").

When we understand a discourse, the content of our understanding implies a difference from the understood discourse. If we reduce the imaginary content of the understanding to its symbolic substratum, we may see that the difference in question lies fundamentally in a signifier. Comprehension adds a signifier that was not included in the comprehended discourse.

When I interpret "love" as "romanticism", my comprehensive interpretation adds "romanticism" to "love" and implies a difference between the interpreted "love" and the comprehended "romanticism". In my comprehension, "love" and "romanticism" may be the same, of course. However, this comprehended sameness is not inherent in the interpreted discourse, but in my interpreting discourse. The identity has nothing to do with Francisco Javier, but it belongs to my comprehension of his discourse, and even to my personal beliefs or pre-comprehensions, as I do not need Francisco Javier to identify "love" and "romanticism". This can be illustrated by considering the exemplary comprehensive interpretation of Ricœurian hermeneutics, in which 'comprehension' must be preceded by 'belief' and 'pre-comprehension' (Ricœur, 1960, pp. 481–488).

By recognizing the necessity of belief and pre-comprehension, Ricœur acknowledges that his comprehensive interpretation depends on faith, preconception and predisposition, bias and prejudice. In this way, Ricœur frankly admits his 'ties with obscurantism' (Lacan, 1966b, p. 210), which can be judged as proof of 'honesty' (Ricœur, 1960, p. 488), but also as evidence of 'obscenity' (Lacan, 1967g, p. 335). In any case, the French philosopher does not hesitate to advocate a 'post-critique faith' and a 'second naïveté' (Ricœur, 1965, p. 37). In this conscious and calculated reaction or regression, one would rationally decide to be naïve by having every faith in one's comprehension.[2] Now, besides *comprehension*, this *faith in comprehension* is the only reason for comprehension, as any 'comprehension' depends only on itself and on this 'faith' (1960, pp. 481–488; 1965, pp. 36–37). This faith creates, sustains and justifies the comprehension itself. Naturally, when we interpret a discourse, we only have to be naïve in order to reach the comprehension that confirms our naïveté. But this phenomenon of autosuggestion has nothing to do with the interpreted discourse. It happens outside discourse, between ourselves and our image in the mirror, in our heart and mind, or, more precisely, in our faith and naïveté.

Knowingly supported by the extra-discursive faith and naïveté of the one who interprets a discourse, the comprehensive hermeneutic interpretation is deliberately positioned in the imaginary space of the mirror. Absorbed by this space, the Ricœurian interpretation is diametrically opposed to the Lacanian one, which can only be absorbed by the real emptiness of the symbolic.[3] This diametrical opposition has been clearly established by Ricœur (1965) and by Lacan (1975–1976):

- From the 'pre-comprehension' and through the faith in 'comprehension', the Ricœurian interpretation leads to an 'emergence of the possible', a 'restoration of sense' and a 'grace of imagination' (Ricœur, 1965, pp. 36–44). In this way, it chooses the 'imaginary' or 'what makes sense' (Lacan, 1975–1976, 13.04.76, p. 131). Its choice is the 'mystification' by the 'illusions and lies of consciousness' (cf. Ricœur, 1965, p. 40).

- From the absence of pre-comprehension and through the 'exercise of suspicion' about 'comprehension', the Lacanian interpretation leads to an 'asceticism of the necessary', a restoration of nonsense and a 'discipline of the real' (Ricœur, 1965, pp. 40–44). In this manner, it decides on the 'real' as 'different' from the 'field of sense' (Lacan, 1975–1976, 13.04.76, p. 134). Its decision is in favour of 'demystification' as the 'elimination of the illusions and lies of consciousness' (Ricœur, 1965, pp. 35–40).

Ricœurian hermeneutic interpretation	*Lacanian psychoanalytic interpretation*
Mystification (imaginary)	Demystification (real)
Faith and grace (possibility)	Suspicion and discipline (necessity)
Comprehension (seizing)	Explanation (unfolding)

The distinction between the comprehensive hermeneutic interpretation and the non-comprehensive psychoanalytic interpretation may be synthetically described as an opposition between mystification and demystification, grace and discipline, possibility and necessity, faith and suspicion in relation to comprehension. Actually, in the Lacanian psychoanalytic interpretation, we give up the idea of comprehending. Nevertheless, in compensation, we may take up the idea of explaining. We may propose an 'explanation' of what we analyze (Lacan, 1962–1963, 12.06.63, pp. 323–336). We may 'explain' what we 'do not understand' (1972–1973, 09.01.73, p. 46). Our *interpretation* may be an *explanation* (from the Latin *explicare*, to unfold). But this timid *explanation* has nothing to do with confident *comprehension* (from *comprehendere*, to grasp). The explanation remains respectfully distant, outlying, in the exterior of the explained discourse. Instead, comprehension pretends to go through the discourse, make a way into what it would mean, break into the consciousness of the speaker and take hold of its content. The supposed comprehension of our fellow men is always disrespectful and impertinent, intrusive and invasive, avid and grasping, voracious and even gluttonous. Fortunately, this comprehension is merely imaginary. The imaginary 'understanding' always amounts to a real 'misunderstanding' (Miller, 1995, p. 9). We cannot really understand our fellow men. The assumption of this impossibility of a real 'understanding' or 'comprehension' is precisely what leads us to make an effort towards 'explanation' (Lacan, 1972–1973, 09.01.73, pp. 45–46). Thus, in a Lacanian psychoanalytic interpretation, we engage in a symbolic explanation precisely because we recognize the merely imaginary character of comprehension.[4]

Unlike comprehension, the explanation does not pretend to *know* what is *expressed* by the interpreted discourse. The explanation does not refer to a knowable and expressible reality, but it refers to the real signifying structure that 'carves out' this 'reality' (Lacan, 1967a, pp. 352–353). This structure is that which must be explained in a Lacanian interpretation. As part of the signifying social structure in itself, the explained structure exists for the one who expresses the discourse and not only for the one who interprets it. Nevertheless, as discussed many times before, the structure in itself does not exist in the same way for both of them. The explained structure is not the same for the position of the one as it is for the position of the other. The same language is not the same for me and for Francisco Javier. Its code is not the same. When I interpret Francisco Javier's discourse, as Badiou would notice, I interpret a 'text' that 'bears its own specific code' and is then 'radically singular' (Badiou & Foucault, 1965, p. 472). Since I could never be in the structural position of the Eperrist, I could never know the structure for his position, the 'code' of *his* 'message', the language of *his* discourse, *his* language, his exteriority, his 'unconscious' (pp. 470–472).

Despite Foucault, the 'message' does not provide us with its 'code' (Badiou & Foucault, 1965, pp. 470–471). Francisco Javier's 'unconscious' does not offer me its 'key' (ibid.). This is why I cannot *seize* or understand anything in it. From the outside of its interiority, I cannot be conscious of anything in it. I can only explain or unfold its exterior structure. But this explanation proves to be just *my* explanation of *the* structure. Since I cannot even know the structure for Francisco Javier's position, my explanation simply interprets the structure for my position. Unlike the imaginary comprehension, this subjective explanation does not pretend to objectively grasp a meaning or penetrate the reality of the Eperrist. The Lacanian explanation does not refer to the 'signified' and does not 'fill an objective function of deciphering' (cf. Barthes, 1964, p. 80). Instead, it fills a subjective function or re-ciphering. It is not a 'deciphering', but rather a re-ciphering that results from a 'decryption of a text whose key is not available' (Badiou & Foucault, 1965, p. 470).

Given that the key of the interpreted discourse is not available, we cannot understand its 'meaning': that is something kept locked away, 'something private, something elusive that we can only compare with the consciousness' of the subject who expresses the discourse (Wittgenstein, 1949, §358, p. 167). Now, in a Lacanian interpretation, we are not interested in this consciousness, but in the unconscious. Therefore, we may confine our interpretation to the exteriority of the signifying social structure, as the public locus of speech, instead of trying to break into the private mental interiority of the subject who expresses the interpreted discourse. As this interiority is concealed, we cannot know the meaning of the words for the subject. We have to ignore what the 'subject' would virtually 'mean' or '*want to say*' (Lacan, 1955–1956, 23.11.55, p. 31). Just like our analysis, our interpretation must be confined to that which is actually '*said*' or '*not said*' in discourse (ibid.).[5]

In a Lacanian interpretation, we must not imagine understanding what the subject would mean, or *would want to say*, in what he says or does not say. We must not know our own imaginary reality by imagining that we know an unknowable reality behind the interpreted discourse. We must not rush at ourselves by rushing towards an understanding that escapes us. We must be aware that 'it is always at the point where we have understood, where we have rushed in to fill the case up with understanding, that we have missed the interpretation that it is appropriate to make or not make' (Lacan, 1955–1956, 23.11.55, p. 31). In truth, as Lacan notes, we never 'know' in retrospect 'what the subject meant' or 'wanted to say' (*a voulu dire*), but we 'know' only 'that he did not say it' (ibid.). We only know that the supposed meaning *of* discourse has not been enunciated *as* discourse. Amazingly, what we understand (the meaning) is precisely that which is not present in what we pretend to understand (the discourse). In actual fact, the supposed signification of a discourse is nothing but a signifier, of course, but a signifier that cannot be present among the signifiers of the interpreted discourse.

From this peculiar point of view, what a subject means or wants to say can only be that which is not said.[6]

Since we know perfectly what is *said* and *not said*, why should we be interested in what the subject *means* or *wants to say* in what he says? Perhaps because 'that which means something is less dangerous' (Barthes, 1957, p. 88). Or perhaps because we want to say in a roundabout way, through our fellow men, that which we do not want to say in a direct way. In any case, *anybody may want to say what we want him to want to say*. All things and persons can be understood as we understand them. Hence the necessity of our 'discipline' (Lacan, 1958d, p. 71), our 'asceticism' (1965a, p. 199), and our 'ascetic' principle that obliges us to limit our 'interpretation' to what is strictly 'necessary' (cf. Ricoeur, 1965, p. 45). In our Lacanian perspective, we must interpret with this principle in mind.[7] On this principle, Lacan criticizes Glover, who 'finds interpretation everywhere, being unable to set any limits to it' (Lacan, 1958d, p. 70). Without any limits, the interpretation 'becomes a sort of phlogiston' (ibid.). It discovers fire in all places. It finds what it looks for everywhere. It comes across the same image in all mirrors. According to Lacan, this comprehensive interpretation 'is manifest in everything that is understood rightly or wrongly, as long as it feeds the flame of the imaginary' (ibid.).

The renunciation of the imaginary flame does not darken our interpretation. When we renounce this flame, we may still work in the light of the interpreted discourse. By the way, this discourse is the only combustible that feeds the imaginary flame. As for understanding, it consists of nothing more than this flame, so it is caused entirely by the combustion of discourse. As Hobbes (1651) observes, 'understanding is nothing else, but conception caused by speech' (I, §4, p. 30). Similarly, from our viewpoint, understanding is nothing but an imaginary cognition determined by the symbolic system of discourse. As a symbolic universe, this system is a universal human environment that surrounds and nourishes the imaginary flames of all of our understandings. These 'imaginary' segments of 'understanding' are thus 'included' in the 'symbolic' sphere of discourse (Lacan, J. 1955–1956, 16.11.55, p. 17). Therefore, when we confine our interpretation to discourse, the imaginary reality of understanding may be legitimately reduced to its truth as an 'element of the symbolic code' (1958b, p. 168). Besides being legitimate, this reduction is advisable, as it makes it possible for us to neutralize, at least to some extent, the imaginary functioning of understanding as a conscious 'screen whose filter impedes the communication of the unconscious message' (ibid.).

Introducing a signifier of an unconscious psychic language and attributing a concept of a conscious psychological metalanguage

While avoiding any kind of comprehension, we may enrich our Lacanian explanation with the open and explicit 'introduction' of signifiers into the interpreted discourse (Lacan, 1957–1958, 11.06.58, p. 444). But the 'introduced' signifiers 'must be allowed by the function of the Other in the possession of the code' (Lacan, 1958d, p. 70). This does not mean that we must have a *conscious knowledge* of the code. However, in our place, the Other must *possess the code.* The signifying social structure must have an *unconscious wisdom* of a code that would enable our introduction of the signifier into the interpreted discourse. When we introduce the signifier "counter-revolution" into Francisco Javier's discourse, for example, our introduction must be permitted by the unconscious wisdom of the structure in which the "new society" of our "revolution" is opposed to "our time" as the time of the "counter-revolution". Once allowed by the structure, our explanatory signifier may be 'introduced into the synchrony of signifiers that come together' (ibid.). The "counter-revolutionary" may thus be included among "our time", the "revolutionary", and the "new society". In this synchrony, our signifier 'makes translation possible' (ibid.). It 'deciphers' for our position the 'diachrony' of the interpreted discourse (ibid.). It may even 'deliver' a 'signified effect' (Miller, 1995, p. 9). It may thus cause the 'advent of the signified' (Lacan, 1958d, p. 71).

Before deciphering and creating an imaginary signified effect, the introduced signifier *re-ciphers* and has a symbolic signifying effect. Put differently, the interpretative introduction of the explanatory signifier has an effect of signifierization on the interpreted discourse. Unlike the secondary conscious effect of signification, this primary unconscious effect of signifierization does not *reproduce a reality* (*réalité*). Nevertheless, it may *produce a truth* (*vérité*). It may have an 'effect of truth' (Lacan, 1970–1971, 13.01.71, p. 14). Actually, by means of the signifierization inherent in the introduction of a signifier, the Lacanian 'interpretation' must aim at 'provoking the truth' (p. 13). It must frankly aim at reaching its own retroactive substantiation, or *verification*, by which the truth (*veritas*) is made (*facere*) by its own consequences.

When I interpret Francisco Javier's discourse, my interpretation cannot yet be true, but it can only become true in the future, in a retroactive way and by its own consequences. These unpredictable consequences may arise in different discursive domains, for example in the interpreted signifiers, whose destiny may be positively transformed by the introduction of *my* signifiers, or in the next words of the Eperrist, who may fruitfully react against an undeserved interpretation, or even in my own work or in the work of my colleagues, which may be productively affected by the hypothetical subversive character of my interpretative method. In any case, the truth of the interpretation resides in its unforeseeable outcome and not in its correspondence with an existent reality. Therefore, when I introduce the signifier "counter-revolutionary", my interpretation may *become* true even if it *is* wrong or inexact in relation to an evidently "consistent revolutionary".[8] Now, for my interpretation to become true, I do not need Francisco Javier to turn into a "counter-revolutionary" or an "inconsistent revolutionary", which seems rather unlikely. To be sure, my interpretation will not be corroborated by a future predictable correspondence (*adequatio*) with a well-known reality, but by a future unpredictable revelation of a still unknown truth (*aletheia*). This truth of my interpretation will not be the "counter-revolutionary" itself, of course, but something in relation to it, and then 'different' than it, and also in 'contradiction' with it (Mao Zedong, 1937, II, p. 60).

Paradoxically, the truth of my interpretation will corroborate my interpretation by contradicting it. Providentially, for the time being, I cannot yet know this truth. I cannot even know if it exists. The truth cannot be retrospectively demonstrated at the moment, but it has to be retroactively established afterwards. Therefore, the truth of my interpretation is somewhere in the future. It cannot exist yet, since my interpretation works precisely with the aim of making it exist in the future. Just as for the Marxian and Marxist interpretations, my Freudian-Lacanian interpretation is thus future-oriented. It treats 'time' as 'a vehicle (*vecteur*) for novelty' (Soler, 2008). It is a *committed interpretation* that tries to 'produce something new' (Lacan, 1958d, p. 71), which may only be the subversive 'truth', as 'that which is always new' (1946, p. 192).

Centred on the novelty of the truth, our future-oriented Freudian-Lacanian interpretation is not really 'turned towards the resurgence of archaic meanings' (cf. Ricœur, 1965, pp. 478–479). Nor is it blocked by the 'regression towards the key-signifiers of the unconscious' (ibid.). Instead, in this unconscious, our interpretation really tends 'towards the emergence of anticipatory figures of our spiritual adventure' (ibid.). Although founded on the past of the interpreted discourse, our interpretation must be turned towards the future advent of its own truth.[9]

Our Lacanian interpretation must be focused on its verification. Now, as a *revelation of an unknown truth*, this verification must not be confused with a *confirmation of known wisdom*, such as that of the 'psychological hypothesis (*hypothèse*)', which Lacan (1965a) describes as a 'mortgage (*hypothèque*) raised by the wisdom-being on the truth-being' (p. 199). Mortgaging the future, the predictable wisdom-being of the hypothesis mortgages an unpredictable truth-being that can only *be* in the future. In other words, the psychological hypothesis functions as wisdom (S1–S2) that prevents its own subversion by exorcizing the unforeseeable novelty of the truth ($\S1–S2). On the contrary, our Lacanian interpretation must be open to this 'truth' and its subversion of 'wisdom' (1970a, pp. 442–443). If this 'wisdom' is 'added to the real' (ibid.), the signifier introduced by our interpretation is 'added' to 'wisdom' (1969–1970, 11.03.70, p. 130) with the aim of revealing the 'truth' *in which* 'wisdom' is affected by the 'real' (1970a, pp. 442–443).

Affected by the real, the 'wisdom' suffers the 'symptom' of the 'truth' (Lacan, 1970a, p. 443). Now, unlike the wisdom itself, the truth does not reside in the enunciated fact, but in a symptomatic gap in the fact. This gap *discloses* the truth of the enunciating act. This is why it concerns a Lacanian interpretation principally concerned with the truth. When I interpret Francisco Javier's discourse by introducing the signifier of the "counter-revolutionary", I am trying to open or clear the gap from which I expect the truth to appear in the wisdom of the structure. If my interpretation proved to be pertinent, the gap would reveal the truth of the proletarianized expressing real subject whose workforce is exploited by the articulating work of the symbolic system. This revelation might take many different forms, such as a symptomatic reaction or retraction of Francisco Javier, a dreamlike assumption of his contradictions, or a Freudian slip or lapse in the evolution of his discourse. The revelation might also occur far away from the Eperrist, for example in a nonsensical turn of my interpretation, or in the subversive incomprehension of my colleagues. In any case, the emergence of the revealed truth has nothing to do with a correspondence between a veiling reality and a psychological hypothesis. Verification through an interpretative signifier such as "inconsistent" is not the same thing as a confirmation of a statement such as "a revolutionary is inconsistent". The former can be accomplished by a "consistent revolutionary" and by anybody else, while the latter necessitates the presence of the supposed reality denoted by the expression "inconsistent revolutionary".

The verification through our interpretative signifier concerns the conflicting relationship between the subject and the signifier, while the confirmation of the hypothetical statement refers to the conciliatory relationship between the hypothesis and its reality, the statement and its meaning, the signifier and its signification. In order to confirm the hypothetical existence of the *inconsistent revolutionary*, we would have to find him somewhere in reality. To find him, we would need to understand who he is and what he looks like. We would need to have a comprehensive idea of his *inconsistency*, for example in terms of *incongruity, absurdity, irrationality, irregularity, volatility, changeability*, etc. We would also need to have an idea of the exact opposite, that is to say, the "consistent revolutionary" interpreted in Francisco Javier's discourse. In this case, our comprehension might include *rationality, regularity, stability, reliability*, and many other things. Unfortunately, all these *things* are nothing more than *words*. They are words taken for meanings. More precisely, they are symbols taken for the reality of the "consistent revolutionary". Likewise, at the root of a psychological hypothesis, there is always a comprehensive interpretation that uses a number of signifiers as if they were the things signified by the interpreted signifiers.

Besides introducing the signifier of the hypothetical statement ("inconsistency"), the comprehensive psychological interpretation surreptitiously introduces many other signifiers (e.g., "incongruity" or "stability") that are treated as realities of a *psychological metalanguage*. Instead, a Lacanian interpretation openly introduces signifiers that are treated as pure signifiers, simple words, and constituent elements of a *psychic language* whose symbolic universe excludes the existence of any kind of psychological metalanguage. Since we cannot leave this exteriority of the structure that we partly share with Francisco Javier, we cannot offer a Lacanian psychological conscious metalanguage composed of realities that would be signified by the psychic unconscious language that articulates the discourse of the Eperrist.

Even when we speak in Lacanese, our language must not claim to be a conscious metalanguage that interprets the unconscious language, but it must accept itself as an unconscious language that is always interpreting itself.[10] Whether as the structure in itself or as the structure for my structural position, this language is the only one at my disposal. From the only viewpoint of my individual position, this language embraces both my interpreting discourse and the interpreted discourse. Actually, when I interpret, it is this language that interprets itself in my place. By interpreting, we do the work of the unconscious, a work of signifierization and re-signifierization. This work is the only one that we can do by interpreting. Our interpretation can only function as the work of an unconscious language that signifierizes or re-signifierizes itself in that which is interpreted. Accordingly, our interpretation cannot function as the work of a conscious metalanguage whose interpreting elements would be the things signified by the interpreted words. This signification is merely imaginary. With this signification, the interpretation cannot be true. To be true and 'reach the real', an interpretation must 'lose its signification' (Lacan, 1972a, p. 487).

The Lacanian interpretation is not supposed to provide the signification of the interpreted discourse. When we bring in the signifier "inconsistency", this is just a signifier *introduced* into Francisco Javier's consistent discourse and not a signification *attributed* to this discourse. Actually, the "inconsistency" does not have a real signification in itself, but only a *symbolic value*, a sense that arises from its opposition to the sense of the "consistency" in the signifying structure. Generating sense, this opposition of sense can be also observed between the "revolutionary" and our "counter-revolutionary", or between the "conviction" and our "obligation". As evidenced by these oppositions, 'the sense arises from the translation of one discourse to another' (Lacan, 1972a, p. 480). It arises from the crossing of the gulf between the structure for the structural position of Francisco Javier and the structure for my position. The fact remains that both structures are the same structure from the viewpoint of my position. They are also the same structure in itself. In either case, both languages are simultaneously the same language. Their respective discourses belong to the same language. From this angle, the sense results from a movement inside language. By contrast, the meaning results from a supposed movement outside language, in an imaginary conscious metalanguage that apparently provides the signification of the signifiers that compose the unconscious language. But this meaning or signification cannot be credited by Lacanian interpreters. Their 'interpretation' is not 'directed' at 'meaning' (1964, 27.05.64, p. 236). At the very most, their 'interpretation is of sense' (1972a, p. 480). But it 'goes against signification' (ibid.). Its regard for signifiers also involves a disregard for signification. It even entails an elimination of it.[11]

Unlike Lacanian interpreters, standard psychologists resolutely believe in signification. To interpret a signifier of the psychic language that surrounds them, they turn to the psychological metalanguage of their theory and they look there for an interpretative concept that supposedly corresponds to the interpreted signifier. Once they find their concept, they sincerely have the impression that 'the interpreted signifier found the signified that suits it' (Miller, 1995, p. 10). They may then 'abandon the original signifier' and keep only 'the new signifier', the one of their supposed metalanguage, which creates for them a 'positive effect of signification' (ibid.). In an interpretation of Francisco Javier's discourse, for instance, a psychologist might throw away the "significance of marriage" and simply retain an "attitude towards marriage". This "attitude" would function as the meaning or signification of the "significance". However, in reality, the "attitude" would be just another signifier surreptitiously introduced by the psychologist into the interpreted discourse.

Comprehensive psychological interpretation	*Lacanian psychoanalytical interpretation*
Imaginary signification	Real signifierization
Attributes a signified concept of a conscious psychological metalanguage	Introduces a signifying element of an unconscious psychic language

If the comprehensive psychological interpretation consisted only in introducing a new signifier into the interpreted discourse, then we might consider it identical to the Lacanian psychoanalytical interpretation. The difference lies in the fact that a Lacanian must know that he is only introducing a signifier of an unconscious psychic language, while a standard psychologist can take this signifier for a concept of a conscious psychological metalanguage whose concepts would be signified by the interpreted signifiers of the unconscious psychic language. Unlike that psychologist, the Lacanian must admit that his interpretative signifier does not give the signification of the interpreted signifier. He must also recognize that his interpretation is not a matter of *imaginary signification*, but a matter of *real signifierization*. He must finally confess that his interpreting work is not really *his*, given that it belongs to the Other, to a language, to a symbolic system, that interprets when the interpreter imagines that he interprets.

The interpreting work is the work of the symbolic system, the work of the unconscious, which uses the workforce of the real subject who carries out the interpretation. The Lacanian interpreter must be aware of this. He must acknowledge his proletarianized condition, as the enunciating workforce of language, which is the same condition of the real subject who expresses the interpreted discourse. When interpreting this discourse, the interpreter must realize that a symbolic system articulates the discourse as well as its interpretation. Actually, the articulating system expresses itself and interprets itself by exploiting consecutively the expressing workforce of one subject and the interpreting workforce of another subject. Therefore, when we interpret, our interpretation is totally determined by the signifying structure of the symbolic system. The interpretations of standard psychologists are also totally determined by the same structure, of course. However, psychologists are not aware of this, and they claim to speak from outside the structure, from the exterior of psychic language, from a neutral psychological metalanguage. Nevertheless, this claim is also determined by the structure, which needs it, just as it needs our complementary critique of it. In fact, the claim and its critique are as complementary as the speaker and the interpreter. This complementarity can be observed everywhere in the structure. Here, logically, everything has to be complementary. Different interpretations also have to be complementary. In spite of Ricœur, they 'do not give rise to conflict'

(Cléro, 2008, p. 151). Far from it, they 'complement one another' (Lacan, 1969–1970, 15.04.70, p. 157).

The imaginary reality of a meaningful content and the real emptiness of the signifying structure

Just like other pieces of the symbolic system, the different interpretations complement one another. After all, they can only be complementary, since they compose the same complete structure in itself. They *are* the same structure for diverse structural positions. They fill their particular functions in the same symbolic functioning. Now, in a Lacanian interpretation, we are not only interested in this symbolic functioning (S1→S2), but also in its real support ($) and its real product (*a*). However, unlike psychological imaginary concepts, these real things cannot be supposedly signified by the psychic signifiers of the symbolic functioning. Since they are real, they cannot compose an imaginary mental metalanguage outside the symbolic universe of language. At the same time, as they are real, they cannot be constituent elements of the same symbolic universe. We can then say that they are *impossible*, since they cannot be either inside the universe or outside it. Nevertheless, despite their impossibility, they certainly do exist. They are actually the only real psychic things that we know. So, they deserve our interest.[12]

In a Lacanian interpretation, we must not be only interested in the symbolic, but also in the real of the symbolic. Just like our analysis, our interpretation must take this real into account. In fact, we cannot analyze or interpret the symbolic independently of the real. We cannot approach a value if we leave its materialization aside. When we analyze or interpret a signifier, we may pay no attention to its signified, its meaning or its signification, but we cannot ignore its literal presence. We cannot disregard this truth of wisdom. We cannot overlook this nonsensical support of sense. As noted above, our 'interpretation' must be also 'directed' towards this 'non-sense of the signifiers' (Lacan, 1964, 27.05.64, p. 236). In our 'interpretation', we may even try to 'reduce' the sense to this 'non-sense' (ibid.). Through this reduction of the symbolic value to its nonsensical real support, we should be able to reveal, at least in part, a particularization of our civilization's universal enormous nonsense, which comprises the articulating real structure of the symbolic, its work, and its exploitation of the expressing real workforce of the enunciating subject, as well as the real production of this work, namely, an object that attracts, hooks, and retains the discontented subject. To 'rediscover' all these 'determinants of the subject's entire behaviour' (ibid.), Lacanian interpretation turns into a sort of experimental method that simply explains what it analyzes, introduces a signifier into what it explains, and waits for the consequences of this introduction. Such a method seems to be even more elementary than the psychological observation of behaviour. While this observation irresistibly tends to give a sense to the observed behaviour, our interpretation tries to recover the behavioural determinants in the purity of their non-sense.[13] In this purity, the behavioural determinants cannot be the mental representations, granted, but they cannot be the discursive representatives either. They can only be the real or literal presences and absences that lie beneath symbolic representatives and imaginary representations.

To approach the determinants of the subject's behaviour, we must not leave the symbolic universe of language. However, in this universe, we must go beneath the sense or symbolic value of the representatives. Even if our interpretation must remain in language, it must separate 'sense' from 'language' (Lacan, 1975, p. 314). Our interest in the linguistic disciplines of 'grammar' and 'equivocal forms' has to be principally motivated by the fact that they 'contradict sense' (ibid.). When we 'interpret', we must try to 'isolate in the subject a kernel of nonsense' (1964, 17.06.64, p. 278). In our interpretation, what must 'count' for more than anything else is not the 'sense' (S1–S2), but a nonsensical 'remainder' (*a*) that cannot be assimilated into 'sense' (1962–1963, 23.01.63, p. 149). At this stage, obviously, our interpretation is no longer an 'interpretation' of 'sense' (1972a, p. 480), but an 'interpretation' of 'nonsense' that must tackle language with only the aim of demonstrating its absurdity (1964, 27.05.64, p. 236). Here, instead of dissolving the absurdity into the supposed strategic functioning of the symbolic system, we must examine closely the absurd functioning, distinguish its individual particularity, and isolate it from any universal rational wisdom. In the end, if possible, we have to look into the irrational truth of the real speaking workforce exploited by the symbolic system with its rational wisdom. To reach this nonsense of sense, we have to explore the real emptiness of the signifying social structure. We have to fathom this logical void that proves to be a space of negativity and impossibility, frustration and privation, lack, acting out, drives, and desires.[14]

The Lacanian interpretation must go beneath wisdom and explore the truth of its real support, granted, but it must also acknowledge the negativity and impossibility of this support. The fact of transcending the symbolic value of sense must not lead us to the imaginary reality of a meaningful content, but rather to the real emptiness of the signifying structure. Directed towards this void, the movement that transcends sense must not give rise to a new transcendent religion. Actually, in Lacanian 'interpretation', the crossing of 'sense' is also a crossing of 'religion' (Lacan, 1979–1980, 18.03.80). If 'religion' systematically employs an 'interpretation' (1967g, p. 335), then the Lacanian interpretation must distinguish itself from this religious interpretation by *piercing* a 'sense' that is 'always religious' (1980, p. 318). When we pierce this sense, nothing remains of the interpretation in the ordinary meaning of the word, of course. However, Lacan explicitly rejects this ordinary meaning by which 'we imagine that interpretation proceeds only through the sense' (1979–1980, 18.03.80). Against this idea, Lacan defends an 'interpretation' whose 'driving force' (*ressort*) is the 'signifier' (ibid.), a signifier that involves the sense, but also nonsense.[15]

The interpretation of discourse as a reinterpretation of an interpretation

In a signifier, we may distinguish between *the sense or symbolic value of the representative* and *the literal and nonsensical presence of its real support*. The former relates *only* to the wisdom of a language, while the latter *also* concerns the truth of the speaking subject. The latter thus *also* concerns an enunciating act ($\$\lozenge a$) and not only the enunciated fact (S1→S2). Put differently, the nonsense resides in the intersection between the being of the subject and the sense of the Other. In effect, it corresponds to the literal junction between a real body and a symbolic system. This can be illustrated by the Lacanian diagram of alienation:

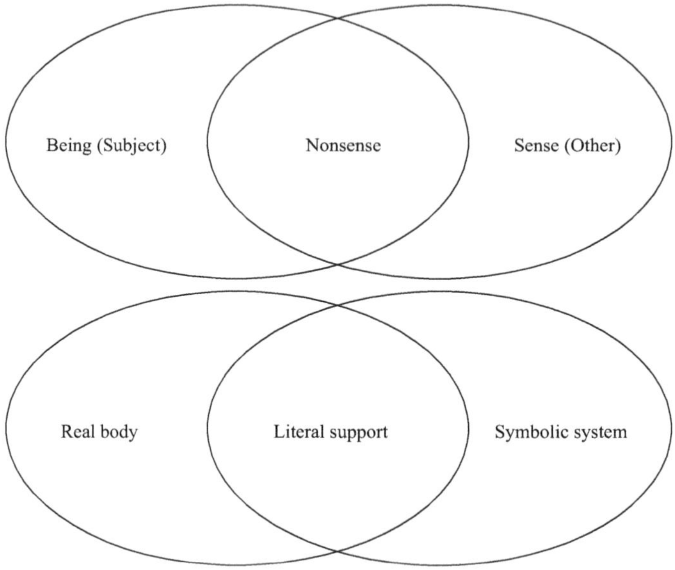

When the interpretation works only with 'sense', this sense is inevitably 'deprived of that part of nonsense' which 'constitutes' the 'unconscious' in 'the realization of the subject' (Lacan, 1964, 27.05.64, p. 211). Deprived of this 'nonsense' as the anchoring subjective 'element' of the 'unconscious' (1970a, p. 435), the interpreted sense arises from a floating spoken discourse without a speaking subject. It relates to an abstract wisdom without a concrete truth. It merely refers to the Other, but not to the subject. Its interpretation elucidates the symbolic system independently of the real being. Thus, neglecting this being of the enunciating act, interpretations in current discursive psychology are often limited to the sense of the enunciated fact. By contrast, a Lacanian interpretation does not 'proceed only through the sense', but it embraces the whole 'signifier', its reproductive sense as well as its subversive nonsense, its symbolic value as well as its literal support, its enunciated fact as well as its enunciating act (1979–1980, 18.03.80).

The Lacanian interpretation may lean towards nonsense, but it must neither forget nor overlook the sense of the interpreted discourse. An exclusive focus on the nonsense would be as narrow and partial as the limited focus on the sense. In fact, if we totally excluded sense from our interpretation, there would not really be an interpretation. Although we reject the ordinary meaning of the interpretation as a pure attribution of sense, an interpretation intrinsically involves a generation of sense. Therefore, when we interpret, our *consideration of the nonsense* cannot mean an *exclusion of the sense.* To be sure, the sense cannot be excluded, since it is *always already there,* not only in our interpreting discourse, but also in the interpreted discourse, which simultaneously functions as an interpreting discourse that is already *making sense.*

Condemned to deal with sense, our interpretation always amounts to a reinterpretation of an interpretation. Logically, the interpreted discourse already involves a previous interpretation, symbolization, and signifierization. Before being interpreted, the signifiers are interpreting. Their signifying structure can then be described as an *interpretative structure.*[16]

Let us take the case of Francisco Javier. In the interpretative structure detected in his discourse, the "familiar obligations" are *interpreted as* "marriage", "love", "monogamy", and "faithfulness". This interpretation may reflect the interpretative move of "our time", in which the 'familiar institution' loses its 'social predominance', which is then transferred to 'marriage' (Lacan, 1938, p. 58). If that is the way it is, then "marriage" can be treated as an interpretation of the "family" by the signifying social structure of "our time". As for this "family", it was already an interpretation of another interpretation of another one, and so on. The interpreted discourse is thus composed of a dense and impenetrable web of interpretations. Each new interpretation condenses, complicates, and obscures the web even further. As Lacan (1970a) points out, 'the more a discourse is interpreted, the more it is confirmed as unconscious' (p. 418).

Besides interpreting, the unconscious makes itself through its interpreting work. It creates itself by interpreting itself and by camouflaging itself in its own perceptible and unintelligible interpretations. In their external materiality composed of words without meaning, these 'interpretations are nothing more than the unconscious' (Miller, 1996c, p. 9). They are the constitution of the unconscious by itself, which is also a concealment of the unconscious by itself. When scientific research leads us to reinterpret the automatic interpretations deployed in discourse, our deliberate reinterpretation contributes to this concealment of the unconscious by itself. It contributes to it by concealing 'the fact that the unconscious' has 'already proceeded through interpretation' (Lacan, 1964, 15.04.64,

p. 146). By concealing this *fact*, our interpretation conceals the fact of the 'unconscious', which is the fact of 'interpretation' (Miller, 1996c, p. 9). This *enunciated fact* is nothing but a fact of language, of a language that 'is already there in every opening, however fleeting it may be, of the unconscious' (Lacan, 1964, 15.04.64, p. 146).

As a *discourse of the Other*, the Lacanian unconscious is an *interpretation of a language*. Once interpreted or articulated by the symbolic system of this language, the interpretation has to be expressed by a real subject. Then it has to be reinterpreted by the symbolic system. The interpretation arouses a reinterpretation. As Miller (1996c) notes, 'interpretation always breeds interpretation' (pp. 9–10). It breeds an interpretation that, in turn, breeds another interpretation, and so on. This is how the symbolic system reproduces itself. It reproduces itself through the work of the unconscious, an interpreting work that always remains unconscious, and which then breeds more interpreting work, since 'deciphering is always ciphering again' (ibid.). The supposed signification is always a signifierization, or, more precisely, a re-signifierization. Without a real conscious signification, each real unconscious re-signifierization entails another unconscious re-signifierization, which entails another, and so on. Each time, there is a reinterpretation of language by language, an auto-reconfiguration of the symbolic system, an auto-reconstitution of the unconscious as the discourse of the Other. Since there is no Other of this Other, there is no one who could become conscious of the unconscious. There is no mind in which the unconscious words may find a real conscious meaning. As for the supposed mental metalanguage of consciousness, it is just an imaginary representation of an unconscious reinterpretation of the same language by the same language. Just as any other reinterpretation, this one is not 'stratified' in relation to the unconscious, but 'it is of the same order'; it belongs to 'the same register'; it is a 'constituent of this register' (Miller, 1996c, p. 10).

Lacanian word-for-word interpretation

There is always continuity between my interpreting discourse and the interpreted discourse. Both are in the same symbolic universe. Both belong to the same structure in itself. Both are deployed in the same structure for my structural position. There must then be a close connection between them. The sense of my interpretation must follow one way or another from the sense of the interpreted discourse. Therefore, to respect the natural order of things, my 'interpretation cannot be bent to any sense' (Lacan, 1964, 27.05.64, p. 233). It cannot be 'open to any sense' (17.06.64, p. 278). Its 'opening' cannot be 'total', but there must be a 'closing' imposed by the word-for-word character of the interpretation and by the limited character of the interpreted discourse (Regnault, 2003–2004, 25.03.04).

The Lacanian interpretation is a word-for-word interpretation. It is thus confined to the interpreted symbolic value of the literal word. From this value, we may introduce a new symbolic value, granted, but this introduction must strictly follow from the interpreted value. The introduced value has to *fall into line* with the interpreted value. *In the Lacanian word-for-word interpretation, the introduced word has to be for the interpreted word. But this does not mean that both words have to be equivalent or share the same symbolic value. Instead, they must have complementary opposed values in the same symbolic system of language. Furthermore, they must function as successive links in the same discursive chain.* Here, between the values of both words, there has to be a *linear* or direct contradiction (S1–S2) that reveals the gap between the exploiting articulating structure (S2/*a*) and the structural position of the exploited expressing workforce ($\S1). To reveal this division of the subject ($) between his alienation in a language (S2/*a*) and his identification with a signifier ($\S1), our interpretation must be *the one* that demonstrates the contradiction which causes it, that is, the difference (S1–S2/*a*) between the subjective *exchange value* (S1) and the predicative *use value* (S2) of a real subject in the symbolic system ($\S1–S2). In its diverse forms, this is *the right interpretation*. It is the interpretation that I want to make of Francisco Javier's discourse, for example, when I contrast the "counter-revolutionary" of "our time" with the "revolutionary" of the "new society". Through this opposition in the enunciated wisdom, my interpretation tries to reveal the subversive truth of the enunciating subject that is hypothetically divided between the terms of the opposition.

The 'right interpretation' is the 'only one' that reveals the 'truth' of the subject (Lacan, 1953b, p. 136). This truth can be revealed by 'only a single series of signifiers' (1964, 27.05.64, p. 233). In this series, there are two main places, one for the interpreter and the signifier that he introduces, another for the interpreted signifier and the one who expresses it. These places cannot depend on the will of the interpreter, since they are pre-determined by the signifying social structure. In this structure, they are simply two structural positions. They are two words, *one word for the other*, the "counter-revolutionary" for the "revolutionary", the "bourgeois ideology" for the "proletarian ideology", one word opposed to the other, one in relation to the other. Between them, there is the 'typical social link' by which, according to Miller (1996a), 'we have a chance to interpret' *word for word* and thereby 'limit the non-dialogue' between subjects (p. 18).

By limiting the non-dialogue between subjects, our word-for-word interpretation may 'impose a limit' on the 'autistic monologue' of 'the Other' (Miller, 1996b, pp. 16–17). When we interpret word for word, there is a sort of dialogue between the word we introduce and the literal word we interpret. Each word represents a subject for the other word. Between both words, there is the only achievable 'intersubjective' relation, namely, the 'intersignifying' one (Lacan, 1970–1971, 13.01.71, p. 10). This structural connection belongs to the signifying social structure. In this structure, it involves a 'social link' between our position and the one 'to which we refer' (Miller, 1996a, pp. 17–18).

By referring to the literal word of the interpreted discourse, our introduction of another word may establish a direct 'relation with the Other' (Miller, 1996a, pp. 17–18). The correlative literal term of this relation is the only precise landmark that may accurately orient our interpretation in the signifying social structure. In this exteriority of the unconscious, the literal word of the interpreted discourse is the only objective reference mark for our interpretation. It is 'the only thing that tidies our absolute semantic solitude' (ibid.). It is 'the only thing that limits our reading of the signifier' (ibid.).

Thanks to our opening to the literal word of the interpreted discourse, we may undertake a 'symbolic interpretation' in the 'hysterical intersubjectivity' of the signifying social structure (Lacan, 1953a, p. 252). Otherwise, if we suffered from the 'resistance' of our 'obsessive intrasubjectivity', our interpretation would be hermetically closed to the literal word (ibid.). Accordingly, our solitary unlimited wisdom would not have any relation to the interpreted wisdom. It would not be able to demonstrate its contradictory sense (S1→S2). Nor would it be able to reveal its nonsensical truth ($\$\lozenge a$). To reveal this truth, our interpretation must be immersed in the interpreted structure that interprets itself. By forming part of this interpreting structure of wisdom, our interpretation may internally demonstrate its intrinsic contradiction of sense and thus expose its nonsensical truth. To expose this nonsense, the sense of our interpretation must be consonant with the sense whose dissonant nonsense has to be exposed. Both senses must be on the same wavelength. Otherwise, the nonsense cannot be isolated.

Complementary incomplete interpretations

By following the sense of the interpreted discourse, we may arrive at the truth of its 'pure nonsense' (Lacan, 1964, 17.06.64, p. 280). We may infer this truth from all kinds of 'irreducible, nonsensical signifying elements' encountered in discourse (ibid.). As the common denominator of these nonsensical elements, the pure nonsense resides in an unavoidable contradiction of sense between the enunciated subject and its non-tautological predicate. For the enunciating subject, this contradiction indicates the difference between his identification with a signifier and his alienation in a language, that is to say, the disparity between his insignificant subjective exchange-value and the significant predicative use-value of his enunciating workforce. As discussed before, this disparity creates a symbolic surplus value that maintains the functioning of a language by giving sense to its discourses. Without this predicative surplus (S2), which interprets the enunciated subject (S1), discourse would be tautological (S1→S1). It would not have any sense, because its sense can only come from the interpretative surplus value produced by the exploitation of the subject's enunciating workforce. But this sense of the surplus value (→S2) implies the nonsense of a surplus-enjoyment ($\rightarrow S2/a$). The exploitation by the system of *wisdom* (S1→S2) entails the nonsensical *truth* of the subject's marginalized corporeal being ($\$\lozenge a$). It entails the marginalization of this real being (a) that is lost by the speaking subject ($\$$) as the literal support of the symbolic system ($\$\backslash S1 \rightarrow S2/a$). Logically, as real enjoyment of the symbolic system by the subject, this real being is a nonsensical experience that cannot be assimilated into sense. It is an excessive truth that overflows wisdom. It cannot be signifierized by language. It cannot be either contained or assimilated by a discursive form. It cannot be either imagined by a cognitive psychology or analyzed by a discursive psychology. To approach this excess, we need a psychoanalytical interpretation.[17]

In the light of our Lacanian psychoanalytical interpretation, the missing real being of the speaking subject appears as a nonsensical excess excluded by the symbolic system that generates sense. As 'pure nonsense', the excessive corporeal being is marginalized in itself in order to become the exploited literal support of the symbol, the real price of the symbolic surplus value, 'the bearer of the infinitization of the value of the subject, not open to all senses, but abolishing them all' (Lacan, 1964, 17.06.64, p. 280). Thus, besides supporting all senses, the nonsensical real being 'kills all senses' (p. 252). It is that which simultaneously undermines and underpins sense. It is the permanent impossibility that motivates the next interpretation by invalidating the last one.

According to Lacan (1964), the real impossibility (*a*) inherent in the symbolic interpretation (S1–S2/*a*) demonstrates the 'absurdity' of the idea that 'all interpretations' are valid or 'possible' (17.06.64, p. 278). *Even if all interpretations are complementary, the only suitable and well-founded interpretation, in a specific structural context, is the one that is motivated by the particular incomplete character of the last interpretation. When the last interpretation is invalidated, the only valid interpretation is the complementary one, the next one, which completes the last one, but which proves also to be incomplete and then justifies another interpretation, and so on.* Now, in this signifying chain, all symbolic interpretations are stimulated by the same 'irreducible nonsense' that nullifies them all (p. 279). In each interpretation, this nonsense corresponds to the real being that cannot be assimilated by the sense of any symbolic interpretation. Each interpretation is incomplete because of this lacking real being (*a*), whose lacking encourages the next interpretation (S1→S2), which will be logically as incomplete as the last one (S1→S2/*a*).[18]

Each interpretation is incomplete. The symbolic value of each one (S1→S2) cannot embrace the missing real being (*a*). Its sense is always partially nonsensical. Therefore, its sense is always partial, deficient, limited. No interpretation can be 'open to all senses' (Lacan, 1964, 17.06.64, p. 280). By assuming this unavoidable closing of sense, the Lacanian interpretation methodically 'imposes limits' on its generation of sense (Miller, 1996b, p. 17). This generation 'includes' strict 'limits' in its 'transformation' of nonsense into sense (Bruno, 1996, p. 104).

Our limited interpretation must not be confused with an 'interpretation of sense' that tries to 'get rid of limits' (Miller, 1996b, p. 17). This *unlimited* interpretation 'imagines' that 'it can abolish the distance' between the nonsensical real being and the 'meaning' of the *sensical* symbolic being (Bruno, 1996, p. 104). In due course, by systematically reducing this distance *in* the imaginary, the interpretation develops into a comprehensive interpretation *of* the imaginary. The missing real being (*a*) is then replaced by an imaginary being [i(*a*)]. When the interpreted discourse is full, its structuring fullness and truthfulness is disregarded and replaced by a meaningful mental content. Otherwise, when the discourse is empty, its 'emptiness' is merely 'filled' with an imaginary 'reality beyond speech' (Lacan, 1953a, p. 246). In any case, the comprehensive interpreter would *understand* the interpreted discourse. He would *understand* it by *elaborating* on it and *completing* it. Here, obviously, the problem is not the elaboration and completion, but the imaginary understanding or comprehension.

The nonsensical remainder of interpretation

All interpretations elaborate on other interpretations. All interpretations complete other interpretations. In the symbolic system, all interpretations are complementary. However, there is always a residue, a missing real being, which cannot be completed or elaborated, interpreted or symbolized.

There is always a nonsensical remainder that prevents a reinterpretation from fully completing the sense of a reinterpreted interpretation. The symbolic value of this sense will be always devoid of the remainder, dispossessed of its real being, corroded by its absence, eroded by its nonsense. Now, unlike a comprehensive interpretation, our Lacanian explanatory interpretation does not aim at eliminating or grasping the remainder. Furthermore, even elaborating and completing, our explanation is not intended for this elaboration and completion. On the contrary, its intention is to reveal the truth of the real being that cannot be assimilated into the symbolic system of language, of language's wisdom, or by any completion or elaboration of discourse. In search of this nonsensical truth, our Lacanian interpretation chooses a 'way of perplexity' instead of the 'way of elaboration' preferred by the comprehensive interpretation (Miller, 1996c, p. 13).

In the way of perplexity, a Lacanian 'interpretation' looks for a nonsensical truth that can only be found in the form of an 'enigma' (Lacan, 1969–1970, 17.12.69, p. 39). This enigma puts together the contradictory terms of discourse. It materializes their contradiction, antagonism, and disagreement. It is itself an expression of this disagreement.[19] It differs from itself. It is intrinsically differing, conflicting, incongruous. It can only generate perplexity or mistakes and misunderstandings. It can only be accurately formulated in paradoxical assertions or in questions without answers. Thus, in Francisco Javier's discourse, the enigma can be illustrated by "marriage" as a "revolutionary activity", the "love" that "leads" to a "dissolution of the couple", or the "familiar obligation" of a "faithfulness from conviction". In the same discourse, the enigma can be also exemplified by some insoluble questions. Why should the "revolutionaries" lend such "importance" to "marriage"? Why should the "new society" be founded on a "monogamous family"? Why can a "revolutionary" only be "consistent" if his "conceptions of marriage" are based on "faithfulness"?

Whether interrogative or paradoxical, the formulation of the enigma gives us an idea of the 'fundamentally equivocal nature of speech', whose double 'function is to cover and to discover' (Lacan, 1953b, p. 140). As spoken wisdom that covers and discovers the nonsensical truth, the formulation of the enigma 'defines', in Lacan (1969–1970), the right 'structure' of 'interpretation' (17.12.69, p. 39). It is the structure of a *discovering covering*, a *half-discovering*, a 'half-saying (*mi-dire*)', a *half-wisdom*, a 'wisdom without wisdom', a 'wisdom as truth' (ibid.). This enigmatic wisdom can be 'gathered in the fabric of discourse' (p. 40). Here, in wisdom, it may be perceived as an incomplete piece of wisdom, a 'wisdom without wisdom', whose enigmatic nature would result from its incomplete character (p. 39). Therefore, to solve the enigma, the 'interpreter' may 'complete' the incomplete wisdom (p. 40). However, in so doing, he would turn his 'interpretation' into a 'lie' (ibid.).

After formulating the enigma through paradoxical assertions or questions without answers, the truthful interpreter must try not to answer or unravel the enigmatic formulations. If he introduces a signifier, the signifier must contribute to the formulation or explanation of the enigma, but it must not be aimed at its comprehension and solution. This solution would be a waste of the enigma. Yet the enigma has to be preserved, since it represents the most important outcome of our interpretation, namely, the truth of the enunciated wisdom that we interpret.

As the truth of an enunciated wisdom, the 'enigma' is a 'matter of enunciation' (Lacan, 1975–1976, 11.05.76, p. 153). In the enigma, the question is 'why' a particular wisdom has been 'enunciated' (ibid.). The question is the enunciating act. Actually, when we formulate the enigma, we are paradoxically enunciating an enunciating act without an enunciated fact. This is why the 'enigma' is 'wisdom as truth' and 'wisdom without wisdom' (Lacan, 1969–1970, 17.12.69, p. 39). It is an enunciated enunciation (*wisdom as truth*) without an enunciated statement (*without wisdom*). It is an enunciated 'enunciation whose enunciated statement is not found' (20.01.76, p. 67). Thus, even if the 'message' is not found, the enigmatic 'essence' of the 'message' is found by our interpretation (Bruno, 1996, p. 102). But this essence has the form of a message. Its truth has the form of wisdom. It is wisdom, but *wisdom without wisdom*, or *wisdom as truth*. In our interpretative 'know-how' (*savoir-faire*), this peculiar 'wisdom' (*savoir*) represents the only 'possibility' to know the 'truth' of wisdom (Lacan, 1976–1977, 18.11.76, p. 13).

The nonsensical truth *of* wisdom can only be known *in* wisdom through the nonsensical sense of an enigma. In Lacan (1973b), such a sense is the 'height of sense' (p. 553). It is '*the* sense of sense' (1974a, p. 562). It is the *nonsensical sense of sense*. Now, since the 'sense' is 'always religious' (1980, p. 318), we can say that an enigma expresses the nonsensical sense of our 'religion' of 'sense' (1979–1980, 18.03.80). It thereby expresses the *unreasonable reason* for this still prevailing religion that compels us to comprehend everything, or give a sense to everything, in order to incorporate everything into a religious totalization in which everything makes sense.[20]

In contrast with the religious totalization of the comprehensive interpretation, the enigma of our Lacanian interpretation reveals a truth that 'makes an objection to the idea of totality' (Lacan, 1974a, p. 562). This truth is itself an objection raised against a total wisdom. This is why it can only arise in the enigmatic form of something that is 'half-said' (1976–1977, 18.11.76, p. 13). The truth can only be half-said ($) because it refers to a real excess ($◊*a*) that overflows the symbolic totality of sense (S1–S2), as well as the imaginary totality of meaning [*ego* | i(*a*)]. Just like the totalitarian sense, this totalitarian 'meaning excludes the real', because 'the real, reluctant to any wording, only allows the half-saying, the *mi-dire* of truth' (Braunstein, 2000, p. 219).

From a Lacanian viewpoint, the 'truth' can only reside in a 'half-saying' (Lacan, 1975–1976, 09.12.75, p. 31). The truth can only be 'half-said' (1976–1977, 18.11.76, p. 13). The 'half-told' (*midit*) is the only thing that can be 'told' in that which is 'posed in truth' by a Lacanian interpretation (1972a, p. 452). Here is an interpretative restriction that must become for us, in our interpretation, a strict methodological rule. It is a rule of self-control and moderation. It compels us to restraint. It requires us to keep silent about some things and leave our interpreting work unfinished. It can be thus described as a *noncompletion principle* that will condition the truthfulness of our interpretation.[21]

Our *noncompletion principle* is fully justified by the fact that we cannot tell the whole truth. There is 'no truth' that 'could be told in the whole' (Lacan, 1973c, p. 310). Therefore, 'to tell the truth, we must not say everything, we must not tell the whole truth, we must tell the not-whole (*pas-toute*) truth' (Regnault, 1987, p. 170). There is only 'the half' of 'the truth' that can be 'told' (Lacan, 1970c, p. 394). Accordingly, we would lie if we claimed to tell the whole truth. In truth, 'we do not succeed in telling the whole truth' (1973a, p. 509). This 'is impossible, materially impossible, words fail us' (ibid.). Since the real cannot be totally symbolized, it 'prevents us from telling the whole truth' (p. 533). It is thus *impossible* to tell the whole truth because of a real being whose fundamental relation to the truth resides precisely in this 'impossibility' (p. 509).

Notes

1. Unlike cognitive psychologists, we are not obliged to 'assemble' the ideal 'pieces of meaning' of the analyzed discourse, as if they were material 'bricks' emerging from discourse and entering our head (cf. Gineste & Le Ny, 2002, p. 105). In a Lacanian Discourse Analysis, we are not obliged to smash our head open with such imaginary material bricks, but we can interpret the real material bricks of discourse in their symbolic exteriority.
2. In social psychology, this *rational second naïveté* corresponds to the 'middle ground between naïveté and formalization' that Ghiglione (1991) proposes in his Propositional Discourse Analysis (p. 34). Like

Ricœur, Ghiglione considers that a new 'sense is co-constructed' in 'each analysis' (ibid.). From a Lacanian viewpoint, one would not understand why the sense would be *co-constructed* and not only *constructed* by the analyst. After all, the proletarianized analyst does all the work here. He gives the sense, as well as the belief, the pre-comprehension, and the comprehension. Why should we conceal his achievements? It is greatly to his credit that he does everything in front of the mirror, that is, everything that happens in the mirror.

3. Our 'task' in a Lacanian Discourse Analysis 'is to work on the line of the Symbolic (working within the domain of the text)', while a Ricœurian 'approaches a text in the hermeneutic mode, as something we can *understand*', so he works 'on the line of the Imaginary (imagining that we interpret from outside of the text)' (Parker, 2005a, p. 177).
4. In opposition to this idea, Parker (1997b) judges it 'better to talk of *understanding* rather than to refer to *explanation* in discursive research' (p. 490). The basis for this assertion is the observation of the 'chaotic and complex unconscious meanings which pervade language' (ibid.). If these contradictory *meanings* really *pervaded language*, then it would be logical to expect 'contradictory understandings' of them (ibid.). However, from my point of view, the *meanings* cannot *pervade* a language that is composed only of *words*. Unlike meanings or significations, these perceptible and explainable words or signifiers are neither intelligible nor comprehensible, as evidenced by the fact that they are not conscious, but unconscious. Now, by speaking of *unconscious meanings*, Parker shows that his opposition to my idea is purely terminological. Since his *meanings* are unconscious, they amount to my *signifiers*, so that their understanding corresponds to an explanation, as there is nothing conscious to understand in them.
5. Thus, together with Billig (1997), we may interpret 'what is not said, but could easily have been, and, indeed, on occasions is almost said' (p. 152). However, we must not therefore understand either that discourse necessarily *means or wants to say* what *it does not say*, or that *it desires* what *it wants to say* and *represses* what *it does not say*. If this were the case, what is not said would always be the 'repressed' meaning of what is said, an indemonstrable meaning composed of banal 'desires', for example 'desires to be rude, to contradict, *to speak one's mind*' (p. 151).
6. It is as if the value of the understood meaning resided in its non-existence within the interpreted discourse. For instance, Bardin (1977) not only recommends us 'to understand a sense' not literally

included in 'communication', but also 'to tear ourselves away from this communication and turn our gaze to another signification', to 'another message that we discover through the first one or close to it' (p. 46). Here Bardin at least recognizes that the understood *signification* is nothing more than *another message*. Therefore, to understand a message, one should not understand it. Instead, one should understand another message, which would be the supposed signification of the first message.

7. Likewise, in a neighbouring perspective, Frosh (2007) adopts the same principle and explicitly asserts that 'limits to making sense, to making connections, have to be set' (p. 638).
8. Actually, to become true, my interpretation may resort to an 'effective lie' that 'makes itself a truth' (Marx, 1843a, pp. 313–316). Despite the lack of 'exactness', my lie may become a 'true story' (pp. 312–313). Like the Marxian truth of 'lies' and 'fables' (ibid.), the Lacanian truth can be found in that which is usually regarded as 'the less true in essence', such as 'dreams', 'symptoms', 'lapses', and 'nonsense' (Lacan, 1956c, p. 407). In any event, 'the truth shows its fictional structure' (1957a, p. 448). This structure may logically operate in our Lacanian interpretations. While interpreting, we may even dare to emulate the wise craziness of dreams or Freudian slips. After all, these formations of the unconscious always prove to be our most pertinent interpretations.
9. Therefore, in a sense, we may conceivably say that our interpretation must not be 'operational', but 'finalist', as it has to be focused on the 'arrival point' (the advent of its own truth), and not on the 'path' from the interpreted 'departure text' to the interpreting 'arrival text' (Todorov, 1977, p. 319).
10. Our interpretative 'proposition' must not be formulated in an 'appropriate metalanguage', but in the only appropriate or inappropriate language at our disposal (c.f. Van Dijk & Kintsch, 1983, p. 112). In this language, our proposition is a sentence among other sentences. It has to be 'taken as' an interpretative sentence added to an interpreted sentence and not 'as the meaning' of the interpreted 'sentence' (ibid.). It must not be 'used to identify the meaning' or the signification (p. 111), but to continue with the process of signifierization.
11. As Anzieu and Martin (1968) observe, the 'attention devoted to each word eliminates the significant content of the message' (p. 194). The authors deplore this elimination. On the contrary, a Lacanian will be rather glad about it. It is remarkable that our attention to words eliminates their meaning. Therefore, to interpret a meaning,

we should preferably be inattentive to the interpreted words of discourse. The fact speaks for itself.

12. They even deserve *a psychology*. However, since they cannot be part of an imaginary mental metalanguage, their psychology cannot be a cognitive psychology. At the same time, as they cannot be pieces of the symbolic system of language, their psychology cannot be a simple discursive psychology. Finally, given that they are not supposedly independent from the symbolic system, their psychology cannot be a resurrection of the old behavioural psychology. Unlike these abstract psychologies that consider only one aspect of the psyche, the study of *real psychic things* should be subordinated to a psychology that would take into consideration the coexistence of the real, the symbolic, and the imaginary (Pavón Cuéllar, 2009). This psychology may approximately correspond to the project of a 'concrete psychology' put forward by Politzer (1928, 1947). Only such a psychology may resist the revival, in current psychology, of two 'fundamental processes of classical psychology' (1928, C, §1, p. 239). On the one hand, the discursive 'formalism', with its 'abstraction' of that which transcends its symbolic form (II, I, p. 86). On the other hand, the cognitive 'realism', with its imaginary reality, the '*sui generis* reality of inner life' (II, I, p. 83).
13. To this end, the Lacanian 'psychoanalytic interpretation' must *return from* psychology rather than go 'beyond psychology' (cf. Billig, 2006a, p. 11). In comparison with our elementary 'psychoanalytic interpretation', the sophisticated 'psychological observation of the behaviour' (ibid.) is further away from that which is observed or interpreted. In a psychological perspective, it is naturally difficult to accept this paradoxical 'distinction' between our down-to-earth 'psychoanalytic interpretation' and the resourceful 'psychological observation' (ibid.).
14. In all of this, Lacanian psychoanalytic interpretation deliberately runs counter to an 'over-strong discursive move' that 'participates in a rationalist fallacy that itself *flattens out* situations of great emotional complexity, or intense feeling' (Frosh, 2002, p. 189). To say 'something' about these *situations*, we need a discourse 'derived from psychoanalysis' (p. 192).
15. Strictly speaking, the Lacanian perspective does not entail a 'scepticism regarding interpretation', but only a 'scepticism regarding interpretation' *in the ordinary meaning of the word* (cf. Braunstein, 2000, p. 218). As Braunstein observes, this 'scepticism' seems to be founded on the idea that 'interpretation' *in the ordinary meaning of the word* is not an 'instrument of liberation with regard to the oppressive repression', but rather

a 'reinforcement of repression through the work and combined action of the Master's and the University's discourses' (ibid.).

16. In social psychology, this *interpretative structure* approximately corresponds to the 'interpretative repertoire' that Potter and Wetherell (1987) propose instead of the 'social representation' (p. 146). Now, unlike this repertoire, our signifying social structure is not exactly a 'system of terms used for characterizing and evaluating actions, events and other phenomena' (p. 149). In the radicalism of the Lacanian perspective, the *interpretative structure* should be rather described as the real structure of the symbolic system that uses us (our enunciating workforce) for constituting everything.
17. On this point, Frosh (1999) observes that 'psychoanalysis attends to the excess, what cannot be held or contained, which keeps cropping up' (p. 386). Now, in a Lacanian interpretation, this real excess can only be reached through the exceeded symbolic form. This form of discourse is the only place in which our interpretation may deal with 'this excess' that 'slips away from discourse' (Frosh, 2002, pp. 192–193).
18. This is how we may explain, in a Lacanian perspective, the situation in which there are 'too many possible interpretations', as well as 'something threatening that gives momentum to all this productivity, undermining meaning at the same time it makes it happen' (Frosh, 2007, p. 644).
19. This enigmatic formulation corresponds to an 'understanding of the nature of discourse as constituted by deadlocks of perspective' in which 'it is the failure of agreement that needs to be displayed rather than an attempt to cover that disagreement over' (Parker, 2005a, p. 176).
20. As it expresses the nonsensical sense of this religion of sense, our enigma may not be unrelated to the 'concealed mystery' of the 'profane religion' of Moscovici (1961, p. 463).
21. This *noncompletion principle* is radically opposed to the 'Gestalt principle' that Hollway and Jefferson (2000) 'try to apply' to the 'understanding' of a 'whole text' (p. 69). As a production of the symbolic system, the real being of the subject might confirm that 'the whole is greater than the sum of the parts' (p. 68). *The whole* certainly produces a remaining *part* that cannot be included in *the sum of the parts*. Nevertheless, this remaining *part* cannot be included in *the whole* either. To be sure, the real surplus-enjoyment (*a*) cannot be included in a symbolic universe composed of no more than values and surplus values (S1→S2/*a*). This is precisely why the remainder is *produced* by being *excluded*. After this exclusion, the whole is paradoxically incomplete. When the interpreter completely 'keeps' the whole 'in mind' (p. 70), he is mentally completing, in the imaginary, that which is really incomplete in the symbolic.

CONCLUSION

According to Lacan (1970a), 'we do not have to learn everything about the truth', since 'one bit is enough' (p. 442). This sufficient *bit of truth* would be 'that which is expressed, in view of the structure, by the idea of having wisdom of a bit of the truth' (ibid.). Following this idea, I have not intended, in this book, to offer wisdom that would embrace the entire truth of that which is analyzed and interpreted. I never tried, for instance, to use the Lacanian concepts in order to exhaust Francisco Javier's discourse. In point of fact, this discourse was not exactly my object of analysis, but an example to illustrate my application of some concepts to discourse analysis. Although the concepts were applied to discourse analysis, they were not really applied to the analyzed discourse. Instead, in the 'reversal' recommended by Regnault (1987, p. 180), the discourse was applied to the concepts, so as to implement their application to analysis, as well as their positioning among other concepts.

In their application, the proposed concepts were situated in a precise position among other concepts belonging to different methods of discourse analysis in social psychology. Implying an alternative method, the application of the Lacanian concepts logically forced me to take a firm stance on the other methods. This stance has been elucidated and justified, at every opportunity, on an ad hoc basis. It is thus dispersed and disseminated all over the footnotes. Let me recompose it now:

- On Propositional Discourse Analysis and other cognitive analyses of content (e.g., Ghiglione et al., 1980, 1985, 1991; Ghiglione, 1997, 2003; Bromberg & Trognon, 2000; Gineste & Le Ny, 2002), I appreciate the richness, vividness and luxuriance of their contribution, but I regret their deliberate confinement in the interiority of a *mind*. By treating this interiority as a merely imaginary reality, I contest the pretension to know the objective meaning of the analyzed discourse, the thinking of the speaking subject, his consciousness and his mental states. I also reject the instrumental conceptions of language as a means of communication, a vehicle of representations, or a tool for the construction of reality.
- On Discursive Psychology with its discourse analysis (e.g., Potter & Wetherell, 1987; Potter, 2003, 2004; Hepburn & Potter, 2003), I share its anti-cognitivist stance, as well as its action orientation, its idea of the performative nature of language, the belief that discourse constructs reality, and the discursive explanation of cognitive entities such as attitudes, categories, and representations. Nevertheless, I censure the reductionism of a Discursive Psychology that only attends to the symbolic and overlooks the real and the imaginary.
- On the current psychoanalytical approaches that react against the reductionism of Discursive Psychology (e.g., Frosh, 1999, 2002, 2007; Frosh, Phoenix & Pattman, 2003; Gough, 2004), I support their will to cross the immanent surface of the enunciated discourse and search the transcendent reasons for the positioning of subjects in discourse. However, in my perspective, this must all be systematically brought back to the symbolic, or, more precisely, to the real of the symbolic, the body of the unconscious, the literal support of the signifier, the enunciating act of the enunciated fact, the expressing workforce and articulating structure of a language.
- On the Psychoanalytic Discursive Psychology of Billig (1997, 1998, 2006b), I have a particularly ambivalent attitude. On the one hand, I accept the acute conceptions of a repressive language

and a dialogic unconscious. On the other hand, I condemn the confidence in the understanding capacity of the analyst, the confusion between the levels of tongue and language, the representation of language as a vehicle that provides the means of repression, the reduction of the unconscious to the outcome of these means in dialogue, and the disregard for both the individual particularity and the real enunciating act of the enunciated fact.

- On the groundbreaking analysis of D'Unrug (1974), I approve its consideration of the real enunciating act, as well as its valuable insights into contradictions and recurrences at the symbolic level of the enunciated fact.
- On the Althusserian-Lacanian Automatic Discourse Analysis of Pêcheux (1969, 1975a, 1975b) and Pêcheux & Fuchs (1975), I have great admiration for its exactness, its strictness, and its pioneering and precursory character. I also think that it still offers substantial theoretical means and methodological possibilities. However, I am wary of a formalism that may involve an absolutization of the symbolic universe and contempt for the real individual subject. In addition, I disagree with the assimilation of language into ideology, the reduction of the intra-discursive individual particularity to the imaginary, and the dissolution of the unconscious into inter-discursive generality.
- On the Lacanian Discourse Analysis of Parker (2000, 2001, 2003, 2005a, 2005b, 2008) and other current applications of Lacan in discourse analysis (e.g., Frosh, 2002; Frosh, Phoenix & Pattman, 2003; Georgaca, 2003, 2005; Hook, 2003, 2008; Branney, 2008), I endorse them, I give my support to their cause and I back their theoretical and methodological enterprise. Nevertheless, when I consider this enterprise with an appraising eye, I become worried about the danger of drifting into new forms of idealism and psychologism, or sociologism, which may respectively entail the desertion of discursive materiality, or the forgetting of the individual particularity of *a language* that is not reducible either to the generality of *the language* or to the social or cultural specificity of *a shared language*.

Like those who precede me, I take a Lacanian stance on other methods of discourse analysis in social psychology. In this psychological field, my psychoanalytical position might also be a new sign that heralds the advent of a concrete psychology such as the one predicted by Politzer (1928, 1947). At the present time, this psychology would distinguish itself from three prevailing abstract psychologies, namely, the *behavioural*, which pays no attention to the symbolic and the imaginary; the *cognitive*, which takes no notice of the real and the symbolic; and the *discursive*, which closes its eyes on the real and the imaginary (Pavón Cuéllar, 2009). Unlike these abstract psychologies, the concrete psychology would not systematically abstract any one of the three 'essential registers of human reality' (Lacan, 1953c, p. 13). Taking the real, the imaginary and the symbolic into consideration, concrete psychology would be complex and multifaceted in its concretion. Furthermore, because of its future-oriented committed involvement in the signifying social structure, it would be social and committed by definition. Now, to find and cement this psychology, we should possibly need, not only the Freudian-Lacanian psychoanalysis, but also the Marxist-Leninist materialism supported by Francisco Javier.

In the expectation of a rather unlikely concrete psychology, I seize the opportunity in this conclusion to congratulate Francisco Javier on his materialism and thank him for *lending* us his revolution, his revolution *in* wisdom, which we borrow from him with the aim of making our subversion, our subversion *of* wisdom. I also take this opportunity to reassure Francisco Javier about our intentions. On the one hand, our subversive enterprise 'is not supposed to consolidate the social order' (Regnault, 2005b, pp. 4–5). On the other hand, even if we may interpret the subjective signifier "revolutionary" and its predicative deployment in "our time", we are 'not at all entitled' to 'interpret' the 'revolutionary practice' itself (Lacan, 1966b, p. 208). This enunciating practice cannot be even 'questioned' by us (Regnault, 2005a, 27.06.05). Our Lacanian interpretation can only deal with the enunciated fact and its relation to the enunciating act, but it cannot question the enunciating act itself. Nor can it justify it, validate it or give a reason for it. Our 'psychology of the unconscious' *is not* 'the philosophy of the revolution' (cf. Gross, 1913a, p. 45). Between both disciplines, there is no simple identity, but rather a complex relation of contradiction, reversal or inversion, and also complementarity. The psychology of revolutionary inconsistency complements the philosophy of the "consistent revolutionary". The Marxist-Leninist revolution might have also complemented a Freudian-Lacanian subversion. Both commitments can even be regarded, in particular cultural environments, as the obverse and the reverse of the same revolt against the same *common sense* that puts on the pleasant masks of cognitivism and liberalism.

Behind its pleasant masks, modern common sense is not as harmless as it looks. This is why Francisco Javier had to be covered with his hood. This may be also the reason why he has been missing for eight years. He is perhaps hiding somewhere, or dead, or in jail. But it is also possible that he is not a revolutionary any longer. It is all the same to me. From my viewpoint, he is still the "consistent revolutionary" of his discourse.

Even though a mortal may always disappear, the subject must stay alive in the structure to which he is subjected. As long as the system functions, the subject must survive and fill his function in the system. He must make his revolution until the deathly silence of his revolutionary discourse. Before this second death, Francisco Javier ($) is not allowed to desert his post (S1) in discourse (S2). As a "consistent revolutionary" ($\S1), he must continue to endure his existential division ($) between his identification with an exchange value (S1) and the alienation of his use value, or enjoyment value (S2), in the symbolic system that exploits his enunciating workforce ($\S1→S2).

The division between the "consistent revolutionary" and "our time" enables Francisco Javier to exist as a "consistent revolutionary" ($\S1) in "our time" (S1→S2). Despite his division, the Eperrist can still be a "consistent revolutionary", at least here in this book, precisely because he bravely assumes the truth of his division ($) and the rather contradictory wisdom of his principles (S1–S2). In this way, he has the courage to be consistent-by-inconsistency. He dares to be his own master by being his own slave. He thus dares to be divided ($) into a 'bipolarity' (S1–S2) that 'betrays itself as essential' for any 'true wisdom' (Lacan, 1970a, p. 425). As long as this true wisdom subsists, its truth has to persist. Francisco Javier has to persevere. He has to be alive.

BIBLIOGRAPHY

Alexandre, V. (1996). Les attitudes: définitions et domaines. In: J.-C. Deschamps & J.-L. Beauvois (Eds.), *Des Attitudes aux Attributions: sur la Construction Sociale de la Réalité* (pp. 23–40). Grenoble: PUG.

Almudever, B. & Le Blanc, A. (2000). La spécificité de l'approche psychosociale au processus de communication. In: N. Roussiau (Ed.), *Psychologie Sociale* (pp. 275–292). Paris: In Press.

Althusser, L. (1964). Freud et Lacan. In: *Écrits sur la Psychanalyse* (pp. 15–53). Paris: STOCK, 1993.

Althusser, L. (1966a). Trois notes sur la théorie de discours. In: *Écrits sur la Psychanalyse* (pp. 111–171). Paris: STOCK, 1993.

Althusser, L. (1966b). Lettres à D. In: *Écrits sur la Psychanalyse* (pp. 55–110). Paris: STOCK, 1993.

Althusser, L. (1976). Sur Marx et Freud. In: *Écrits sur la Psychanalyse* (pp. 226–249). Paris: STOCK, 1993.

Anzieu, D. (1981). *Le Corps de l'Œuvre.* Paris: Gallimard.

Anzieu, D. & Martin, J.-Y. (1968). *La Dynamique des Groupes Restreints.* Paris: PUF, 2003.

Antaki, C. (1994). *Explaining and Arguing: The Social Organization of Accounts.* London: Sage.

Antaki, C. (2006). Producing a cognition. *Discourse Studies*, 8 (1): 9–15.

Arnauld, A. & Lancelot. C. (1676). *Grammaire Générale et Raisonnée.* Bruxelles: Olms, 1973.

Arnauld, A. & Nicole, P. (1683). *La Logique ou l'Art de Penser.* Paris: Flammarion, 1970.

Arrivé, M. (1994). *Langage et Psychanalyse.* Paris: PUF.

Augustine (400). *Les Confessions.* J. Trabucco (Trans.). Paris: Flammarion, 1964.

Austin, J.L. (1955). *How to Do Things with Words.* Cambridge, MA: Harvard University Press, 2000.

Ayerza, J. (1992). Hidden prohibitions and the pleasure principle (interview with Slavoj Žižek), *Flash Art.* http://www.lacan.com/perfume/zizek.htm (accessed 15 September 2008).

Badiou, A. (1998). *Abrégé de Métapolitique.* Paris: Seuil.

Badiou, A. & Foucault, M. (1965). Philosophie et psychologie. In: M. Foucault, *Dits et Écrits I* (pp. 466–476). Paris: Gallimard, 2000.

Bakhtin, M. (1934). Du discours romanesque. In: *Esthétique et Théorie du Roman* (pp. 83–233), D. Olivier (Trans.). Paris: Gallimard, 1975.

Bakhtin, M. (1938). Formes du temps et du chronotope dans le roman. In: *Esthétique et Théorie du Roman* (pp. 235–398). D. Olivier (Trans.), Paris: Gallimard, 1975.

Bardin, L. (1977). *L'analyse de Contenu.* Paris: PUF.

Barthes, R. (1957). *Mythologies.* Paris: Seuil, 1970.

Barthes, R. (1964). Éléments de sémiologie. In: *L'Aventure Sémiologique* (pp. 17–84). Paris: Seuil, 1985.

Beauvois, J.L. (1997). Introduction. In: J.-P. Leyens & J.-L. Beauvois (Eds.), *L'ère de la Cognition* (pp. 7–22). Grenoble: PUG.

Beauvois, J. & Joule, J. (1981). *Soumission et Idéologies.* Paris: PUF.

Berger, P.L. & Luckmann, T. (1966). *The Social Construction of Reality.* New York: Anchor, 1967.

Benveniste, E. (1956). Remarques sur la fonction du langage dans la découverte freudienne. In: *Problèmes de Linguistique Générale I* (pp. 75–87). Paris: Gallimard, 1966.

Benveniste, E. (1958a). De la subjectivité dans le langage. In: *Problèmes de Linguistique Générale I* (pp. 258–266). Paris: Gallimard, 1966.

Benveniste, E. (1958b). Catégories de pensée et catégories de langue. In: *Problèmes de Linguistique Générale I* (pp. 63–74). Paris: Gallimard, 1966.

Benveniste, E. (1968). Structure de la langue et structure de la société. In: *Problèmes de Linguistique Générale II* (pp. 91–102). Paris: Gallimard, 1974.

Billig, M. (1987). *Arguing and Thinking. A Rhetorical Approach to Social Psychology*. Cambridge: Cambridge University Press.

Billig, M. (1997). The dialogic unconscious: Psychoanalysis, discursive psychology and the nature of repression. *British Journal of Social Psychology, 36*: 139–159.

Billig, M. (1998). Dialogic repression and the Oedipus complex: Reinterpreting the Little Hans Case. *Culture & Psychology, 4*: 11–47.

Billig, M. (2006a). Lacan's Misuse of Psychology. Evidence, Rhetoric and the Mirror Stage. *Theory, Culture & Society, 23* (4): 1–26.

Billig, M. (2006b). A Psychoanalytic Discursive Psychology: from consciousness to unconsciousness. *Discourse Studies, 8* (1): 17–24.

Boehme, J. (1623). *Mysterium Magnum*, N. Berdiaeff (Trans.). Paris: Aubier-Montaigne, 1978.

Branney, P. (2008). Subjectivity, Not Personality: Combining Discourse Analysis and Psychoanalysis. *Social and Personality Psychology Compass, 2* (2): 574–590.

Braunstein, N. (2000). Construction, Interpretation and Deconstruction in Contemporary Psychoanalysis. In: J.M. Rabaté (Ed.), *Lacan in America* (pp. 191–221). New York: Other.

Bromberg, M. (2004). Contrat de communication et co-construction de sens. In: *Psychologie Sociale et Communication* (pp. 95–108). Paris: Dunod.

Bromberg, M. & Trognon, A. (2000). La psychologie sociale de l'usage du langage. In: N. Roussiau (Ed.), *Psychologie Sociale* (pp. 293–312). Paris: In Press.

Bronckart, J.-P. (1985). *Le Fonctionnement du Discours.* Neuchâtel: Delachaux et Niestlé.

Bruno, P. (1996). L'interprétation encore et toujours. In: *La Passe* (pp. 101–106). Toulouse: Presses Universitaires du Mirail, 2003.

Butler, J. (1997). *Le Pouvoir des Mots. Politique du Performatif*, C. Nordmann (Trans.). Paris: Amsterdam, 2004.

Camus, O. (1999). Les interactions langagières. In: J.-P. Pétard (Ed.), *Psychologie Sociale* (pp. 259–316). Rosny: Bréal.

Champagnol, R. (1993). *Signification du Langage*. Paris: PUF.

Chauchat, H. (1999). Du fondement social de l'identité du sujet. In: H. Chauchat & A. Durand-Delvigne (Eds.), *De l'Identité du Sujet au Lien Social* (pp. 7–26). Paris: PUF.

Chomsky, N. (1975). *Reflections on Language*. New York: Pantheon.

Cléro, J.-P. (2008). *Dictionnaire Lacan*. Paris: Ellipses.

Condillac, E. (1746). *Essai sur l'Origine des Connaissances Humaines.* Genève: Slatkine, 1970.

Cottet, S. (1987). Je pense où je ne suis pas, je suis où je ne pense pas. In: G. Miller (Ed.), *Lacan* (pp. 13–29). Paris: Bordas.

Damourette, J. & Pichon, E. (1911). *Des Mots à la Pensée, Essai de Grammaire de la Langue Française*. Paris: Artrey, 1968.

Debord, G. (1955). Introduction à une critique de la géographie urbaine. *Les Lèvres Nues, 6*. http://www.larevuedesressources.org/article.php3?id_article = 33 (accessed 24 July 2007).

Debord, G. (1967). *La Société du Spectacle*. Paris: Gallimard (Folio), 2006.

Deleuze, G. (1969). *Logique du Sens*. Paris: Minuit, 1982.

Deleuze, G. & Guattari, F. (1972). *L'Antiœdipe*. Paris: Minuit.

Derrida, J. (1967). *De la Grammatologie*. Paris: Minuit, 2002.

Derrida, J. (1972). *Positions*. Paris: Minuit.

Derrida, J. (1975). Le facteur de la vérité. In: *La Carte Postale de Socrate à Freud* (pp. 439–524). Paris: Flammarion, 1980.

Derrida, J. (1992). Pour l'amour de Lacan. In: *Résistances de la Psychanalyse* (pp. 55–88). Paris: Galilée, 1996.

Descartes, R. (1640). *Méditations Métaphysiques*. Paris: Flammarion, 1979.

Deutsch, M. & Krauss, R.M. (1972). *Les Théories en Psychologie Sociale*. Paris: Mouton.

Diderot, D. (1774). Jacques le Fataliste. In: *Œuvres Romanesques* (pp. 493–780). Paris: Garnier, 1962.

Doise, W. (1982). *L'Explication en Psychologie Sociale*. Paris: PUF.

Dreyfuss, J.-P., Jadin, J.-M. & Ritter, M. (1999). *Qu'est-ce que l'Inconscient? L'Inconscient Structuré comme un Langage*. Strasbourg: Arcanes.

Dunker, C.I.L. (2008). La psychanalyse en son temps. *Mensuel, 35*: 85–88.

Dunker, C.I.L. & Parker, I. (2009). How to be Secretly Lacanian in Anti-Psychoanalytic Qualitative Research, or Socio-Critical Models and Methods in Qualitative Research: Four Psychoanalytic Instances, and Strategies for their Sublation. *Annual Review of Critical Psychology*, 7, 52–71. http://www.discourseunit.com/arcp/7.htm (accessed 6 January 2010).

D'Unrug, M.-C. (1974). *Analyse de Contenu et Acte de Parole, de l'Énoncé à l'Énonciation*. Paris: Editions Universitaires.

Eggs, E. (1999). Ethos aristotélicien, conviction et pragmatique moderne. In: R. Amossy (Ed.), *Images de Soi dans le Discours* (pp. 31–59). Lausanne: Delachaux et Niestlé.

Evans, D. (1996). *An Introductory Dictionary of Lacanian Psychoanalysis*. London: Routledge.

Festinger, L. & Aronson, E. (1960). Éveil et réduction de la dissonance dans les contextes sociaux. In: C. Facheux & S. Moscovici (Eds.), *Psychologie Sociale Théorique et Expérimentale*. Paris: Mouton, 1971.

Flament, C. & Rouquette, M.-L. (2003). *Anatomie des Idées Ordinaires*. Paris: Colin.

Flaubert, G. (1852). Lettre à L. Colet. In: *Correspondance III* (pp. 51–55). Paris: Conard, 1926.

Foucault, M. (1966). *Les Mots et les Choses*. Paris: Gallimard, 2002.

Foucault, M. (1972). Table ronde. In: *Dits et Écrits I* (pp. 1184–1207). Paris: Gallimard, 2000.

Foucault, M. (1975). La mort du père. In: *Dits et Écrits I* (pp. 1602–1607). Paris: Gallimard, 2000.

Freud, S. (1910). Des sens opposés dans les mots primitifs. In: *Essais de Psychanalyse Appliquée* (pp. 59–67), M. Bonaparte (Trans.). Paris: Gallimard, 1933.

Freud, S. (1912). Lettre du 04.07.12. In: S. Freud & L. Binswanger, *Correspondance* (pp. 159–161), R. Menahem & M. Strauss (Trans.). Paris: Calmann-Lévy, 1995.

Freud, S. (1939). *Moïse et la Religion Monothéiste*, C. Heim (Trans.). Paris: Gallimard, 1989.

Frosh, S. (1999). What is outside discourse? *Psychoanalytic Studies*, *1*: 381–391.

Frosh, S. (2002). Enjoyment, Bigotry, Discourse and Cognition. *British Journal of Social Psychology*, *41*: 189–193.

Frosh, S. (2007). Disintegrating Qualitative Research. *Theory & Psychology*, *17* (5): 635–653.

Frosh, S., Phoenix, A. & Pattman, R. (2003). Taking a Stand: Using Psychoanalysis to Explore the Positioning of Subjects in Discourse. *British Journal of Social Psychology*, *42*: 39–53.

Gaonac'h, D. & Passerault, J.-M. (1998). Le langage. In: J.L. Roulin (Co-ord.), *Psychologie Cognitive* (pp. 327–384). Rosny: Bréal.

Genette, G. (1976). *Mimologiques, Voyage en Cratylie*. Paris: Seuil.

Georgaca, E. (2003). Exploring Signs and Voices in the Therapeutic Space. *Theory & Psychology*, *13* (4): 541–560.

Georgaca, E. (2005). Lacanian psychoanalysis and the subject of social constructionist psychology: Analysing subjectivity in talk. *International Journal of Critical Psychology*, *14*: 74–94.

Ghiglione, R. (1997). La psychologie sociale cognitive de la communication. In: J.-P. Leyens & J.-L. Beauvois (Eds.), *L'Ère de la Cognition* (pp. 225–251). Grenoble: PUG.

Ghiglione, R. (2003). Discours et persuasion. In: S. Moscovici (Ed.), *Psychologie Sociale* (pp. 473–498). Paris: PUF.

Ghiglione, R. & Blanchet, A. (1991). *Analyse de Contenu et Contenus d'Analyse*. Paris: Dunod.

Ghiglione, R., Beauvois, J.-L., Chabrol, C. & Trognon, A. (1980). *Manuel d'Analyse de Contenu*. Paris: Colin.

Ghiglione, R., Matalon, B. & Bacri, N. (1985). *Les Dires Analysés: l'Analyse Propositionnelle du Discours*. Saint-Denis: Presses Universitaires de Vincennes.

Gineste, M.-D. & Le Ny, J.-F. (2002). *Psychologie Cognitive du Langage*. Paris: Dunod.

Goffman, E. (1981). *Façons de Parler*, A. Kihm (Trans.). Paris: Minuit, 1987.

Gough, B. (2004). Psychoanalysis as a resource for understanding emotional ruptures in the text: The case of defensive masculinities. *British Journal of Social Psychology, 43*: 245–267.

Goutas, N., Girandola, F. & Minary, J.P. (2003). Le Sentiment d'Injustice Subie: un nouveau regard sur l'agression. *Revue Internationale de Psychologie Sociale, 16* (2): 125–149.

Gramsci, A. (1930). Cahier 6. In: *Cahiers de Prison* (pp. 11–161), G. Fulchignoni (Trans.). Paris: Gallimard, 1978.

Gramsci, A. (1931). Cahier 7. In: *Cahiers de Prison* (pp. 163–246), G. Fulchignoni (Trans.). Paris: Gallimard, 1978.

Gramsci, A. (1932). Cahier 12. In: *Cahiers de Prison* (pp. 305–347), G. Fulchignoni (Trans.). Paris: Gallimard, 1978.

Gramsci, A. (1934). Cahier 13. In: *Cahiers de Prison* (pp. 412–413), G. Fulchignoni (Trans.). Paris: Gallimard, 1978.

Gross, O. (1913a). Comment surmonter la crise culturelle? In: *Révolution sur le Divan* (pp. 45–47), J. Étoré (Trans.). Paris: Solin, 1988.

Gross, O. (1913b). À propos d'une nouvelle éthique. In: *Révolution sur le Divan* (pp. 55–57), J. Étoré (Trans.). Paris: Solin, 1988.

Gross, O. (1919). Le formation intellectuelle du révolutionnaire. In: *Révolution sur le Divan* (pp. 102–108), J. Étoré (Trans.). Paris: Solin, 1988.

Habermas, J. (1981). *Théorie de l'Agir Communicationnel*, J.-M. Ferry (Trans.). Paris: Fayard, 1987.

Habermas, J. (1984). *Sociologie et Théorie de Langage*, R. Rochlitz (Trans.). Paris: Colin, 1995.

Habermas, J. (1988). *La Pensée Postmétaphysique*, R. Rochlitz (Trans.). Paris: Colin.

Harré, R. (1985). Grammaire et lexiques, vecteurs des représentations sociales. In: D. Jodelet (Ed.), *Les Représentations Sociales* (pp. 131–151). Paris: PUF, 1997.

Harré, R., Clarke, D. & De Carlo, N. (1985). *Motives and Mechanisms. An Introduction to the Psychology of Action*. London: Methuen.

Hayes, G. (2003). Walking the streets: Psychology and the flâneur. *Annual Review of Critical Psychology, 3*: 50–66. http://www.discourseunit.com/arcp/3.htm (accessed 29 October 2008).

Hegel, G.W.F. (1807). *Phénoménologie de l'Esprit*, J. Hyppolite (Trans.). Paris: Aubier, 1941.

Hegel, G.W.F. (1820). *Principes de la Philosophie du Droit*, J.-F. Kervegan (Trans.). Paris: PUF, 1998.

Helmholtz, H. (1878). Die Tatsachen in der Wahrnehmung. In: *Philosophische Vorträge und Aufsätze* (pp. 247–282). Berlin: Akademie, 1971.

Hepburn, A. & Potter, J. (2003). Discourse analytic practice. In: C. Seale, D. Silverman, J. Gubrium & G. Gobo (Eds.), *Qualitative Research Practice* (pp. 180–196). London: Sage.

Hermosa Andújar, A. (2006). Legitimidad y Conservación de la Polis en Aristóteles. *Deus Mortalis, 5*: 35–70.

Hitlin, S. (2003). Values as the Core of Personal Identity. *Social Psychology Quarterly, 66* (2): 118–137.

Hobbes, T. (1651). *Leviathan*. Cambridge: Cambridge University Press.

Hollway, W. & Jefferson, T. (2000). *Doing Qualitative Research Differently. Free Association, Narrative and the Interview Method*. London: Sage.

Hook, D. (2003). Language and the flesh: psychoanalysis and the limits of discourse. London: LES Research Online. http://eprints.lse.ac.uk/archive/958 (accessed 8 September 2008).

Hook, D. (2008). Absolute Other: Lacan's *Big Other* as Adjunct to Critical Social Psychological Analysis. *Social and Personality Psychology Compass, 2* (1): 51–73.

Humboldt, W. (1820). La recherche linguistique comparative. In: *Introduction à l'Œuvre sur le Kavi et Autres Essais* (pp. 71–96), P. Caussat (Trans.). Paris: Seuil, 1974.

Humboldt, W. (1821). De l'influence de la diversité de caractère des langues sur la littérature et la culture de l'esprit. In: *Sur le Caractère National des Langues et Autres Écrits sur le Langage* (pp. 120–129), D. Thouard (Trans.). Paris: Seuil, 2000.

Humboldt, W. (1822). Sur le caractère national des langues. In: *Sur le Caractère National des Langues et Autres Écrits sur le Langage* (pp. 130–165), D. Thouard (Trans.). Paris: Seuil, 2000.

Humboldt, W. (1834). Introduction à l'œuvre sur le Kavi. In: *Introduction à l'Œuvre sur le Kavi et Autres Essais* (pp. 143–420), P. Caussat (Trans.). Paris: Seuil, 1974.

Jakobson, R. (1929). Réponse. In: *Le Cercle de Prague* (pp. 59–60). Paris: Seuil, 1969.

Jakobson, R. (1936). La transformation poétique. In: *Le Cercle de Prague* (pp. 95–97). Paris: Seuil, 1969.

Jakobson, R. (1949). L'aspect phonologique et l'aspect grammatical du langage. In: *Essais de Linguistique Générale* (pp. 161–175), N. Ruwer (Trans.). Paris: Minuit, 1963.

Jakobson, R. (1957). Les embrayeurs, les catégories verbales et le verbe russe. In: *Essais de Linguistique Générale* (pp. 176–196), N. Ruwer (Trans.). Paris: Minuit, 1963.

Janis, I.L. (1973). Groupthink. In: W.A. Lesko (Ed.), *Readings in Social Psychology* (pp. 328–333). Boston: Allyn and Bacon, 1993.

Jodelet, D. (1984). Représentation sociale: phénomènes, concept et théorie. In: S. Moscovici (Ed.), *Psychologie Sociale* (pp. 357–378). Paris: PUF.

Josselin, F. (2006). Mais où est donc passée la plus-value? *Mensuel, 12*: 47–52.

Juignet, P. (2003). Lacan, le symbolique et le signifiant. *Cliniques Méditerranéennes, 68*: 131–144.

Kaës, R. (1985). Psychanalyse et représentation sociale. In: D. Jodelet (Ed.), *Les Représentations Sociales* (pp. 87–114). Paris: PUF, 1997.

Kant, E. (1781). *Critique de la Raison Pure*, B. Pacaud (Trans.). Paris: PUF, 2001.

Kintsch, W. & Van Dijk, T. (1978). Toward a Model of Discourse Comprehension and Production. *Psychological Review, 85*: 363–394.

Kleist, H. (1806). *De l'Élaboration Progressive des Idées par la Parole*, A. Longuet Marx (Trans.). Paris: Fayard, 2003.

Kleist, H. (1811). Lettre d'un poète à un autre. In: *De l'Élaboration Progressive des Idées par la Parole* (pp. 31–35), A. Longuet Marx (Trans.). Paris: Fayard, 2003.

Lacan, J. (1938). Les complexes familiaux. In: Lacan, 2001, pp. 23–84.

Lacan, J. (1946). Propos sur la causalité psychique. In: Lacan, 1999a, pp. 150–192.

Lacan, J. (1950). Intervention au Congrès mondial de psychiatrie. In: Lacan, 2001, pp. 127–130.

Lacan, J. (1953a). Fonction et champ de la parole et du langage en psychanalyse. In: Lacan, 1999a, pp. 235–321.

Lacan, J. (1953b). Discours de Rome. In: Lacan, 2001, pp. 133–164.

Lacan, J. (1953c). Symbolique, imaginaire et réel. In: *Des Noms-du-Père* (pp. 11–63). Paris: Seuil, 2005.

Lacan, J. (1953–1954). *Le Séminaire. Livre I. Les Écrits Techniques de Freud.* Paris: Seuil, 1998.

Lacan, J. (1955–1956). *Le Séminaire. Livre III. Les Psychoses.* Paris: Seuil, 1981.

Lacan, J. (1956a). Le séminaire sur *La lettre volée.* In: Lacan, 1999a, pp. 11–61.

Lacan, J. (1956b). Réponse au commentaire de Jean Hyppolite sur la *Verneinung* de Freud. In: Lacan, 1999a, pp. 379–397.

Lacan, J. (1956c). La chose freudienne. In: Lacan, 1999a, pp. 398–433.

Lacan, J. (1957a). La psychanalyse et son enseignement. In: Lacan, 1999a, pp. 434–456.

Lacan, J. (1957b). L'instance de la lettre dans l'inconscient. In: Lacan, 1999a, pp. 490–526.

Lacan, J. (1956–1957). *Le Séminaire. Livre IV. La Relation d'Objet.* Paris: Seuil, 1994.

Lacan, J. (1957–1958). *Le Séminaire. Livre V. Les Formations de l'Inconscient.* Paris: Seuil, 1998.

Lacan, J. (1958a). La signification du phallus. In: Lacan, 1999b, pp. 163–174.

Lacan, J. (1958b). La psychanalyse vraie, et la fausse. In: Lacan, 2001, pp. 165–174.

Lacan, J. (1958c). Remarque sur le rapport de D. Lagache. In: Lacan, 1999b, pp. 124–162.

Lacan, J. (1958d). La direction de la cure. In: Lacan, 1999b, pp. 62–123.

Lacan, J. (1958e). D'une question préliminaire à tout traitement possible de la psychose. In: Lacan, 1999b, pp. 9–61.

Lacan, J. (1958–1959). *Le Séminaire. Livre VI. Le Désir et son Interprétation.* Unpublished.

Lacan, J. (1959). À la mémoire d'Ernest Jones: Sur sa théorie du symbolisme. In: Lacan, 1999b, pp. 175–195.

Lacan, J. (1959–1960). *Le Séminaire. Livre VII. L'Éthique de la Psychanalyse.* Paris: Seuil, 1986.

Lacan, J. (1960a). Subversion du sujet et dialectique du désir dans l'inconscient freudien. In: Lacan, 1999b, pp. 273–308.

Lacan, J. (1960b). Position de l'inconscient. In: Lacan, 1999b, pp. 309–330.

Lacan, J. (1960–1961). *Le Séminaire. Livre VIII. Le Transfert*. Paris: Seuil, 2001.

Lacan, J. (1961). Maurice Merleau-Ponty. In: Lacan, 2001, pp. 175–184.

Lacan, J. (1961–1962). *Le Séminaire. Livre IX. L'Identification*. Unpublished.

Lacan, J. (1962–1963). *Le Séminaire. Livre X. L'Angoisse*. Paris: Seuil, 2004.

Lacan, J. (1964). *Le Séminaire. Livre XI. Les Quatre Concepts Fondamentaux de la Psychanalyse*. Paris: Seuil, 1973.

Lacan, J. (1965a). Problèmes cruciaux de la psychanalyse, compte rendu du séminaire 1964–1965. In: Lacan, 2001, pp. 187–189.

Lacan, J. (1965b). Hommage fait à Marguerite Duras. In: Lacan, 2001, pp. 191–197.

Lacan, J. (1966a). D'un syllabaire après coup. In: Lacan, 1999b, pp. 196–202.

Lacan, J. (1966b). Réponses à des étudiants en philosophie. In: Lacan, 2001, pp. 203–211.

Lacan, J. (1966c). Petit discours à l'ORTF. In: Lacan, 2001, pp. 221–226.

Lacan, J. (1966–1967). *Le Séminaire. Livre XIV. La Logique du Fantasme*. Unpublished.

Lacan, J. (1967a). De la psychanalyse dans ses rapports avec la réalité. In: Lacan, 2001, pp. 351–359.

Lacan, J. (1967b). Proposition du 9 octobre 1967 sur la psychanalyse de l'École. In: Lacan, 2001, pp. 243–260.

Lacan, J. (1967c). La psychanalyse. Raison d'un échec. In: Lacan, 2001, pp. 341–350.

Lacan, J. (1967d). Proposition du 9 octobre 1967 sur la psychanalyse de l'École. In: Lacan, 2001, pp. 243–260, 575–591.

Lacan, J. (1967e). Discours à l'École Freudienne de Paris. In: Lacan, 2001, pp. 261–282.

Lacan, J. (1967f). La logique du fantasme. In: Lacan, 2001, pp. 323–328.

Lacan, J. (1967g). La méprise du sujet supposé savoir. In: Lacan, 2001, pp. 329–240.

Lacan, J. (1968–1969). *Le Séminaire. Livre XVI. D'un Autre à l'Autre*. Paris: Seuil, 2006.

Lacan, J. (1969). Préface aux *Écrits* en livre de poche. In: Lacan, 2001, pp. 387–392.

Lacan, J. (1969–1970). *Le Séminaire. Livre XVII. L'Envers de la Psychanalyse.* Paris: Seuil, 1991.
Lacan, J. (1970a). Radiophonie. In: Lacan, 2001, pp. 403–448.
Lacan, J. (1970b). Liminaire. In: Lacan, 2001, pp. 592–596.
Lacan, J. (1970c). Préface à une thèse. In: Lacan, 2001, pp. 393–402.
Lacan, J. (1970–1971). *Le Séminaire. Livre XVIII. D'un Discours qui ne Serait pas du Semblant.* Paris: Seuil, 2008.
Lacan, J. (1971). Lituraterre. In: Lacan, 2001, pp. 11–20.
Lacan, J. (1971–1972). *Le Séminaire. Livre XIX. Ou Pire.* Unpublished.
Lacan, J. (1972a). L'étourdit. In: Lacan, 2001, pp. 449–496.
Lacan, J. (1972b). Avis au lecteur japonais. In: Lacan, 2001, pp. 497–499.
Lacan, J. (1972c). Ou pire ... (compte rendu). In: Lacan, 2001, pp. 547–552.
Lacan, J. (1972d). Du discours psychanalytique (conférence à Milan). Unpublished.
Lacan, J. (1972–1973). *Le Séminaire. Livre XX. Encore.* Paris: Seuil, 1999.
Lacan, J. (1973a). Télévision. In: Lacan, 2001, pp. 509–547.
Lacan, J. (1973b). Introduction à l'édition allemande des Écrits. In: Lacan, 2001, pp. 553–560.
Lacan, J. (1973c). Note italienne. In: Lacan, 2001, pp. 307–312.
Lacan, J. (1973d). Intervention dans la séance de travail 'Sur la passe'. *Lettres de l'École Freudienne, 15*: 185–193.
Lacan, J. (1973e). Conférence au Musée de la science et de la technique de Milan. In: *Lacan in Italia 1953–1978* (pp. 58–77). Milan: La Salamandra, 1978.
Lacan, J. (1974a). Préface à *L'éveil du printemps.* In: Lacan, 2001, pp. 561–564.
Lacan, J. (1974b). La troisième, intervention au Congrès de Rome. *Lettres de l'École Freudienne, 16*: 186–187.
Lacan, J. (1974–1975). *Le Séminaire. Livre XXII. R.S.I.* Unpublished.
Lacan, J. (1975). Peut-être à Vincennes. In: Lacan, 2001, pp. 313–316.
Lacan, J. (1975–1976). *Le Séminaire. Livre XXIII. Le Sinthome.* Paris: Seuil.
Lacan, J. (1976–1977). *Le Séminaire. Livre XXIV. L'Insu que Sait de l'Une-bévue s'Aile à Mourre.* Unpublished.
Lacan, J. (1977–1978). *Le Séminaire. Livre XXV. Le Moment de Conclure.* Unpublished.
Lacan, J. (1979). Joyce le symptôme. In: Lacan, 2001, pp. 565–570.
Lacan, J. (1979–1980). *Le Séminaire. Livre XXVII. Dissolution.* Unpublished.

Lacan, J. (1980). Lettre de dissolution. In: Lacan, 2001, pp. 317–320.

Lacan, J. (1999a). *Écrits I*. Paris: Seuil-Points.

Lacan, J. (1999b). *Écrits II*. Paris: Seuil-Points.

Lacan, J. (2001). *Autres Écrits*. Paris: Seuil.

Laclau, E. (2000a). *La Guerre des Identités*, C. Orsoni (Trans.). Paris: La découverte.

Laclau, E. (2000b). Identity and Hegemony: The Role of Universality in the Constitution of Political Logics. In: J. Butler, E. Laclau, and S. Žižek, *Contingency, Hegemony, Universality: Contemporary Dialogues on the Left* (pp. 44–89). London: Verso.

Lakhdari, S. (2003). Nation, représentations, inconscient. *Outre-terre, 3*: 281–306.

LaPiere, R.T. (1934). Attitudes vs. Actions. In: W.A. Lesko (Ed.), *Readings in Social Psychology* (pp. 96–103). Boston: Allyn and Bacon, 1993.

Le Bihan, A. (2009). Discours et lien social. *Mensuel, 40*: 54–67.

Leclaire, S. & Laplanche, J. (1961). L'inconscient, une étude psychanalytique. *Les Temps Modernes, 183*: 81–129.

Leibniz, G.W. (1704). *Nouveaux Essais sur l'Entendement Humain*. Paris: Flammarion, 1990.

Lenin, V. (1908). Matérialisme et empiriocriticisme. In: *Œuvres 14* (pp. 13–375). Paris: Editions Sociales, 1962.

Lenin, V. (1913). Les trois sources et les trois parties constitutives du marxisme. In: *Œuvres 19* (pp. 13–18). Paris: Editions Sociales, 1967.

Lenin, V. (1915). Sur la question de la dialectique. In: *Œuvres 38* (pp. 339–347). Paris: Éditions Sociales, 1971.

Lewin, K. (1931). Le conflit dans les modes de pensée aristotélicien et galiléen dans la psychologie contemporaine. In: *Psychologie Dynamique* (pp. 23–64), M. Faucheux (Trans.). Paris: PUF, 1959.

Locke, J. (1690). *An Essay Concerning Human Understanding*. London: Thomas Tegg, 1841.

Malone, K.R. (2000). Subjectivity and the address to the Other. *Theory & Psychology, 10* (1): 79–86.

Mao Zedong (1937). De la contradiction. In: *Les Transformations de la Révolution* (pp. 47–104). Paris: Union générale d'éditions, 1970.

Martinet, A. (1960). *Éléments de Linguistique*. Paris: Colin, 1970.

Martinot, D. (1997). Le soi. In: J.-P. Leyens & J.-L. Beauvois (Eds.), *L'Ère de la Cognition* (pp. 39–42). Grenoble: PUG.

Marx, K. (1843a). Interdiction de la Leipziger Allgemeine Zeitung. In: *Œuvres Philosophie* (pp. 311–317), M. Rubel (Trans.). Paris: Gallimard, 1982.

Marx, K. (1843b). Critique de la Philosophie Politique de Hegel. In: *Œuvres Philosophie* (pp. 863–1018), M. Rubel (Trans.). Paris: Gallimard, 1982.

Marx, K. (1844). La question juive. In: *Œuvres Philosophie* (pp. 347–381), M. Rubel (Trans.). Paris: Gallimard, 1982.

Marx, K. (1845). Thèses sur Feuerbach. In: *Œuvres Philosophie* (pp. 1029–1033), M. Rubel (Trans.). Paris: Gallimard, 1982.

Marx, K. (1846). L'idéologie allemande. In: *Œuvres Philosophie* (pp. 1037–1325), M. Rubel (Trans.). Paris: Gallimard, 1982.

Marx, K. (1847). Misère de la philosophie. In: *Œuvres* (pp. 102–176), M. Rubel (Trans.). París: Gallimard, 1963.

Marx, K. (1867). *Le Capital, livre I,* J. Roy (Trans.). Paris: Flammarion, 2006.

Mathesius, V., Mukarovsky, J., Troubetzkoy, N.-S. & Jakobson, R. (1929). Les thèses de 1929. In: *Le Cercle de Prague* (pp. 19–49). Paris: Seuil, 1969.

Melman, C. (2007). *L'homme sans Gravité*. Paris: Denoël.

Melo, A. (2000). *Categorias e Objectos, Inquérito Semiótico Transcendental.* Lisbon: INCM.

Mill, J.S. (1843). *A System of Logic, Ratiocinative and Inductive.* New York: Harper, 1867.

Miller, J.-A. (1988). Sept remarques sur la création. *La Lettre Mensuelle, 68*: 11–13.

Miller, J.-A. (1995). Le plus-de-dire. *La Cause Freudienne, 30*: 7–14.

Miller, J.-A. (1996a). La pulsion est parole. *Quarto, 60*: 9–20.

Miller, J.-A. (1996b). Le monologue de l'apparole. *La Cause Freudienne, 34:* 7–18.

Miller, J.-A. (1996c). L'interprétation à l'envers. *La Cause Freudienne, 32*: 7–14.

Miller, J.-A. (1999). Les six paradigmes de la jouissance. *La Cause Freudienne, 43*: 7–29.

Miller, J.-A. (2002). L'ex-sistence. *La Cause Freudienne, 50*: 7–25.

Miller, J.-A. (2003). Lacan et la politique. *Cités, 16*: 105–123.

Miller, J.-A. (2005). Notice de fil en aiguille. In: *Le Sinthome* (pp. 199–247). Paris: Seuil.

Miller, J.-A. (2005–2006). *Orientation Lacanienne III, 8.* Unpublished.

Miller, J.-A. (2006–2007). *Orientation Lacanienne III, 9.* Unpublished.

Miller, J.-A. (2007–2008). *Orientation Lacanienne III, 10.* Unpublished.

Milner, J.-C. (1978). *L'amour de la Langue.* Paris: Seuil.

Milner, J.-C. (1983). *Les Noms Indistincts.* Paris: Seuil.

Mininni, G. (1994). Le nom de la chose: une analyse diatextuelle des stylèmes mass-médiatiques dans l'écriture politique populaire. In: A. Trognon & J. Larrue (Eds.), *Pragmatique du Discours Politique* (pp. 127–151). Paris: Colin.

Moliner, P. (1995). A Two-dimensional Model of Social Representations. *European Journal of Social Psychology, 25* (1): 27–40.

Moliner, P. (2001). Formation et stabilisation des représentations sociales. In: P. Moliner (Ed.), *La Dynamique des Représentations Sociales* (pp. 15–42). Grenoble: PUG.

Moliner, P. & Vidal, J. (2003). Stéréotype de la catégorie et noyau de la représentation sociale. *Revue Internationale de Psychologie Sociale, 16* (1): 157–176.

Moscovici, S. (1961). *La Psychanalyse, son Image et son Public.* Paris: PUF, 1976.

Moscovici, S. (1985). *L'Âge des Foules.* Bruxelles: Complexe.

Moscovici, S., Lage, E. & Naffrechoux, M. (1969). Influence of a Consistent Minority on the Responses of a Majority in a Color Perception Task. In: M. Hewstone et al. (Eds.), *The Blackwell Reader in Social Psychology* (pp. 527–543). Oxford: Blackwell, 1997.

Muchielli, R. (1974). *L'Analyse de Contenu.* Paris: ESF, 1998.

Mukarovsky, J. (1929). Formalisme russe, structuralisme tchèque. In: *Le Cercle de Prague* (pp. 54–60). Paris: Seuil, 1969.

Newcomb, T.M., Turner, R.H. & Converse, P.E. (1965). *Manuel de Psychologie Sociale,* A.-M. Touzard (Trans.). Paris: PUF, 1970.

Nietzsche, F. (1887). *Le Gai Savoir,* H. Albert (Trans.). Paris: Laffont, 1993.

Oliveira, C. (2004). O capitalista ri: uma leitura d'O Capital de Marx em Lacan. *A Psicanálise & os Discursos, 34–35*: 85–92.

Parker, I. (1992). *Discourse Dynamics: Critical Analysis for Social and Individual Psychology.* London: Routledge.

Parker, I. (1994). Reflexive Research and the Grounding of Analysis: Social Psychology and the Psy-complex. *Journal of Community & Applied Social Psychology, 4*: 244–245.

Parker, I. (1997a). The Unconscious State of Social Psychology. In: T. Ibáñez & L. Íñiguez (Eds.), *Critical Social Psychology* (pp. 157–168). London: Sage.

Parker, I. (1997b). Discourse Analysis and Psycho-Analysis. *British Journal of Social Psychology, 36*: 479–495.

Parker, I. (2000). Looking for Lacan: virtual psychology. In: K. Malone & S. Friedlander (Eds.), *The Subject of Lacan: A Lacanian Reader for Psychologists* (pp. 331–344). New York: SUNY.

Parker, I. (2001). Lacan, Psychology and the Discourse of the University. *Psychoanalytic Studies, 3,* (1): 67–77.

Parker, I. (2003). Jacques Lacan, Barred Psychologist. *Theory & Psychology, 13*: 95–115.

Parker, I. (2005a). Lacanian discourse analysis in psychology: Seven theoretical elements. *Theory & Psychology, 15*: 163–182.

Parker, I. (2005b). Lacanian ethics in psychology: Seven paradigms. In: A. Gülerce, A. Hofmeister, I. Steauble, G. Saunders & J. Kaye (Eds.), *Contemporary Theorizing in Psychology: Global Perspectives* (pp. 233–241). Concord: Captus.

Parker, I. (2008). Psychoanalytic Theory and Psychology: Conditions of Possibility for Clinical and Cultural Practice. *Theory & Psychology, 18* (2): 147–165.

Pascal, B. (1662). *Pensées.* Paris: Garnier-Flammarion, 1976.

Pavón Cuéllar, D. (2005). La Chose en cause. *Lettre Mensuelle, 242*: 13–15.

Pavón Cuéllar, D. (2006). El concepto de sociedad civil: examen de su actual elaboración teórica. *Dilema, 9*(2): 57–79.

Pavón Cuéllar, D. (2007a). El individuo y su división, precedentes filosóficos, místicos y religiosos de una idea lacaniana. *Dilema, 11*(2): 25–48.

Pavón Cuéllar, D. (2007b). Enfermar e sublimar, psicanálise e filosofia crítica. *Revista da Facultade de Letras da Universidade do Porto, 25*(2): 23–45.

Pavón Cuéllar, D. (2009). Untying Real, Imaginary and Symbolic: A Lacanian Criticism of Behavioural, Cognitive and Discursive Psychologies. *Annual Review of Critical Psychology,* 7, 33–51. http://www.discourseunit.com/arcp/7.htm (accessed 6 January 2010).

Pavón Cuéllar, D. (forthcoming). La conciencia del inconsciente, una vinculación entre dos términos opuestos. *Devenires.*

Pavón Cuéllar, D. & López Albertos, M. (1998). *Zapatismo y Contrazapatismo: Cronología de un Enfrentamiento.* Buenos Aires: Turalia.

Pavón Cuéllar, D. & Sabucedo Cameselle, J.M. (2009). El concepto de sociedad civil: breve historia de su elaboración teórica. *Araucaria, 21*: 67–96.

Pavón Cuéllar, D. & Vega, M.L. (1998). O EPR cercado polo siléncio. *Outrasvozes, 11*: 18–19.

Pavón Cuéllar, D. & Vega, M.L. (1999a). Aproximación al Ejército Popular Revolucionario. *Resumen Latinoamericano, 39*: 19.

Pavón Cuéllar, D. & Vega, M.L. (1999b). EPR, EZLN, ERPI, sem espaços de participaçom política. *Abrente, 13*: 10–11.

Pavón Cuéllar, D. & Vega, M.L. (2003). Aproximaciones al EPR. *La Hora*, 490: 1–8.

Pêcheux, M. (1969). *Analyse Automatique de Discours*. Paris: Dunod.

Pêcheux, M. (1975a). Introduction. *Langages, 37*: 3–6.

Pêcheux, M. (1975b). *Les Vérités de La Palice. Linguistique, Sémantique, Philosophie*. Paris: Maspero.

Pêcheux, M. & Fuchs, C. (1975). Mises au point et perspectives à propos de l'analyse automatique de discours. *Langages, 37*: 7–80.

Peirce, C.S. (1897). Ground, Object and Interpretant. In: *Collected Papers II* (pp. 134–136). Cambridge, MA: Harvard University Press, 1974.

Peirce, C.S. (1903). Principles of Philosophy. In: *Collected Papers I* (pp. 1–393). Cambridge, MA: Harvard University Press, 1974.

Pichon-Rivière, E. (1975). Pichon-Rivière habla sobre Jacques Lacan. *Actualidad Psicológica, 12*, 133: 8–11.

Pichon-Rivière, E. & Quiroga, A.P. (1972). Del Psicoanálisis a la Psicología Social. *Corriente Praxis*, 20.02.06. http://www.corrientepraxis.org.ar/spip.php?article199 (accessed 9 May 2008).

Plekhanov, G. (1892). Avertissement et notes pour la traduction russe d'Engels (1892). In: *Œuvres philosophiques* (pp. 399–450), J. Cathala (Trans.). Moscow: Progrès, 1961.

Politzer, G. (1928). *Critique des Fondements de la Psychologie. La Psychologie et la Psychanalyse*. Paris: PUF, 1968.

Politzer, G. (1947). *La Crise de la Psychologie Contemporaine*. Paris: Éditions sociales.

Potter, J. (2003). Discourse analysis and discursive psychology. In: P.M. Camic, J.E. Rhodes & L. Yardley (Eds.), *Qualitative Research in Psychology: Expanding Perspectives in Methodology and Design* (pp. 73–94). Washington: American Psychological Association.

Potter, J. (2004). Discourse analysis. In: M. Hardy & A. Bryman (Eds.), *Handbook of Data Analysis* (pp. 607–624). London: Sage.

Potter, J. & Wetherell, M. (1987). *Discourse and Social Psychology. Beyond Attitudes and Behaviour*. London: Sage.

Ragland-Sullivan, E. (1992). The Paternal Metaphor: A Lacanian Theory of Language. *Revue Internationale de Philosophie, 180*: 49–92.

Recanati, F. (1981). *Les Énoncés Performatifs: Contribution à la Pragmatique.* Paris: Minuit.

Regnault, F. (1987). Ces calembredaines dont fourmillent les textes analytiques. In: G. Miller (Ed.), *Lacan* (pp. 167–182). Paris: Bordas.

Regnault, F. (2003–2004). *Séminaire Parva Clinica.* Unpublished.

Regnault, F. (2005a). *Séminaire Le Marx de Lacan.* Unpublished.

Regnault, F. (2005b). Le Marx de Lacan. *Lettre mensuelle, 242*: 4–6.

Resweber, J.-P. (1998). Une question. *Le Portique, 2.* http://leportique.revues.org/document322.html (accessed 16 April 2006).

Ricœur, P. (1960). *Philosophie de la Volonté. La Symbolique du Mal.* Paris: Aubier.

Ricœur, P. (1965). *De l'Interprétation. Essai sur Freud.* Paris: Seuil.

Rimé, B. (1984). Langage et communication. In: S. Moscovici (Ed.), *Psychologie Sociale* (pp. 415–446). Paris: PUF.

Roberts, C. (1999). Discourse. In: R.A. Wilson & F.C. Keil (Eds.), *The MIT Enciclopedia of the Cognitive Sciences* (pp. 231–233). Cambridge, MA: MIT.

Rousseau, J.-J. (1781). *Essai sur l'Origine des Langues.* Paris: Nizet, 1969.

Rouzel, J. (2003). L'usager de l'action sociale. *Vie Sociale et Traitements, 77*: 29–35.

Saint-Martin, L.-C. (1775). *Des Erreurs de la Vérité ou les Hommes Rappelés au Principe Universel de la Science.* Hildesheim: Olms, 1975.

Sapir, E. (1921). *Language. An Introduction to the Study of Speech.* New York: Harcourt, 1949.

Sapir, E. (1931a). Le langage. In: *Linguistique* (pp. 29–64), J.-E. Boltanski (Trans.). Paris: Gallimard, 1991.

Sapir, E. (1931b). Communication. In: D.G. Mandelbaum (Ed.), *Selected Writings of Edward Sapir* (pp. 104–109). Berkeley, CA: University of California.

Sapir, E. (1933). The Nature of Language. In: D.G. Mandelbaum (Ed.), *Selected Writings of Edward Sapir* (pp. 3–82). Berkeley, CA: University of California.

Sartre, J.-P. (1944). *Huis Clos.* Paris: Folio-Gallimard, 1947.

Saussure, F. (1916). *Cours de Linguistique Générale.* Paris: Payot, 1995.

Schaff, A. (1964). *Langage et Connaissance,* C. Brendel (Trans.). Paris: Anthropos, 1969.

Schepens, P. (2002). Textes, Discours, Sujet, *Semen*, 14. http://semen.revues.org/document2430.html (accessed 7 November 2007).

Searle, J.R. (1969). *Speech Acts: An Essay in the Philosophy of Language*. Cambridge: Cambridge University Press.

Searle, J.R. (1995). *La Construction de la Réalité Sociale*, C. Tiercelin (Trans.). Paris: Gallimard, 1998.

Sextus Empiricus. *Against the Logicians*, R.G. Bury (Trans.). Cambridge, MA: Harvard University Press.

Sharma, D. (1998). The Discursive Voice of Psychoanalysis: A Case for Culturally Constituted Defenses. *Culture & Psychology*, 4: 49–64.

Soler, C. (1987). Une thérapeutique pas comme les autres. In: G. Miller (Ed.), *Lacan* (pp. 137–151). Paris: Bordas.

Soler, C. (1991). Incidence politique du psychanalyste. *Revue de l'École de la Cause Freudienne, Actes, 19*: 59–62.

Soler, C. (2005). Du parlêtre. *Mensuel, 8*: 9–17.

Soler, C. (2006). Pertes et profits. *Mensuel, 14*: 33–42.

Soler, C. (2008). La psychanalyse dans son temps et le temps de la psychanalyse. *Mensuel, 30*. http://www.champlacanienfrance.net/IMG/pdf/Mensuel30_CSoler.pdf (accessed 23 January 2009).

Soueix, A. (1989). Le discours du capitaliste. In: *Marx et Lenin, Freud et Lacan, Actes du Deuxième Colloque de La Découverte Freudienne*. Toulouse: Mirail, 1992.

Spinoza, B. (1674). *Éthique*, C. Appuhn (Trans.). Paris: Garnier, 1965.

Stalin, J. (1938). Le matérialisme dialectique et le matérialisme historique. In: *Oeuvres XIV* (pp. 200–231). Paris: NBE, 1977.

Stalin, J. (1950a). A propos du marxisme en linguistique I (*Pravda*, 20.06.50). In: L.-J. Calvet (Ed.), *Marxisme et Linguistique* (pp. 147–179). Paris: Payot, 1977.

Stalin, J. (1950b). A propos du marxisme en linguistique II (*Bolchevik*, 29.06.50). In: L.-J. Calvet (Ed.), *Marxisme et Linguistique* (pp. 179–183). Paris: Payot, 1977.

Taguieff, P.-A. (1987). *La Force du Préjugé: Essai sur le Racisme et ses Doubles*. Paris: La Découverte.

Tajfel, H. (1982). *Human Groups and Social Categories*. Cambridge: Cambridge University Press.

Tocqueville, A. (1840). *De la Démocratie en Amérique*. Paris: Gallimard, 1961.

Todorov, T. (1977). *Théories du Symbole*. Paris: Seuil.

Todorov, T. (1978). *Symbolisme et Interpretation*. Paris: Seuil.

Touraine, A. (1993). Le racisme aujourd'hui. In: M. Wieviorka (Ed.), *Racisme et Modernité* (pp. 23–41). Paris: La Découverte.

Van Dijk, T.E. & Kintsch, W. (1983). *Strategies of Discourse Comprehension*. Orlando, FL: Academic.

Wagner, W. (2001). Le coping symbolique, les représentations et la construction sociale. In: A.-M. Costalat-Founeau (Ed.), *Identité Sociale et Langage* (pp. 81–129). Paris: Harmattan.

Wieviorka, M. (1991). *L'Espace du Racisme*. Paris: Seuil.

Wittgenstein, L. (1921). *Tractatus Logico-Philosophicus*, P. Klossowski (Trans.). Paris: Gallimard, 1961.

Wittgenstein, L. (1949). *Recherches Philosophiques*, F. Dastur et al. (Trans.). Paris: Gallimard, 2004.

Wittgenstein, L. (1969). *Grammaire Philosophique*, M.-A. Lescourret (Trans.). Paris: Gallimard, 2001.

Žižek, S. (1999a). From *Passionate Attachments* to Dis-Identification. *UMBR(a)*. http://www.lacan.com/zizekpassionate.htm (accessed 3 September 2007).

Žižek, S. (1999b). Psychoanalysis and Post-marxism. The Case of Alain Badiou. *The South Atlantic Quarterly, 97* (2): 235–261. http://www.lacan.com/zizek-badiou.htm (accessed 15 September 2007).

Žižek, S. (2000). From Proto-Reality to the Act. *Center for Theology and Politics*. http://www.lacan.com/zizproto.htm (accessed 15 September 2007).

Žižek, S. (2003). L'*homo sacer*, comme objet du discours de l'université. *Cités, 16*: 25–41.

Žižek, S. (2006). Jacques Lacan's Four Discourses. *Lacan.com*. http://www.lacan.com/zizfour.htm (accessed 21 September 2007).

INDEX

For Product Safety Concerns and Information please contact our EU representative GPSR@taylorandfrancis.com
Taylor & Francis Verlag GmbH, Kaufingerstraße 24, 80331 München, Germany

www.ingramcontent.com/pod-product-compliance
Ingram Content Group UK Ltd.
Pitfield, Milton Keynes, MK11 3LW, UK
UKHW021512250926
475702UK00043B/240

* 9 7 8 0 3 6 7 3 2 4 6 3 6 *